Managing Chronic Pain

Editor

CHARLES E. ARGOFF

MEDICAL CLINICS
OF NORTH AMERICA

www.medical.theclinics.com

Consulting Editors
DOUGLAS S. PAAUW
EDWARD R. BOLLARD

January 2016 • Volume 100 • Number 1

ELSEVIER

1600 John F. Kennedy Boulevard • Suite 1800 • Philadelphia, Pennsylvania, 19103-2899

http://www.theclinics.com

MEDICAL CLINICS OF NORTH AMERICA Volume 100, Number 1
January 2016 ISSN 0025-7125, ISBN-13: 978-0-323-41340-4

Editor: Jessica McCool
Developmental Editor: Alison Swety

Medical Clinics of North America (ISSN 0025-7125) is published bimonthly by Elsevier Inc., 360 Park Avenue South, New York, NY 10010-1710. Months of publication are January, March, May, July, September, and November. Business and editorial offices: 1600 John F. Kennedy Boulevard, Suite 1800, Philadelphia, PA 19103-2899. Periodicals postage paid at New York, NY, and additional mailing offices. Subscription prices are USD $260.00 per year (US individuals), $531.00 per year (US institutions), $100.00 per year (US Students), $320.00 per year (Canadian individuals), $690.00 per year (Canadian institutions), $200.00 per year (Canadian and foreign students), $390.00 per year (foreign individuals), and $690.00 per year (foreign institutions). To receive student/resident rate, orders must be accompanied by name of affiliated institution, date of term, and the signature of program/residency coordinator on institution letterhead. Orders will be billed at individual rate until proof of status is received. Foreign air speed delivery is included in all Clinics' subscription prices. All prices are subject to change without notice. **POSTMASTER:** Send address changes to *Medical Clinics of North America*, Elsevier Health Sciences Division, Subscription Customer Service, 3251 Riverport Lane, Maryland Heights, MO 63043. **Customer Service: Telephone: 1-800-654-2452** (U.S. and Canada); **1-314-447-8871** (outside U.S. and Canada). **Fax: 314-447-8029.** E-mail: **journalscustomerserviceusa@elsevier.com** (for print support); **journalsonlinesupport-usa@elsevier.com** (for online support).

Reprints. For copies of 100 or more of articles in this publication, please contact the Commercial Reprints Department, Elsevier Inc., 360 Park Avenue South, New York, NY 10010-1710. Tel.: 212-633-3874; Fax: 212-633-3820; E-mail: reprints@elsevier.com.

Medical Clinics of North America is also published in Spanish by McGraw-Hill Interamericana Editores S. A., P.O. Box 5-237, 06500 Mexico, D.F., Mexico.

Medical Clinics of North America is covered in *MEDLINE/PubMed (Index Medicus), Current Contents, ASCA, Excerpta Medica, Science Citation Index,* and *ISI/BIOMED.*

PROGRAM OBJECTIVE
The goal of the *Medical Clinics of North America* is to keep practicing physicians up to date with current clinical practice by providing timely articles reviewing the state of the art in patient care.

TARGET AUDIENCE
All practicing physicians and other healthcare professionals.

LEARNING OBJECTIVES
Upon completion of this activity, participants will be able to:
1. Review the pathophysiology of chronic pain, and discuss possible methods of pain prevention.
2. Discuss the benefits and drawbacks of opioid therapy for chronic pain, and review alternative pharmaceutical and non-pharmaceutical treatment plans.
3. Recognize treatments and management strategies for pain due to chronic conditions such as osteoarthritis, chronic headaches, and neuropathy.

ACCREDITATION
The Elsevier Office of Continuing Medical Education (EOCME) is accredited by the Accreditation Council for Continuing Medical Education (ACCME) to provide continuing medical education for physicians.

The EOCME designates this enduring material for a maximum of 15 *AMA PRA Category 1 Credit*(s)™. Physicians should claim only the credit commensurate with the extent of their participation in the activity.

All other health care professionals requesting continuing education credit for this enduring material will be issued a certificate of participation.

DISCLOSURE OF CONFLICTS OF INTEREST
The EOCME assesses conflict of interest with its instructors, faculty, planners, and other individuals who are in a position to control the content of CME activities. All relevant conflicts of interest that are identified are thoroughly vetted by EOCME for fair balance, scientific objectivity, and patient care recommendations. EOCME is committed to providing its learners with CME activities that promote improvements or quality in healthcare and not a specific proprietary business or a commercial interest.

The planning committee, staff, authors and editors listed below have identified no financial relationships or relationships to products or devices they or their spouse/life partner have with commercial interest related to the content of this CME activity:

Charles E. Argoff, MD; Miroslav Backonja, MD; Jaime L. Baratta, MD; Kyle M. Baumbauer, PhD; Benjamin R. Beal, MD; David Beausang, MD; Edward R. Bollard, MD, DDS, FACP; Abigail Brooks, PharmD, BCPS; Kenneth D. Candido, MD; Martin D. Cheatle, PhD; Rebecca Dale, DO; Ravi Desai, DO; Andrew Dubin, MD; Eric Emanski, MD; Ryan C. Guay, DO, MBA; Jessica W. Guite, PhD; Robert Carter Wellford Jones III, MD, PhD; Alan David Kaye, MD, PhD; Mark A. Knaub, MD; Nebojsa Nick Knezevic, MD, PhD; Courtney Kominek, PharmD, BCPS, CPE; Andras Laufer, MD; Erin Lawson, MD; Renee C.B. Manworren, PhD, APRN, BC, PCNS-BC, FAAN; Nathan Patrick, MD; Thien C. Pham, B.S, PharmD; Michelle Poliak-Tunis, MD; John-Paul J. Pozek, MD; Beth S. Russell, PhD; Heather Smith, BA; Brett Stacey, MD; Angela R. Starkweather, PhD, ACNP-BC, CNRN, FAAN; David Walk, MD; Mark S. Wallace, MD; Youngwon Youn, BA; Erin E. Young, PhD.

The planning committee, staff, authors and editors listed below have identified financial relationships or relationships to products or devices they or their spouse/life partner have with commercial interest related to the content of this CME activity:

Gerald M. Aronoff, MD is on the speakers' bureau for, and a consultant/advisor for, XenoPort, Inc.; Kaleo, Inc.; Teva Pharmaceutical Industries Ltd.; Pernix Therapeutics; Purdue Pharma L.P.; Pfizer Inc.; and Mallinckrodt.
Robert A. Duarte, MD is on the speakers' bureau for, and a consultant/advisor for, Allergan.
Grace Forde, MD is on the speakers' bureau for Allergan.
Jeffrey Fudin, BS, PharmD, FACP, FCCP, FASHP is on the speakers' bureau for AstraZeneca and Millenium Health; is a consultant/advisor for AstraZeneca, Zogenix, Inc., and Millenium Health; and has stock ownership in Remitigate, LLC.
Julie G. Pilitsis, MD, PhD is a consultant/advisor for, with research support from Medtronic; Boston Scientific Corporation; and St. Jude, and has research support from the National Institutes of Health.
Noah Rosen, MD is on the speakers' bureau for Allergan, a consultant/advisor for Allergan; Avanir Pharmaceuticals, Inc.; and Curelator, Inc., and has stock ownership in Curelator, Inc.

Eugene R. Viscusi, MD is a consultant/advisor for AcelRx Pharmaceutics, Inc.; AstraZeneca; Mallinckrodt; The Medicines Company; Merck & Co., Inc.; Pacira Pharmaceuticals; Salix Pharmaceuticals, Inc.; and Trevena, Inc.

UNAPPROVED/OFF-LABEL USE DISCLOSURE

The EOCME requires CME faculty to disclose to the participants:

1. When products or procedures being discussed are off-label, unlabelled, experimental, and/or investigational (not US Food and Drug Administration [FDA] approved); and
2. Any limitations on the information presented, such as data that are preliminary or that represent ongoing research, interim analyses, and/or unsupported opinions. Faculty may discuss information about pharmaceutical agents that is outside of FDA-approved labelling. This information is intended solely for CME and is not intended to promote off-label use of these medications. If you have any questions, contact the medical affairs department of the manufacturer for the most recent prescribing information.

TO ENROLL

To enroll in the *Medical Clinics of North America* Continuing Medical Education program, call customer service at 1-800-654-2452 or sign up online at http://www.theclinics.com/home/cme. The CME program is available to subscribers for an additional annual fee of USD $295.

METHOD OF PARTICIPATION

In order to claim credit, participants must complete the following:

1. Complete enrolment as indicated above.
2. Read the activity.
3. Complete the CME Test and Evaluation. Participants must achieve a score of 70% on the test. All CME Tests and Evaluations must be completed online.

CME INQUIRIES/SPECIAL NEEDS

For all CME inquiries or special needs, please contact elsevierCME@elsevier.com.

MEDICAL CLINICS OF NORTH AMERICA

Contributors

CONSULTING EDITORS

DOUGLAS S. PAAUW, MD, MACP
Professor of Medicine, Division of General Internal Medicine, Rathmann Family Foundation Endowed Chair for Patient-Centered Clinical Education; Medicine Student Programs, Professor of Medicine, University of Washington School of Medicine, Seattle, Washington

EDWARD R. BOLLARD, MD, DDS, FACP
Professor of Medicine, Associate Dean of Graduate Medical Education, Designated Institutional Official, Department of Medicine, Penn State–Hershey Medical Center, Penn State University College of Medicine, Hershey, Pennsylvania

EDITOR

CHARLES E. ARGOFF, MD
Professor of Neurology, Albany Medical College, Director, Comprehensive Pain Center, Albany Medical Center, Albany, New York

AUTHORS

GERALD M. ARONOFF, MD
Diplomate, American Board of Psychiatry and Neurology; Diplomate, American Board of Pain Medicine; Medical Director, Carolina Pain Associates, PA, Charlotte, North Carolina

MIROSLAV BACKONJA, MD
Emeritus Professor, Department of Neurology, University of Wisconsin-Madison, Madison, Wisconsin

JAIME L. BARATTA, MD
Department of Anesthesiology, Thomas Jefferson University, Philadelphia, Pennsylvania

KYLE M. BAUMBAUER, PhD
School of Nursing, The Center for Advancing Management of Pain, University of Connecticut, Storrs, Connecticut; Department of Neuroscience, University of Connecticut Health Center, Farmington, Connecticut; Institute for Systems Genomics, University of Connecticut Health Center, Farmington, Connecticut

BENJAMIN R. BEAL, MD
Assistant Professor, Division of Pain Medicine, Department of Anesthesiology, University of California, San Diego, San Diego, California

DAVID BEAUSANG, MD
Department of Anesthesiology, Thomas Jefferson University, Philadelphia, Pennsylvania

ABIGAIL BROOKS, PharmD, BCPS
Clinical Pharmacy Specialist, Pain Management, Minneapolis VA Health Care System, Minneapolis, Minnesota

KENNETH D. CANDIDO, MD
Chairman, Clinical Professor, Department of Anesthesiology, Advocate Illinois Masonic Medical Center, University of Illinois, Chicago, Illinois

MARTIN D. CHEATLE, PhD
Director, Pain and Chemical Dependency Program, Center for Studies of Addiction, Perelman School of Medicine, University of Pennsylvania, Philadelphia, Pennsylvania

REBECCA DALE, DO
Acting Assistant Professor, Pain Medicine Fellowship Director, Anesthesiology and Pain Medicine, Harborview Medical Center, University of Washington, Seattle, Washington

RAVI DESAI, DO
Anesthesiology Resident, Department of Anesthesiology, Advocate Illinois Masonic Medical Center, Chicago, Illinois

ROBERT A. DUARTE, MD
Director, Pain Center, Cushing Neuroscience Institute, North Shore–LIJ Health System, Great Neck, New York

ANDREW DUBIN, MD
Professor, Department of Physical Medicine and Rehabilitation, Albany Medical College, Albany, New York

ERIC EMANSKI, MD
Department of Orthopaedic Surgery, Penn State–Milton S. Hershey Medical Center, Hershey, Pennsylvania

GRACE FORDE, MD
Director of Neurological Services, North American Partners in Pain Management, Department of Pain Medicine, Valley Stream, New York

JEFFREY FUDIN, BS, PharmD, FACP, FCCP, FASHP
Diplomate, American Academy of Pain Management; Clinical Pharmacy Specialist, Pain Management, Director, PGY2 Pain and Palliative Care Pharmacy Residency, Stratton VA Medical Center, Albany, New York; Adjunct Associate Professor of Pharmacy Practice and Pain Management, Western New England University College of Pharmacy, Springfield, Massachusetts; Adjunct Associate Professor of Pharmacy Practice and Pain Management, Albany College of Pharmacy and Health Sciences, Albany, New York; Adjunct Assistant Professor of Pharmacy Practice, University of Connecticut School of Pharmacy, Storrs, Connecticut

RYAN C. GUAY, DO, MBA
Department of Anesthesiology, Albany Medical Center, Albany, New York

JESSICA W. GUITE, PhD
Department of Pediatrics, University of Connecticut School of Medicine, Farmington, Connecticut; Connecticut Children's Center for Community Research (C3R), Hartford, Connecticut; Pediatric Psychology, Hartford Hospital/The Institute of Living, Hartford, Connecticut; Division of Pain and Palliative Medicine, Connecticut Children's Medical Center, Hartford, Connecticut; Pediatric Psychology, Hartford Hospital/Institute of Living, Hartford, Connecticut

ROBERT CARTER WELLFORD JONES III, MD, PhD
Assistant Professor of Anesthesiology, Center for Pain Medicine, University of California, San Diego, San Diego, California

ALAN DAVID KAYE, MD, PhD
Chairman, Professor, Departments of Anesthesiology and Pharmacology, LSU Health Science Center, Louisiana State University School of Medicine, New Orleans, Louisiana

MARK A. KNAUB, MD
Assistant Professor, Department of Orthopaedic Surgery; Chief of Adult Spine Service, Penn State–Milton S. Hershey Medical Center, Hershey, Pennsylvania

NEBOJSA NICK KNEZEVIC, MD, PhD
Vice Chair for Research and Education, Clinical Assistant Professor, Department of Anesthesiology, Advocate Illinois Masonic Medical Center; Department of Anesthesiology, University of Illinois, Chicago, Illinois

COURTNEY KOMINEK, PharmD, BCPS, CPE
Clinical Pharmacy Specialist, Pain Management, Harry S. Truman Memorial Veterans' Hospital, Columbia, Missouri

ANDRAS LAUFER, MD
Department of Anesthesiology, Albany Medical Center, Albany, New York

ERIN LAWSON, MD
Director of Pain Management, Lexington Brain and Spine Institute, Lexington, South Carolina; Voluntary Faculty, Center for Pain Medicine, University of California, San Diego, San Diego, California

RENEE C.B. MANWORREN, PhD, APRN, BC, PCNS-BC, FAAN
Department of Pediatrics, University of Connecticut School of Medicine, Farmington, Connecticut; School of Nursing, The Center for Advancing Management of Pain, University of Connecticut, Storrs, Connecticut; Division of Pain and Palliative Medicine, Connecticut Children's Medical Center, Hartford, Connecticut

NATHAN PATRICK, MD
Department of Orthopaedic Surgery, Penn State–Milton S. Hershey Medical Center, Hershey, Pennsylvania

THIEN C. PHAM, BS, PharmD
PGY2 Pharmacy Resident, Pain and Palliative Care, Stratton VA Medical Center, Albany, New York

JULIE G. PILITSIS, MD, PhD
Department of Neurosurgery, Albany Medical Center, Albany, New York

MICHELLE POLIAK-TUNIS, MD
Assistant Professor, Department of Orthopedics and Rehabilitation, University of Wisconsin School of Medicine and Public Health, Madison, Wisconsin

JOHN-PAUL J. POZEK, MD
Department of Anesthesiology, Thomas Jefferson University, Philadelphia, Pennsylvania

NOAH ROSEN, MD
Residency Director, Associate Professor, Neurology; Associate Professor, Psychiatry; Director, North Shore Headache Center, Cushing Neuroscience Institute, Hofstra North Shore LIJ Medical Center, Hempstead, New York

BETH S. RUSSELL, PhD
Human Development and Family Studies, University of Connecticut, Storrs, Connecticut

HEATHER SMITH, BA
Department of Neurosurgery, Albany Medical Center, Albany, New York

BRETT STACEY, MD
Anesthesiology and Pain Medicine, Professor, Medical Director, UW Center for Pain Relief, University of Washington, Seattle, Washington

ANGELA R. STARKWEATHER, PhD, ANCP-BC, CNRN, FAAN
School of Nursing, The Center for Advancing Management of Pain, University of Connecticut, Storrs, Connecticut

EUGENE R. VISCUSI, MD
Department of Anesthesiology, Thomas Jefferson University, Philadelphia, Pennsylvania

DAVID WALK, MD
Associate Professor, Department of Neurology, University of Minnesota, Minneapolis, Minnesota

MARK S. WALLACE, MD
Professor, Division of Pain Medicine, Department of Anesthesiology, University of California, San Diego, San Diego, California

YOUNGWON YOUN, BA
Department of Neurosurgery, Albany Medical Center, Albany, New York

ERIN E. YOUNG, PhD
School of Nursing, The Center for Advancing Management of Pain, University of Connecticut, Storrs, Connecticut; Institute for Systems Genomics, University of Connecticut Health Center, Farmington, Connecticut; Department of Genetics and Genome Sciences, University of Connecticut Health Center, Farmington, Connecticut

Contents

Background

> Chronic pain has multiple mechanisms that result in pain amplification and maintenance, including central and peripheral sensitization and altered modulation of pain perception. Assessment of pain requires comprehensive assessment of symptoms and signs, suspected pain mechanisms, and the patient's biopsychosocial context. Multiple validated measures exist for the assessment of pain symptoms, pain-related disability, psychological impact of pain, and candidacy for opioid management.

> Chronic postsurgical pain (CPSP) is a distressing disease process that can lead to long-term disability, reduced quality of life, and increased health care spending. Although the exact mechanism of development of CPSP is unknown, nerve injury and inflammation may lead to peripheral and central sensitization. Given the complexity of the disease process, no novel treatment has been identified. The preoperative use of multimodal analgesia has been shown to decrease acute postoperative pain, but it has no proven efficacy in preventing development of CPSP.

> We discuss the complex features of the pathophysiology of chronic pain and the implications for treatment and provide an overview of nociceptive processes, neuropathic pain, cold hyperalgesia, peripheral nerve injury, wind-up pain, central sensitization, and common clinical presentation and diagnostic criteria. Advanced medicine has proven that chronic pain need not involve any structural pathology as pain is a complex biopsychosocial experience. Treatment of the specific mechanisms responsible for pain should be aimed at preventing and or reducing dysfunctional neuro-plasticity resulting from poorly controlled chronic pain. Further study

is needed to reduce the probability and of persistent changes that cause chronic pain.

Chronic Pain Treatment Approaches

Chronic pain affects nearly one-third of the American population. Chronic pain can lead to a variety of problems for a pain sufferer, including developing secondary medical problems, depression, functional and vocational disability, opioid abuse, and suicide. Current pain care models are deficient in providing a necessary comprehensive approach. Most patients with chronic pain are managed by primary care clinicians who are typically ill prepared to effectively and efficiently manage these cases. A biopsychosocial approach to evaluate and treat chronic pain is clinically and economically efficacious, but unique delivery systems are required to meet the challenge of access to specialty care.

Most patients with chronic pain receive multimodal treatment. There is scant literature to guide us, but when approaching combination pharmacotherapy, the practitioner and patient must weigh the benefits with the side effects; many medications have modest effect yet carry significant side effects that can be additive. Chronic pain often leads to depression, anxiety, and deconditioning, which are targets for treatment. Structured interdisciplinary programs are beneficial but costly. Interventions have their place in the treatment of chronic pain and should be a part of a multidisciplinary treatment plan. Further research is needed to validate many common combination treatments.

Patients with chronic pain can be challenging to manage and historically providers have relied on opiates to treat pain. Recent studies have brought into question the safety and efficacy of chronic opiate therapy in the non-cancer population. There is a vast amount of literature to support the use of nonsteroidal anti-inflammatory medications, antidepressants, anticonvulsants, topical agents, cannabinoids, and botulinum toxin either in conjunction with or in lieu of opioids. Intrathecal drug delivery systems can deliver some of these medications directly to their primary site of action while minimizing the side effects seen with systemic administration.

This article provides a broad overview regarding intent to initiate and consider ongoing chronic opioid therapy (COT) for treatment of chronic noncancer pain (CNCP). COT should be an individualized decision based on a comprehensive evaluation, assessment, and monitoring. It is imperative that providers discuss various risks and benefits of COT initially and at follow-up visits, and continue appropriate monitoring and follow-up at regular intervals. The decision to initiate or continue opioid therapy is based on clinical judgment; however, it is understood that opioid and other medication therapy represent one piece of the complete treatment plan for patients with CNCP.

Invasive analgesic therapies provide an alternative to medical management of chronic pain. With the increasing incidence of chronic pain not only in the United States but worldwide, more therapies have evolved to address the growing need for pain relief options. These therapies include spinal injections, nerve blocks, radiofrequency ablation, neurostimulation, and intrathecal drug delivery.

Common Chronic Pain Conditions

Headaches are a very common disorder, more common than asthma and diabetes combined. Migraine is the most common headache disorder, but it remains underdiagnosed and therefore undertreated. The treatment of migraines is divided into acute and prophylaxis. Patients who are experiencing 8 or more headache days a month or those who experience disability with their headaches as determined by the Migraine Disability Assistance Score or MIDAS should be placed on prophylaxis.

Osteoarthritis (OA) is a common problem in society and can lead to significant disability and impairment of a patient's capacity to perform activities of daily living. The focus of this article is various treatment options for the management of OA, with emphasis on conservative management. The emphasis is on the role of exercise, pharmacology, intra-articular joint injections, and bracing options in the management of OA.

Neuropathic pain (NP) arises from injuries or diseases affecting the somatosensory component of the nervous system at any level of the peripheral or central nervous system. NP is diagnosed based on common neurologic signs and symptoms. NP is best treated with a combination

of multiple therapeutic approaches, and treatments include conservative, complementary, medical, interventional, and surgical treatment
modalities. Goals of treatment are the same as in pain management
and include improvement in pain control and in coping skills as well
as restoration of functional status. Most patients with NP benefit most
from an individualized, multimodal approach that emphasizes both
pain and function.

Low back pain is an extremely common presenting complaint that occurs
in upward of 80% of persons. Treatment of an acute episode of back
pain includes relative rest, activity modification, nonsteroidal anti-
inflammatories, and physical therapy. Patient education is also imperative,
as these patients are at risk for further future episodes of back pain.
Chronic back pain (>6 months' duration) develops in a small percentage
of patients. Clinicians' ability to diagnose the exact pathologic source of
these symptoms is severely limited, making a cure unlikely. Treatment of
these patients should be supportive, the goal being to improve pain and
function.

Research has typically focused on otherwise healthy adults with chronic
pain conditions; however there are distinct groups of individuals with
increased vulnerability for chronic pain. These groups are defined by age
and life circumstances associated with increased risk of injury and less
effective pain treatment. Chronic pain is challenging to manage and a significant health issue in pediatric, geriatric, and drug abuser populations.
This article focuses on psychosocial, physiologic, and genetic mechanisms underlying chronic pain in these populations, and highlights the
need for interdisciplinary teams to manage chronic pain with personalized
multimodal approaches for those with greatest risk.

Emerging Treatment

Platelet-rich plasma (PRP) has the potential to regenerate tissues and
decrease pain through the effects of bioactive molecules and growth factors present in alpha granules. Several PRP preparation systems are available with varying end products, doses of growth factors, and bioactive
molecules. This article presents the biology of PRP, the preparation of
PRP, and the effects PRP-related growth factors have on tissue healing
and repair. Based on available evidence-based literature, the success of

PRP therapy depends on the method of preparation and composition of PRP, the patient's medical condition, anatomic location of the injection, and the type of tissue injected.

Foreword

The Management of Chronic Pain: What Do We Know, What Do We Do, and How Should We Redesign Our Comprehensive Assessment and Treatment in order to Provide for More Patient-Centered Care?

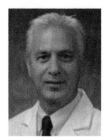

Edward R. Bollard, MD, DDS, FACP
Consulting Editor

The discussion of the management of chronic pain is a daily occurrence for the practicing generalist, whether it be on rounds in the inpatient setting or in busy outpatient clinics. Our patients are exposed to information and advertisements pertaining to modalities directed at the treatment of chronic pain every day. The media addressing both the overutilization and underutilization of various pain management strategies are pervasive; therefore, it is essential that the physician caring for patients with chronic pain has a considerable understanding, as well as a working knowledge, of the pathophysiology, psychosocial aspects, pharmacology, and evidence supporting other treatment options in the comprehensive plan for chronic pain management.

In this issue of *Medical Clinics of North America*, Dr Charles E. Argoff and his colleagues provide insight into the current understanding of chronic pain: from the taxonomy of these conditions, to how one may transition from acute to chronic pain and the implications for treatment, to various modalities to address treatment strategies—including the novel platelet-rich plasma—to the common medical conditions in patients that frequently present to our practices with complaints of "chronic pain." Specific populations at risk for chronic pain, as well as the potential adverse effects of treating the pain in these populations, are presented in the article by Dr Baumbauer

Med Clin N Am 100 (2016) xvii–xviii
http://dx.doi.org/10.1016/j.mcna.2015.10.002
0025-7125/16/$ – see front matter © 2016 Published by Elsevier Inc.

and colleagues. Finally, a frank discussion and review of guidelines for the utilization of narcotics and the potential of abuse in prescribing this pharmacologic intervention are presented.

Chronic pain can be frustrating to the practitioner, who has gaps in the breadth and depth of knowledge that is needed to assess, diagnose, and manage it. We hope the articles in this issue will go a long way in reducing these knowledge gaps, resulting in more advanced, comprehensive, safe, and effective care for our patients.

Edward R. Bollard, MD, DDS, FACP
Department of Medicine
Penn State–Hershey Medical Center
Penn State University College of Medicine
500 University Drive
PO Box 850 (Mail Code H039)
Hershey, PA 17033-0850, USA

E-mail address:
ebollard@hmc.psu.edu

Preface

Yes, You Can Manage Chronic Pain

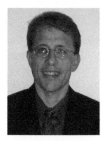

Charles E. Argoff, MD
Editor

Many readers may be aware of the frequently quoted estimated number of American adults who experience chronic pain annually—a staggering estimate of 100 million people! Many of you may also recognize that this number exceeds the number of American adults who are treated for diabetes, cardiovascular diseases, and cancer COMBINED on an annual basis. I wish that someone could then explain the rationale underlying why so few American medical schools require or even offer significant undergraduate medical education in pain management and why so few graduate medical education programs truly train their residents in pain management!

The truth is that "pain" is the number one reason a person seeks medical attention. Although acute pain may be considered in many instances an expected consequence of a medical condition or procedure, chronic pain is never a welcome condition and, in fact, chronic pain is associated with unwelcome anatomic and physiologic changes in a person's peripheral and/or central nervous system. All too often this not only results in the experience of ongoing pain itself but also in the loss of function and impaired quality of life. How tragic it is then that more health care providers are not typically adequately trained: to recognize the mechanisms and types of chronic pain, to institute means to prevent acute pain from becoming chronic, to appropriately diagnose chronic painful conditions, to institute a multimodal patient-centered treatment program, and to recognize that chronic pain is a chronic disease that requires ongoing management, re-evaluation, and monitoring to optimize outcomes.

I am so pleased to serve as guest editor for this issue of *Medical Clinics of North America*. I hope that the reader will appreciate this issue as a comprehensive group of related articles that emphasize the need to understand, to the fullest extent possible, the mechanism(s) of a person's chronic pain, as well as the varied medical conditions associated with chronic pain and the multiple ways in which individuals with chronic pain can be treated. I apologize to the reader for not including even more topics, but I was informed that there were space limits! The reader of this issue will see the

Med Clin N Am 100 (2016) xix–xx
http://dx.doi.org/10.1016/j.mcna.2015.10.001
0025-7125/16/$ – see front matter © 2016 Published by Elsevier Inc.

medical.theclinics.com

richness of the science underlying the mechanisms of chronic pain in addition to the numerous evidence-based medical and nonmedical therapies that we can offer to our patients. I am grateful to every author in this issue, whose outstanding contributions will interest you and I have no doubt further stimulate your interest in the young and rapidly growing medical subspecialty of pain management. As you read this issue, please become empowered and enthusiastic about managing chronic pain in your practice—aiding in the relief of suffering is the foundation of being a health care provider—and please remember, "Yes, you can manage chronic pain."

Charles E. Argoff, MD
Albany Medical College
Comprehensive Pain Center
Albany Medical Center
43 New Scotland Avenue
MC 70
Albany, NY 12208, USA

E-mail address:
argoffc@mail.amc.edu

Background

Chronic Pain Management

An Overview of Taxonomy, Conditions Commonly Encountered, and Assessment

David Walk, MD[a],*, Michelle Poliak-Tunis, MD[b]

KEYWORDS

- Chronic pain • Mechanisms of pain • Pain assessment

KEY POINTS

- Chronic pain has multiple mechanisms that result in pain amplification and maintenance, including central and peripheral sensitization and altered modulation of pain perception.
- Assessment of pain requires comprehensive assessment of symptoms and signs, suspected pain mechanisms, and patient's biopsychosocial context.
- Multiple validated measures exist for the assessment of pain symptoms, pain-related disability, psychological impact of pain, and candidacy for opioid management.

Chronic pain is a substantial health problem, both in its prevalence and its impact. The prevalence of chronic pain in a 12-month period has been estimated at 43% of the US population and 38% worldwide.[1] Institute for Health Metrics and Evaluation data rank low back pain seventh among global causes of disability-adjusted life-years, and, if combined, low back and neck pain would rank third.[2] Among US adults, the reported prevalence of chronic pain ranges from 2% to 40%, with a median of 15%.[3] In 2009, a National Health Interview Survey demonstrated that during a 3-month period, 16% of adults reported having a migraine or severe headache, 15% pain in the neck area, 28% pain in lower back, and 5% pain in the jaw or face.[3]

The impact and prevalence of chronic pain are themselves evidence of limitations in managing pain. In 2011, the Institute of Medicine released a report entitled, *Relieving Pain in America: A Blueprint for Transforming Prevention, Care, Education, and Research*, that outlined disparities between the impact of pain and current investments in all domains listed in their subtitle.[4] It addressed reasons for these disparities as well as possible solutions. This article outlines the current evidence for chronic pain

Disclosures: None.
[a] Department of Neurology, University of Minnesota, 420 Delaware Street Southeast, MMC 295, Minneapolis, MN 55455, USA; [b] Department of Orthopedics and Rehabilitation, University of Wisconsin School of Medicine and Public Health, Madison, WI, USA
* Corresponding author.
E-mail address: walkx001@umn.edu

Med Clin N Am 100 (2016) 1–16
http://dx.doi.org/10.1016/j.mcna.2015.09.005   medical.theclinics.com

as a disease, taxonomies of pain, and an approach to the assessment of painful conditions. Subsequent articles in this issue delve in greater depth into these topics individually.

THE EXPERIENCE OF PAIN

Pain is defined as "an unpleasant sensory and emotional experience associated with actual or potential tissue damage, or described in terms of such damage."[5] This definition indicates several things about pain. First, it combines a sensory perception with an unpleasant emotional experience. These are distinct aspects of pain that reflect distinct pathways of activation of somatosensory and limbic cerebral cortex.[6] These 2 pathways can be uncoupled in pathology. In pain asymbolia, a rarely described syndrome that can be a consequence of injury to insular cortex, patients accurately describe nociceptive stimulation as painful but do not perceive it as unpleasant. Furthermore, the attention-motivational component of the pain experience, which results in withdrawal from painful stimuli and protection of the affected area, is absent in pain asymbolia, indicating that the responsible lesion interrupts both the emotional and motivational aspects of the experience of pain.[7] Second, pain descriptors are commonly words that describe tissue damage. This seems appropriate, because physiologic pain is initiated by stimulation of nociceptors, which are transducing elements on nerve terminals that only initiate an action potential in the context of a stimulus capable of inducing tissue damage. Finally, this definition specifies that pain is an experience and, therefore, is both subjective and does not have an obligate correspondence with nociceptive stimulation. Pain can only be measured as it is reported.

That said, the report of pain as a symptom may be a surrogate for a wide variety of concerns, only one of which is a desire for pain relief. People who present with pain as a chief complaint may be motivated to seek help because of fear, anxiety, loss of life roles, disrupted sleep, functional and occupational disability, dependency, addiction, or other factors. Even if not explicitly acknowledged as goals of therapy separate from pain relief itself, these state, trait, and situational factors can influence reported pain severity itself.

THE BIOLOGY OF CHRONIC PAIN

There is a growing body of evidence that chronic pain can exist as a disease state. This concept is supported by both clinical and preclinical evidence. In the clinical realm, several distinct pain syndromes have been demonstrated to present with a consistent symptom complex, no evident end-organ pathology, and reproducible differences from healthy control subjects in psychophysical, neurophysiological, or functional neuroimaging studies.[8,9] This literature suggests that these conditions are disorders of somatosensory and pain signaling in the nervous system. Preclinical evidence in animal models of chronic inflammation or nerve injury provide robust models of peripheral and central sensitization modulated by second messenger systems and epigenetic modifications responding to repetitive nociceptor stimulation.[10] This supports the view that acute pain conditions can, in certain circumstances, lead to sensitization that persists well after acute tissue injury has resolved or exacerbates pain perception in the context of chronic nociceptor stimulation. These data are further buttressed by identification of genetic and epigenetic factors that may predispose to sensitization of nociceptive pathways in the nervous system.[11,12]

The concept that chronic pain can exist as a pathologic state, or that in some cases physiologic mechanisms can result in maladaptive sensitization in conditions with chronic nociceptive stimulation, has profound implications for clinicians engaged in pain management. At minimum these findings suggest that management approaches designed for acute, self-limited pain are likely to prove inadequate or even inappropriate for the treatment of chronic pain. It is not yet clear how best to apply this emerging knowledge in the clinical arena. It is clear, however, that this will not be applied successfully without re-educating health care providers and the general public, among whom the view remains prevalent that pain is an unfiltered direct reporter of the presence and severity of local tissue injury.

PAIN TAXONOMY

Pain can be classified along a broad range of axes. The International Association of the Study of Pain issued a coding system in 1994 that promulgated the description of pain according to regions, organ systems, temporal characteristics, intensity, and etiology.[13] In clinical practice it is customary to categorize a patient's condition in all these domains but not necessarily using this schema. This article provides an overview along only 2 axes: first, a pain taxonomy according to mechanisms of chronic pain as distinguished from pain due to acute tissue injury, and second, a pain taxonomy according to commonly applied clinical categories. The former is provided as an introduction to the scientific basis of conceptualizing chronic pain as a medical disorder with unique pathophysiologic mechanisms that distinguish it from acute pain that happens to be long-lasting. The latter is designed as an overview of chronic pain diagnostic categories because they are typically triaged in the clinical environment. Several mechanistic categories are relevant in each clinical category.

Taxonomy of Chronic Pain I: Mechanisms of Chronic Pain as a Medical Disorder

Acute pain is a physiologic phenomenon precipitated when stimuli that result in potential tissue injury result in signal transduction in nociceptors, resulting in turn in the generation of an action potential from that peripheral nociceptor to cells in the spinal cord or, in the case of head and facial pain, brainstem. The signal is transmitted to the thalamus and cerebral cortex via polysynaptic pathways that are subject to physiologic modulation. Chronic pain is distinct from acute pain not only by virtue of its duration but also because of several mechanisms that can sustain and amplify pain after acute events in tissues innervated by nociceptors. These mechanisms include peripheral and central sensitization, alterations in descending modulation, and deafferentation.

Sensitization is an important factor in chronic pain because it is a mechanism to pathologically sustain and amplify pain. Peripheral nociceptors in skin, joints, tendons, and viscera have physiologically determined stimulation thresholds that assure accurate reporting of the location and severity of potential tissue injury. For example, a cutaneous heat nociceptor initiates an action potential only when tissue is warmed to a temperature of greater than or equal to 43°C. The firing rate, which codes for intensity, is slow at this threshold temperature, and rises as the skin temperature rises. Exposure to inflammatory mediators or sustained nociceptor stimulation, however, can result in transient modulation, principally via phosphorylation, of membrane receptors and ion channels that sensitize the nociceptor. Repeated stimulation can also lead to post-translational modifications resulting in increased receptor and channel gene expression that result in turn in sustained nociceptor sensitization.[10]

Electrophysiologically, these changes results in generation of a nociceptor action potential on exposure to warming to less than 43°C and to a pathologic increase in firing frequency. Clinically, this can manifest as allodynia (pain due to a stimulus that does not normally evoke pain) or hyperalgesia (increased pain from a stimulus that normally evokes pain).[14] Sensitization can also occur in second-order neurons in the dorsal horn of the spinal cord; hence, both peripheral and central sensitization can occur in the context of sustained tissue inflammation or injury, predisposing to chronic pain even after healing or improvement of local tissue injury. Other postulated mechanisms of peripheral and central sensitization include alterations in sympathetic modulation of nociceptive input, phenotypic switch of non-nociceptors to express nociceptive characteristics, and effects of activated glia on dorsal horn neurons.[15–17]

The potent role of descending modulation was first dramatically shown by the demonstration of stimulation-induced analgesia in 1969, wherein brainstem stimulation enabled abdominal surgery without anesthetic agents and without resultant pain behaviors.[18] It has since become clear that centers in the periaqueductal gray (PAG) and rostroventral medulla (RVM) modulate the intensity of peripheral nociceptive transmission via descending modulation of dorsal horn neurons. Modulation is believed to be bidirectional, with either amplification or attenuation of pain as clinically possible. Although the PAG and RVM are critical output pathways of descending modulation, the PAG receives inputs from several cortical regions that likely can influence descending modulation in both pronociceptive and antinociceptive ways.[19]

It has long been known that injury to nociceptive pathways can, seemingly paradoxically, predispose to pain. Thus, a proportion of patients who suffer thalamic infarction develop, after a delay of several months on average, a chronic pain state perceived as involving the deafferented body areas. Deafferentation may be a relevant mechanism in some cases of pain with severe peripheral neuropathy or spinal cord injury. And, finally, in the setting of loss of both peripheral tissues and nociceptors – amputation – pain can develop in a phantom limb. Studies using functional MRI suggest that phantom limb pain is related to alterations in the cortical map of the homunculus in somatosensory cortex, as if pain is the default mechanism for sensory mislabeling.[20]

The aforementioned neural mechanisms of chronic pain represent pathologic, or maladaptive physiologic, responses to injury. Although they are all neural mechanisms, they are relevant to chronic pain from all etiologies. In addition, glial activation[21] and tissue inflammation can contribute to the maintenance of chronic pain. Finally, pain, as a symptom, can be a surrogate for distress – either mechanistically – that is, pain presenting as a biomarker of psychosocial disruption – or linguistically – that is, pain used as the chief complaint when in fact the chief concern is fear, disability, loss of physical independence, or loss of life roles due to a painful condition.

Taxonomy of Chronic Pain II: Clinical Pain Categories

Most readers find the clinical taxonomy that follows more familiar than the aforementioned mechanistic taxonomy, but the various mechanisms of chronic pain are relevant, to varying degrees, in each clinically based pain category. Put simply, it is incumbent on the pain diagnostician to address both complementary questions, "where does it hurt" (clinical taxonomy) and "why does it hurt" (mechanistic taxonomy).

This discussion begins with 2 unique categories based on possibly distinct mechanisms: neuropathic pain and fibromyalgia. Information gleaned from preclinical and clinical research in these areas has transformed understanding of chronic pain. A brief overview of several categories is then provided, based on organ system or region: musculoskeletal, spinal, headache, visceral, pelvic, and vascular pain. One unique category finishes this discussion: cancer pain. This is a mixed classification schema; however, it reflects the divisions in diagnostic categories that in actual practice drive patient referrals to particular medical specialties or subspecialties within pain medicine.

Neuropathic pain

Neuropathic pain has been defined as "pain arising as a direct consequence of a lesion or disease affecting the somatosensory system."[22] It is, therefore, distinct from other forms of chronic pain in that the pain generator is a disturbance in the nociceptive reporting system rather than a disturbance in innervated tissues. That said, neuropathic pain shares with other chronic pain states some of the postulated mechanisms of chronic pain, such as the potential for pronociceptive modulation and modification of nerve terminals as a consequence of repeated stimulation. Unlike other chronic pain categories, however, neuropathic pain has some distinct features that follow from the presence of neurologic dysfunction. First, as demonstrated clinically by neuropathic pain symptom inventory validation data,[23,24] allodynia and hyperalgesia are probably more prevalent in neuropathic pain than in some other chronic pain categories, such as musculoskeletal pain. Second, spontaneous sensory phenomena, such as paresthesias and sharp, shooting pains, are in particular characteristic of neuropathic pain. This has mechanistic face validity: metabolically challenged neurons, as, for example, in diabetic neuropathy, may at times not have sufficient energy stores to maintain adequate activity of the sodium-potassium pump, resulting in a pathologic elevation of the resting membrane potential and increase likelihood of spontaneous depolarization and generation of an action potential. Demyelinated axons, as can occur in chronic inflammatory demyelinating neuropathy, entrapment neuropathy (median nerve entrapment at the carpal tunnel), or post-traumatic neuralgia, are prone to ectopic and ephaptic discharges and to depolarization provoked by mechanical deformation, a strong indicator of a neuropathic etiology as in Tinel sign. Finally, a unique feature of neuropathic pain is the presence of sensory deficits; both negative and positive sensory phenomena are nearly universally present in neuropathic pain states and, conversely, normal sensory thresholds to small-fiber and large-fiber modality testing should put a diagnosis of neuropathic pain in question. Hence, examining the patient is essential.

Common neuropathic pain states are painful diabetic neuropathy, postherpetic neuralgia, trigeminal neuralgia, posttraumatic neuralgia, spinal cord injury pain, and central poststroke pain. Common medical causes of painful neuropathy are frank diabetes and impaired glucose tolerance in the context of the metabolic syndrome, chemotherapy-induced neuropathy, alcoholic neuropathy, and the infectious neuropathies caused by HIV and chronic hepatitis C infection with cryoglobulinemia.

Fibromyalgia and related disorders

Fibromyalgia is a well-characterized syndrome of widespread muscle tenderness exacerbated by physical activity and associated with multiple discrete areas of tenderness to pressure in the absence of muscle or joint pathology. Fibromyalgia is of particular scientific interest because of accumulating evidence that it is associated with impaired descending modulation of afferent input or, more specifically, conditioned pain modulation. As such it is a painful state possibly related to augmented sensory processing but is not clearly neuropathic, not clearly inflammatory, and not purely nociceptive. Impaired conditioned pain modulation in fibromyalgia has been demonstrated in psychophysical paradigms,[25,26] and abnormal cortical modulation of pain has been demonstrated using functional imaging.[27] Fibromyalgia is associated with a high incidence of fatigue, sleep disturbance, and symptoms of cognitive inefficiency.

PAIN CATEGORIES BASED ON ORGAN SYSTEM OR REGION

In many patients with regional pain syndromes, the primary diagnostic challenge is to determine the degree to which the chief complaint reflects local organ system pathology; occupational, postural, or lifestyle-related causes; neuropathic pain; or pain due to impaired pain modulation as is believed to occur in fibromyalgia. Fibromyalgia has provided the model for disorders of pain modulation that present as organ-based or region-based syndromes and have historically been termed functional disorders. Using diffuse noxious inhibitory controls, functional imaging, and other research tools of central pain modulation, a clearer understanding of these conditions is now emerging.

The following is a brief outline of pain categories based on organ system or region.

Musculoskeletal Pain

Musculoskeletal pain is pain in the moving parts of the human organism. Motion occurs across joints but also involves the ligaments, muscles, and the tendons that link the contractile apparatus (muscle) to the center of movement (joint). The central differentiation in joint pain diagnosis is between inflammatory joint disease and osteoarthritis. A well-recognized differentiating symptom is the presence of morning stiffness with gradual resolution over minutes to hours, common in inflammatory arthritis, as opposed to joint pain that develops reproducibly with activity and weight bearing, because is prominent in osteoarthritis. Inflammatory modulators of pain can be present in both but are primary in inflammatory arthritides. Distinct from joint pain, musculoskeletal pain can reflect a variety of specific impingement or overuse syndromes that are suggested in the history or by specific provocative maneuvers.

Myofascial Pain

Myofascial pain is characterized by localized tenderness in muscle at rest, often concentrated at defined trigger points. Literature exists to support the conflicting, or perhaps complementary, hypotheses that myofascial pain reflects local pathology as well as disturbances of pain modulation in the central nervous system.[28,29]

Spinal Pain

Neck and low back pain are complex disorders because of the interaction of musculoskeletal, articular, radicular, myofascial, postural, and occupational factors. Careful clinical evaluation of each is therefore needed. It has long been recognized that structural pathology on spine imaging is prevalent in asymptomatic individuals,[30] and clinical correlation is, therefore, of particular importance in evaluation of pain referenced to the spine.

Headache

As with other chronic pain conditions, it is critical to determine whether structural intracranial pathology is present. This can readily be established with a neurologic history and examination. Prevalent headache syndromes include migraine and its variants, analgesic rebound headache, and muscle contraction headache syndromes, including cervicogenic headache.

Vascular Pain

Vascular pain syndromes are limited in number and include claudication syndromes, characterized by ischemic pain associated with muscular activity (usually in the lower limbs) that is relieved at rest, rest pain due to severe limb ischemia, and the intermittent pain associated with Raynaud disease (an isolated phenomenon) and Raynaud syndrome (Raynaud symptoms in the context of systemic inflammatory disease).

Visceral and Pelvic Pain

Visceral pain is distinct in that the adequate stimulus (that is, the stimulus that is transduced into an action potential) in small diameter axons in the gut is visceral distention; the types of tissue injury that cause pain in skin and other somatic tissues do not cause pain in the gut. Chronic visceral pain can develop as a consequence of a wide variety of gastrointestinal disorders. Among the most prevalent and difficult to manage is chronic pancreatitis, in which pain is often the most disabling feature. There is evidence of a combination of local organ pathology, nociceptor sensitization, and altered pain modulation in chronic pancreatitis, and management often requires a multidisciplinary approach as in other chronic pain conditions.[31]

Visceral pain without evident gastrointestinal pathology is common, and the most prevalent such syndrome is irritable bowel syndrome. Irritable bowel syndrome has been associated with evidence of alterations in pain modulation.[32]

Pelvic pain involves a wide variety of diagnostic and etiologic categories, including both somatic and visceral pain generators. First, identifiable pathology in the gastrointestinal, genitourinary, or pelvic organs needs to be identified and treated. In some cases myofascial or musculoskeletal pelvic floor dysfunction can be identified and treated with physical therapy. Prior surgery or childbirth can result in neuropathic injury. Pelvic pain syndromes that are often not associated with identifiable local organ pathology and are difficult to treat include prostate pain syndrome and vulvodynia.

Cancer Pain

Cancer pain is a special case in that there are several distinct chronic pain syndromes prevalent in cancer, including bone pain from metastases, local pain from mass lesions, pain from complications of surgery and radiation therapy, and neuropathic pain from chemotherapy.

ASSESSMENT OF PAIN

To comprehensively assess a patient's pain symptoms, it is important to characterize the pain syndrome by mechanism, organ system, and syndrome when possible. As discussed previously, there may be a combination of postulated generators, such as nociceptive, inflammatory, sensitization, and cortical modulation.[33] Accordingly, obtaining a thorough history is critical when evaluating a patient with chronic pain.

To properly assess chronic pain, a complete history should include an individual's medical history and specific pain-related questions. The provider should first investigate the location of the pain; whether or not the pain radiates; the intensity, characteristics, or quality of the pain; duration, onset, and changes since onset; whether or not the pain is constant or intermittent; any breakthrough pain; exacerbating or triggering factors; and lastly any relieving factors.[34] The provider should then inquire about any specific events in the patient's past (if known) linked to the onset of the pain. If a patient is unable to provide clear descriptors of the nature of the pain, prompts may assist the patient in describing the sensation of the pain. Examples of descriptors include sharp, dull, stabbing, shooting, burning, electrical, or pulsating.[34]

Numerous medical comorbidities can accompany and contribute to chronic pain. Although it is important to address chronic pain in isolation, it is also imperative to treat the underlying medical condition to prevent worsening pain complaints and medical complications. These medical comorbidities often include but are certainly not limited to diabetes, cancer, hypertension, chronic alcohol use, obesity, depression, psychiatric disorders, and chronic tobacco use.[35] Moreover, postural and mechanical mechanisms and poor workplace ergonomic environments can also have a dramatic impact on pain symptoms and treatment.

A patient's emotional and psychological state is another major factor in chronic pain control and management.[36] So too are social, occupational, and environmental factors that may influence pain perception and management and are thus important to consider when evaluating a patient with chronic pain.[37]

At the onset of treatment, a provider treating people with chronic pain must also be mindful of the importance of setting realistic expectations. Managing chronic pain can result in strain to a patient-provider relationship[38] and it is, therefore, imperative that realistic goals are defined early to allow for potential setbacks and course corrections. Patients often enter the provider-patient relationship with an expectation of complete pain relief. Because such outcomes are the exception rather than the rule, the entire care team should strive for open and transparent communication with patients regarding pain treatment outcomes, including that the process of treating pain is often a long-term, iterative undertaking.[39] Incongruent expectations not only are personally unpleasant for patient and provider but also can have negative medical consequences and exacerbate a patient's symptoms.

PAIN ASSESSMENT INSTRUMENTS

There are many established approaches for assessing pain beyond the medical history and examination. Perhaps the most instructive is the pain diagram, in which a patient is instructed to demonstrate areas and types of pain on a body outline. The pain diagram can, in an elegant fashion, not only allow a patient to provide the chief complaint in a pictorial representation but also indicate immediately to a provider the likely diagnosis, by virtue of indicating the pain type and areas affected by pain (**Fig. 1**).

Pain intensity has become a standard pain reporting tool and the universally recognized tool for reporting pain as the fifth vital sign in the general medical clinic. There are several ways for a patient to report pain intensity. The 3 most commonly used methods to quantify the pain are verbal rating scales, numeric rating scales and visual analog scales.[40]

Verbal Rating Scales

Verbal rating scales use adjectives or phrases to characterize the pain. Each adjective or phrase is assigned a number according to its rank.

Numeric Rating Scales

Numeric rating scales consist of a series of numbers rating pain intensity, typically from 0 to 10 or 0 to 100, with 0 being "no pain" and 10 or 100 "the worst pain imaginable."

Visual Analog Scales

Visual analog scales usually consist of a line, 10 cm long, with verbal anchors on each end, such as "no pain" and "worst pain imaginable." The patient is instructed to place

A

Please use colored markers to indicate location and type of your pain on the diagram below:

Yellow = aching
Blue = burning
Red = stabbing
Black = numbness
Green = tingling/pins & needles
Orange = hurts to touch
Purple = other_____

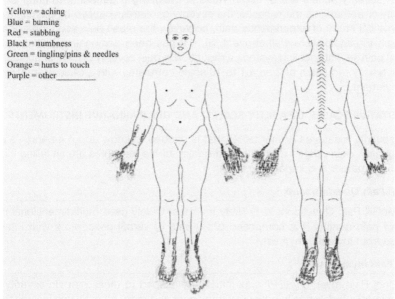

B

Please use colored markers to indicate location and type of your pain on the diagram below:

Yellow = aching
Blue = burning
Red = stabbing
Black = numbness
Green = tingling/pins & needles
Orange = hurts to touch
Purple = other_____

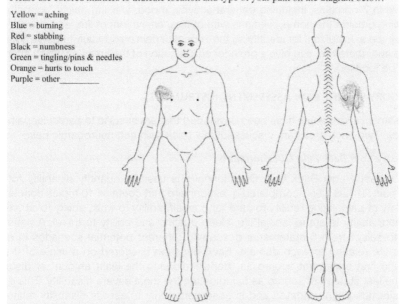

Fig. 1. Pain diagrams from patients with (*A*) painful sensory neuropathy and (*B*) postherpetic neuralgia. (*Courtesy of* Sehgal N, MD, Madison, WI.)

a mark on the line indicating pain severity, which can then be measured in millimeters, which more closely approximates a continuous measure of pain severity.

Pain severity scales are of some value in providing a general indication of pain severity or perhaps, in many cases, the severity of distress caused by pain. In a psychophysical study of experimental pain, however, the mean pain scores reported at the pain threshold were well above 1/10.[41] It has been demonstrated that using a 0 to 10 pain severity scaling system, a reduction in pain severity of 33% or an absolute pain intensity reduction of 2 on a 1 to 10 scale correlates with a clinically meaningful improvement.[42]

QUALITATIVE SCALES, DISABILITY SCALES, AND DISCRIMINATIVE INSTRUMENTS

Pain severity measures do not tell all that is needed to know about a person's pain. Pain quality, pain-related disability, and quality-of-life measures are all telling indicators of the nature and impact of pain.

McGill Pain Questionnaire

The McGill Pain Questionnaire is likely the most widely used multidimensional measure of pain quality. It is composed of 20 sets of verbal descriptors with intensity labeled from lowest to highest.[43]

Brief Pain Inventory

The Brief Pain Inventory (BPI) was initially developed to measure pain severity and pain-related interference in patients with cancer and more recently has included non-cancer pain patients. The most commonly used version of this scale uses an 11-point numeric rating scale where 0 = no interference and 11 = complete pain-related interference in 7 domains, including general activity, mood, walking ability, normal work including outside the home, relations with others, enjoyment of life, and sleep.[44] The BPI can be a useful tool for identifying the impact of pain on clinically important life domains and, therefore, can give a provider an indication of the areas on which attention need be focused.[45]

CATEGORY-SPECIFIC PAIN ASSESSMENT INSTRUMENTS

Assessment instruments have been developed that are specific to particular pain categories. Two such areas are discussed: low back pain and neuropathic pain.

Oswestry Low Back Pain Questionnaire

The Oswestry Low Back Pain Questionnaire is used to quantify disability for low back pain. This is a self-completed questionnaire that contains 10 topics concerning intensity of pain, lifting, ability to care for oneself, ability to walk, ability to sit, sexual function, ability to stand, social life, sleep quality, and ability to travel. A patient is able to select from 6 statements describing different potential scenarios in a patient's life relating to each domain. Each question is scored on a scale of 0 to 5, with the first statement scored as 0 and indicating the least amount of disability and the last statement scored as 5, indicating the most severe disability. This questionnaire has been validated and is used commonly to assess disability related to low back pain.[46]

Neuropathic Pain Assessment Tools

Several instruments have been designed for the purpose of discriminating neuropathic from non-neuropathic pain, the description and monitoring of neuropathic pain symptoms, or both. These include the Neuropathic Pain Scale, the Neuropathic Pain Questionnaire, and the Douleur Neuropathique 4 (DN4) questionnaire.[23,24,47] All include similar self-reported questionnaires inquiring about the presence of positive (spontaneous burning, paresthesias, hyperalgesia, or allodynia) and negative (reduced perception of tactile, thermal, or punctate stimuli) sensory symptoms, and some include limited examination components. Discriminative instruments generally indicate the presence of neuropathic pain if both positive and negative sensory symptoms are present, particularly if the positive symptoms are of the nature discussed previously. The Neuropathic Pain Questionnaire multiplies the numeric score provided in response to each question by a constant specific for that question; the sum of the values thus obtained indicates that the pain is likely non-neuropathic if it is less than 0 and likely neuropathic if it is greater than 0. Such tools are not intended to replace clinical judgment but do have the benefit of accelerating history taking, providing responses that can be monitored over the course of treatment, and providing a pretest probability for the pain category and even cause in advance of a medical evaluation.

ASSESSING RISK AND BENEFIT OF OPIOID THERAPY

Opioid therapy can be a valuable component of pain management but also carries risk of numerous potential adverse effects as well as tachyphylaxis, dependency, addiction, misuse, and diversion. In addition, appropriate monitoring of opioid therapy introduces added complexity to a patient's care plan. Therefore, several instruments have been designed to assist the practitioner in assessing risks, and, in some cases benefits, of opioid therapy.[48]

Screener and Opioid Assessment for Patients with Pain

Screener and Opioid Assessment for Patients with Pain (SOAPP) is a scientifically validated tool that is self-administered and is designed for use by patients who are receiving, or under consideration for, long-term opioid therapy for management of chronic pain. This tool allows physicians to better gauge the likelihood of opioid misuse or abuse.[49]

Opioid Risk Tool

The Opioid Risk Tool (ORT) is a self-administered 5-question assessment. It assesses the subject for features known to correlate with risk of opioid use, including personal or family history of substance abuse, history of preadolescent sexual abuse, depression, attention-deficit disorder, obsessive-compulsive disorder, bipolar disorder, and schizophrenia. It helps predict who is at high risk of exhibiting aberrant behaviors associated with opioid abuse or addiction.[50]

Diagnosis, Intractability, Risk, Efficacy

Diagnosis, Intractability, Risk, Efficacy (DIRE) score assesses the risk of opioid abuse and suitability of candidates for long-term opioid therapy. It comprises 7 items. Unlike SOAPP and ORT, DIRE is an assessment completed by the provider and is designed to assess potential benefit and risk of opioid therapy.[51]

ASSESSMENTS OF PSYCHOLOGICAL STATE AND TRAIT IN PAIN MANAGEMENT

As discussed previously, assessment of psychological factors is critical in pain management. In some centers this is performed routinely by a psychologist or other mental health professional with subspecialty experience in pain management. Assessment of anxiety and depression, using either a mental health evaluation or standard inventories of these comorbidities, is valuable. In addition, validated instruments of some pain-related mental health states and traits exist. These include the Pain Anxiety Symptoms Scale,[52] which assesses severity of pain-related anxiety, and the Pain Catastrophizing Scale. Pain catastrophizing has been conceptualized as "an exaggerated negative orientation toward noxious stimuli"[53] and reflects a substantially disabling outcome of chronic pain in many people in pain. Application of the Pain Catastrophizing Scale can identify individuals in whom addressing this aspect of their pain experience may be as important as providing analgesia per se.

PUTTING IT ALL TOGETHER: A SAMPLE PAIN MANAGEMENT CONSULTATION
Chief Complaint

"My back hurts."

History of Present Illness

Mr Smith is a 48-year-old man with past medical history of diabetes, obesity, and depression who presents as a new patient consultation to a chronic pain clinic for management of his back pain complaints. He states his pain began 20 years ago; however, he is unsure of any inciting event or trauma prior to the initiation of his complaints. His pain has gradually worsened over the past 20 years. He describes his pain in his low back as a sharp, aching feeling and denies any radicular symptoms into his lower extremities. The pain is intermittent, worse with back extension, and alleviated by sitting or lying down. Currently he describes his pain as 3/10; however, it may increase up to 7/10 while he is working or extending his back. He had radiographs performed and MRI ordered by his primary care physician due to the chronicity of his complaints for which he was told he had degenerative changes. He tried physical therapy, chiropractic care, and massage techniques, none of which provided long-lasting benefit for his pain complaints. He was prescribed nonsteroidal anti-inflammatory drugs, muscle relaxants, and opiate medications intermittently over the past 20 years and states some alleviation of his pain in the past with use. He has never undergone injections for his pain complaints. He denies any bowel or bladder changes, any unintentional weight loss, saddle anesthesia, or weakness in his extremities.

Past Medical History

Diabetes mellitus, obesity, and hypertension.

Past Surgical History

Denies.

Psychiatric History

Reactive depression 8 years ago and on medication since; denies prior psychiatric hospitalization, thoughts of self-harm, or anhedonia.

Social History

He works full time as an electrician. He states working does make his pain symptoms worse. At the end of his workday he returns home only to get in bed due to the severity of his pain. Although he is independent in performing his instrumental activities of daily living, he is unable to help with any household chores at home due to his pain complaints. He is married with 2 children, ages 23 and 25. He quit tobacco use 5 years ago. He denies any alcohol use or illicit drug use. He is unable to perform regular exercise due to his back pain complaints. He believes his pain is interfering with his daily life and would like to find ways to improve his function given his current pain level.

Medications

Insulin for his diabetes mellitus, lisinopril for his hypertension, and fluoxetine for his depression.

Allergies

No known drug allergies.

Focused Physical Examination

Gait: Normal without the use of an assistive device. He was able to walk on his toes and heels without difficulty.

Back: No abnormalities noted on inspection. Full lumbar flexion and extension only mildly limited due to pain. Pain on palpation of his lumbar paraspinal muscles and over sacroiliac joints bilaterally. Pain on lumbar extension and twisting (facet loading) bilaterally and reproduced his pain complaints. Straight leg raise was negative bilaterally. Flexion, abduction, external rotation, and extension was positive bilaterally; however, it did not reproduce his pain complaints.

Strength: 5/5 Bilateral lower extremities.

Sensation: Intact to light touch in bilateral lower extremities.

Reflexes: 2+ and symmetric in bilateral patellae and Achilles

No ankle clonus was elicited and Babinski was negative bilaterally.

Fibromyalgia tender points: 4/18.

Brief Pain Inventory

Average pain 5/10 over past 24 hours (range 3–6); estimates 30% relief from medications. Pain interference greater than 4/10 in general activity, walking, and normal work; less than 4/10 in other domains.

McGill Pain Questionnaire

A score of 30 of 78 (higher scores correlate with more severe pain).

Oswestry Low Back Pain Questionnaire

15/50 or 30%.

Opioid Risk Tool

3

Medical Diagnosis

1. Lumbar facet joint pain
2. Myofascial pain
3. Sacroiliac joint pain

Treatment Recommendations

1. Would recommend reinitiation of physical therapy for biomechanical recommendations, stretching, and a graded home exercise program
2. Medications: short-term trial of nonsteroidal anti-inflammatory drugs and a muscle relaxant because the patient describes benefit in the past. Switch his current

selective serotonin reuptake inhibitor to a balanced serotonin norepinephrine reuptake inhibitor to help with both mood and pain.
3. Injections: will perform lumbar facet injections and/or medial branch blocks
4. Pain psychology evaluation of psychological state and traits, to better assess psychosocial impact of pain and to educate regarding strategies for self-care and relaxation exercises and to reinforce realistic functional expectations and goals
5. Patient may be a candidate for long-acting opioid therapy in the future, depending on response to initial interventions.
6. Follow-up in 2 months

REFERENCES

1. Tsang A, Von Korff M, Lee S, et al. Common chronic pain conditions in developed and developing countries: gender and age differences and comorbidity with depression-anxiety disorders. J Pain 2008;9(10):883–91.
2. GBD 2010 Heat Map. 2015. Available at: http://vizhub.healthdata.org/irank/heat.php. Accessed May 13, 2015.
3. Gaskin DJ, Richard P. The economic costs of pain in the United States. J Pain 2012;13(8):715–24.
4. Institute of Medicine. Relieving pain in America: a blueprint for transforming prevention, care, education, and research. 2011. Available at: https://www.iom.edu/Reports/2011/Relieving-Pain-in-America-A-Blueprint-for-Transforming-Prevention-Care-Education-Research.aspx. Accessed May 11, 2015.
5. IASP taxonomy. 1994. Available at: http://iasp-pain.org/Taxonomy?navItemNumber=576#Pain. Accessed April 06, 2015.
6. Almeida TF, Roizenblatt S, Tufik S. Afferent pain pathways: a neuroanatomical review. Brain Res 2004;1000(1–2):40–56.
7. Berthier M, Starkstein S, Leiguarda R. Asymbolia for pain: a sensory-limbic disconnection syndrome. Ann Neurol 1988;24(1):41–9.
8. Keszthelyi D, Troost FJ, Masclee AA. Irritable bowel syndrome: methods, mechanisms, and pathophysiology. Methods to assess visceral hypersensitivity in irritable bowel syndrome. Am J Physiol Gastrointest Liver Physiol 2012;303(2):G141–54.
9. Williams DA, Gracely RH. Biology and therapy of fibromyalgia. Functional magnetic resonance imaging findings in fibromyalgia. Arthritis Res Ther 2006;8(6):224.
10. Costigan M, Scholz J, Woolf CJ. Neuropathic pain: a maladaptive response of the nervous system to damage. Annu Rev Neurosci 2009;32:1–32.
11. Young EE, Lariviere WR, Belfer I. Genetic basis of pain variability: recent advances. J Med Genet 2012;49(1):1–9.
12. Bali KK, Kuner R. Noncoding RNAs: key molecules in understanding and treating pain. Trends Mol Med 2014;20(8):437–48.
13. Topics and Codes. Topics and Codes. Available at: http://www.iasp-pain.org/files/Content/ContentFolders/Publications2/ClassificationofChronicPain/Part_I-Scheme+Topics.pdf. Accessed May 06, 2015.
14. LaMotte RH, Thalhammer JG, Torebjork HE, et al. Peripheral neural mechanisms of cutaneous hyperalgesia following mild injury by heat. J Neurosci 1982;2(6):765–81.
15. Janig BR. The role of the sympathetic nervous system in pain processing. The pain system in normal and pathological states: a primer for clinicians. 1st edition. Seattle (WA): IASP Press; 2004. p. 193–210.

16. Neumann S, Doubell TP, Leslie T, et al. Inflammatory pain hypersensitivity mediated by phenotypic switch in myelinated primary sensory neurons. Nature 1996; 384(6607):360–4.
17. Milligan ED, Watkins LR. Pathological and protective roles of glia in chronic pain. Nature reviews. Neuroscience 2009;10(1):23–36.
18. Reynolds DV. Surgery in the rat during electrical analgesia induced by focal brain stimulation. Science 1969;164(3878):444–5.
19. Fields H. State-dependent opioid control of pain. Nature reviews. Neuroscience 2004;5(7):565–75.
20. Karl A, Birbaumer N, Lutzenberger W, et al. Reorganization of motor and somatosensory cortex in upper extremity amputees with phantom limb pain. J Neurosci 2001;21(10):3609–18.
21. Alfonso Romero-Sandoval E, Sweitzer S. Nonneuronal central mechanisms of pain: glia and immune response. Prog Mol Biol Translational Sci 2015;131: 325–58.
22. Treede RD, Jensen TS, Campbell JN, et al. Neuropathic pain: redefinition and a grading system for clinical and research purposes. Neurology 2008;70(18): 1630–5.
23. Bouhassira D, Attal N, Alchaar H, et al. Comparison of pain syndromes associated with nervous or somatic lesions and development of a new neuropathic pain diagnostic questionnaire (DN4). Pain 2005;114(1–2):29–36.
24. Krause SJ, Backonja MM. Development of a neuropathic pain questionnaire. Clin J Pain 2003;19(5):306–14.
25. Julien N, Goffaux P, Arsenault P, et al. Widespread pain in fibromyalgia is related to a deficit of endogenous pain inhibition. Pain 2005;114(1–2):295–302.
26. Staud R, Robinson ME, Vierck CJ Jr, et al. Diffuse noxious inhibitory controls (DNIC) attenuate temporal summation of second pain in normal males but not in normal females or fibromyalgia patients. Pain 2003;101(1–2):167–74.
27. Lopez-Sola M, Pujol J, Wager TD, et al. Altered functional magnetic resonance imaging responses to nonpainful sensory stimulation in fibromyalgia patients. Arthritis Rheumatol 2014;66(11):3200–9.
28. Niddam DM, Chan RC, Lee SH, et al. Central representation of hyperalgesia from myofascial trigger point. Neuroimage 2008;39(3):1299–306.
29. Kuan TS. Current studies on myofascial pain syndrome. Curr Pain Headache Rep 2009;13(5):365–9.
30. Boden SD, McCowin PR, Davis DO, et al. Abnormal magnetic-resonance scans of the cervical spine in asymptomatic subjects. A prospective investigation. J Bone Jointt Surg 1990;72(8):1178–84.
31. Bouwense SA, de Vries M, Schreuder LT, et al. Systematic mechanism-orientated approach to chronic pancreatitis pain. World J Gastroenterol 2015; 21(1):47–59.
32. Brandesi S, Mayer EA. Irritable bowel syndrome. Science of pain. Boston: Elsevier; 2009.
33. Benzon HT. Essentials of pain medicine. 3rd edition. Philadelphia: Elsevier/Saunders; 2011.
34. Assessment and management of chronic pain. 2013. Available at: https://www.icsi.org/guidelines__more/catalog_guidelines_and_more/catalog_guidelines/catalog_neurological_guidelines/pain/. Accessed May 12, 2015.
35. Makris UE, Higashi RT, Marks EG, et al. Ageism, negative attitudes, and competing co-morbidities - why older adults may not seek care for restricting back pain: a qualitative study. BMC Geriatr 2015;15:39.

36. Kadimpati S, Zale EL, Hooten MW, et al. Associations between Neuroticism and depression in relation to catastrophizing and pain-related anxiety in chronic pain patients. PLoS One 2015;10(4). e0126351.
37. Pizzo PA, Clark NM. Alleviating suffering 101–pain relief in the United States. N Engl J Med 2012;366(3):197–9.
38. Matthias MS, Krebs EE, Bergman AA, et al. Communicating about opioids for chronic pain: a qualitative study of patient attributions and the influence of the patient-physician relationship. Eur J Pain 2014;18(6):835–43.
39. Dima A, Lewith GT, Little P, et al. Patients' treatment beliefs in low back pain: development and validation of a questionnaire in primary care. Pain 2015; 156(8):1489–500.
40. Hjermstad MJ, Fayers PM, Haugen DF, et al. Studies comparing Numerical Rating Scales, Verbal Rating Scales, and Visual Analogue Scales for assessment of pain intensity in adults: a systematic literature review. J Pain Symptom Manage 2011;41(6):1073–93.
41. Kelly KG, Cook T, Backonja MM. Pain ratings at the thresholds are necessary for interpretation of quantitative sensory testing. Muscle Nerve 2005;32(2): 179–84.
42. Farrar JT, Portenoy RK, Berlin JA, et al. Defining the clinically important difference in pain outcome measures. Pain 2000;88(3):287–94.
43. Melzack R, Stein C, Mendl G. The McGill pain questionnaire. Available at: http://www.cebp.nl/?NODE=77&SUBNODE=1136. Accessed May 12, 2015.
44. Atkinson TM, Rosenfeld BD, Sit L, et al. Using confirmatory factor analysis to evaluate construct validity of the Brief Pain Inventory (BPI). J Pain Symptom Manage 2011;41(3):558–65.
45. Cleeland CS. Brief pain inventory. Pain Inventory; 1991. Available at: http://www.mdanderson.org/education-and-research/departments-programs-and-labs/departments-and-divisions/symptom-research/symptom-assessment-tools/brief-pain-inventory.html. Accessed May 12, 2015.
46. Gronblad M, Hupli M, Wennerstrand P, et al. Intercorrelation and test-retest reliability of the Pain Disability Index (PDI) and the Oswestry Disability Questionnaire (ODQ) and their correlation with pain intensity in low back pain patients. Clin J Pain 1993;9(3):189–95.
47. Galer BS, Jensen MP. Development and preliminary validation of a pain measure specific to neuropathic pain: the neuropathic pain scale. Neurology 1997;48(2): 332–8.
48. Moore TM, Jones T, Browder JH, et al. A comparison of common screening methods for predicting aberrant drug-related behavior among patients receiving opioids for chronic pain management. Pain Med 2009;10(8): 1426–33.
49. Butler S. The screener and opioid assessment for patients with pain (SOAPP). New Hampshire Medical Society.
50. LR W. Opiod Risk Tool. Predicting aberrant behaviors in opioid-treated patients: preliminary validation of the opioid risk tool. 2005. Available at: http://www.opioidrisk.com/node/1203. Accessed May 11, 2015.
51. Belgrade MJ, Schamber CD, Lindgren BR. The DIRE score: predicting outcomes of opioid prescribing for chronic pain. J Pain 2006;7(9):671–81.
52. McCracken LM, Zayfert C, Gross RT. The pain anxiety symptoms scale: development and validation of a scale to measure fear of pain. Pain 1992;50(1):67–73.
53. Sullivan MJL, Bishop S, Pivik J. The pain catastrophizing scale: development and validation. Psychol Assess 1995;7:524–32.

The Acute to Chronic Pain Transition

Can Chronic Pain Be Prevented?

John-Paul J. Pozek, MD[a],*, David Beausang, MD[b],
Jaime L. Baratta, MD[a], Eugene R. Viscusi, MD[b]

KEYWORDS

- Chronic postsurgical pain • Neuropathic pain • Quantitative sensory testing
- Central sensitization • Peripheral sensitization • Ketamine • Gabapentinoids

KEY POINTS

- Chronic postsurgical pain (CPSP) is defined as an unpleasant sensory and emotional experience that persists for 3 to 6 months after surgery.
- There are multiple risk factors for the development of CPSP. These include patient-specific and procedure-specific factors.
- Quantitative sensory testing (QST), psychomimetic testing, and postoperative Verbal Rating Scale and Numerical Pain Scale scores have shown promise for prediction of development of CPSP.
- The mechanism for development of CPSP is currently unknown, but is likely due to peripheral and central sensitization that can occur after persistent acute pain.
- Multimodal analgesia significantly reduces acute postoperative pain, but has yet to be proven to decrease incidence of CPSP. This may be due to inadequate duration of therapy.

INTRODUCTION

Chronic postsurgical pain (CPSP) is defined as the persistence of pain at least 3 months after a surgical procedure. Emphasis is placed on the relation to surgical intervention, as pain attributed to malignancy or infection is not included. Persistence of pain can be a distressing process, leading to increased health care spending and reduced quality of life.[1] **Table 1** identifies incidence of CPSP with common surgical procedures. When these percentages are applied to the estimated volumes of these procedures, we can see that many patients are at risk.[1]

[a] Department of Anesthesiology, Thomas Jefferson University, Gibbon Building, Suite 8280, 111 South 11th Street, Philadelphia, PA 19107, USA; [b] Department of Anesthesiology, Thomas Jefferson University, Gibbon Building, Suite 8490, 111 South 11th Street, Philadelphia, PA 19107, USA
* Corresponding author.
E-mail address: John-Paul.Pozek@jefferson.edu

Med Clin N Am 100 (2016) 17–30
http://dx.doi.org/10.1016/j.mcna.2015.08.005   **medical.theclinics.com**

Table 1
Incidence of chronic postsurgical pain following common procedures

Surgical Type	Incidence of Chronic Postsurgical Pain, %	US Surgical Volumes, 1000s
Amputation	57–62	159
Breast surgery	27–48	479
Thoracotomy	52–61	Unknown
Herniorrhaphy	19–40	609
Coronary artery bypass graft	23–39	598
Cesarean delivery	12	220

Data from Kehlet H, Jensen TS, Woolf C. Persistent postsurgical pain: risk factors and prevention. Lancet 2006;367:1618–25.

Research in the topic has intensified since Crombie and colleagues[2] first described the conversion of acute to chronic pain in 1998. Current studies have focused on identifying risk factors to predict CPSP, elucidating the mechanism, and building analgesic strategies to avoid conversion of acute to chronic pain.

RISK FACTORS FOR DEVELOPMENT OF CHRONIC POSTSURGICAL PAIN

Numerous studies determined risk factors for the development of CPSP. These risk factors are both patient-specific and surgery-specific, as summarized in **Fig. 1**.

Demographic Factors

Risk of developing CPSP is associated with younger patient age and female gender. In the surgical treatment of breast cancer, younger women present with larger breast masses, increased postoperative pain, and develop CPSP more frequently than older patients.[3] A study by Smith and colleagues[4] showed that 65% of women aged 30 to 49 had persistent pain after mastectomy compared with 40% in the 50 to 69 age group and only a quarter of patients older than 70. This trend of increased development of CPSP in younger populations is also seen after hernia repairs.[5]

Gender exhibits importance in the development of CPSP. Katz and colleagues[6] demonstrated that women are at a greater risk than men for both acute and persistent

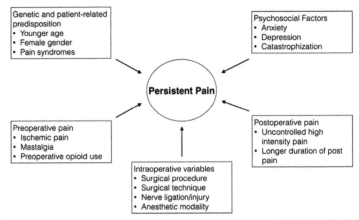

Fig. 1. Risk factors for CPSP following surgery. (*Data from* Refs.[3–6,17,19,20,22,23,25,26,28–33,39])

postoperative pain. Other demographic factors, such as employment, housing status, and marital status have not been shown to contribute to the development of CPSP.

Genetic Factors

The interpatient variation with regard to sensitivity and perception of pain has led to attempts at identifying genetic components that increase the risk of CPSP. Genotypic variations of Na^+ channels, μ-opioid receptors, and GTP cyclohydrolase have been studied,[7–9] along with genetic explanations for the variations in cyclo-oxygenase-2 (COX-2) and nonsteroidal anti-inflammatory drug responses.[10]

Single-nucleotide polymorphisms are hypothesized to inhibit the activity of catechol-o-methyltransferase (COMT) and increase sensitivity to pain. Early studies found a correlation between polymorphisms and the development of chronic temporomandibular arthralgia.[11] However, the role of COMT variation in predicting postoperative pain has more recently come into question. In a study by Kambur and colleagues,[12] polymorphisms in COMT had only weak associations with increased sensitivity to heat and cold pain. Clinical applicability of COMT polymorphisms was not shown, as these patients did not demonstrate increased postoperative opioid consumption.

Experimentation on mice suggests that development of neuropathic pain after a nerve injury has a strong heritable component.[13] This has yet to be investigated in the human population, but a study reviewing chronic pain after cardiac surgery yielded intriguing results. Patients with chronic pain after cardiac surgery were more likely to experience pain in both sternotomy and saphenectomy sites rather than at each site separately.[14] Devor[15] hypothesized that this is evidence of a heritable component for development of CPSP.

Psychosocial Factors

The role of depression and anxiety is well documented in patients with chronic nonsurgical pain. Becker and colleagues[16] found that 60% of patients with chronic pain reported psychiatric comorbidities. This led to a shift in theories about chronic pain from a strictly biomedical model to a biopsychosocial one, integrating biological and psychological variables. Evidence regarding psychosocial factors in the development of CPSP has been mixed.

Katz and colleagues[6] identified preoperative anxiety as a risk factor for development of pain for up to 30 days after breast surgery. In patients with mastectomy, persistent pain was more prevalent in patients with preoperative anxiety and depression.[17] Depression has also been seen as an independent risk factor for patients developing CPSP after hip and knee replacement.[18] Still other studies found no evidence that preoperative anxiety and depression significantly predict postoperative pain.[19]

An exaggerated pessimism regarding postoperative pain, or a tendency to catastrophize pain, may be seen as a risk factor for CPSP. Peters and colleagues[20] demonstrated that fear of surgery was associated with more pain, poorer recovery, and decreased quality of life. Catastrophism of pain correlates positively with development of phantom pain up to 2 years after amputation.[21]

Disease States

Multiple pain syndromes, such as fibromyalgia, migraine headaches, irritable bowel syndrome (IBS), irritable bladder, and Reynaud syndrome, are associated with the development of CPSP. Studies show that IBS, headaches, and preexisting lower back pain are risk factors for chronic pain after herniorrhaphy.[22,23] The presence of fibromyalgia and its effect on development of CPSP is an area of interest. A study of patients with CPSP after hysterectomy found that many women complained of preoperative pain in the head, neck, shoulders, and lower back. These locations of pain are commonly found in fibromyalgia. In a recent study, patients undergoing hip arthroplasty were given a survey on fibromyalgia, and those with higher scores suggestive of fibromyalgia were found to have increased postoperative opioid consumption.[24]

Preoperative Pain

The presence of pain before surgery or untreated pain is a risk factor for development of CPSP. Multiple studies regarding postherniotomy pain show preoperative pain and functional impairment significantly increase risk for development of CPSP.[5,19]

Development of phantom and stump pain after amputation has been associated with preoperative ischemic pain in the affected extremity.[25] This can be applied to thoracic surgery, as well as patients requiring opioids preoperatively had a significantly higher risk of developing chronic pain than those who did not require opioids.[26] In surgery for breast cancer, patients with mastalgia preoperatively exhibited a higher risk of developing phantom breast pain.[27] This has not been demonstrated for all surgeries, as preoperative hip pain did not correlate with the development of CPSP after arthroplasty.

Surgical Factors

Surgical decisions, such as technique, incision location, and expertise, affect the risk for development of CPSP. Duration of surgery of more than 3 hours is associated with increased risk of developing CPSP, as well as poorer outcomes in general.[20] A surgical provider's experience with the specific procedure may play a role in the development of CPSP. A study by Tasmuth and colleagues[17] found that the development of CPSP is more common in hospitals with lower volume for breast procedures and less-experienced staff.

Because neural injury may lead to nerve dysfunction, surgical technique targeted at avoiding nerve injury has been proposed to decrease the incidence of CPSP. Postoperative pain following hysterectomies is less with Pfannensteil incisions versus midline.[28] Furthermore, thoracotomy by the anterolateral approach results in less nerve damage and chronic pain than the posterolateral approach.[29] Furthermore, suturing through ribs has been shown to avoid direct nerve compression, possibly leading to decreased CPSP.[30] Nonetheless, elective division of the ilioinguinal nerve during hernia repair does not appear to lead to development of CPSP.[31]

Aasvang and colleagues[19] demonstrated significantly reduced persistent postherniotomy pain with laparoscopic versus open herniotomy. This is hypothesized to be due to significantly lower risk of nerve injury with laparoscopy, as well as glue fixation and the use of lightweight mesh. Increased incidence of CPSP also occurs in open cholecystectomies versus laparoscopic.[32] Surgical procedure influences the development of CPSP in breast surgery as well. In one study, 53% of patients reported chronic pain after mastectomy with reconstruction by implant compared with 31% with mastectomy and 22% after breast reduction.[33]

Studies conclude a combination of surgical intervention with adjuvant therapy, such as radiation and chemotherapy, to be an independent risk factor for the development of chronic pain after breast cancer surgery.[34] However, the need for adjuvant therapy may signify advanced disease, a confounding factor that may be leading to increased pain.

Anesthetic Factors

Currently, there is no correlation between anesthetic medications and an increased risk of developing CPSP, but choice of anesthetic modality and analgesic techniques may play a role in avoiding the conversion of acute to chronic pain. No positive correlation has been identified between the frequently used anesthetic agents sevoflurane, desflurane, and propofol and development of postoperative pain.[35] The use of high-dose opioids for analgesia counterintuitively demonstrated hyperalgesia, increasing postoperative pain intensity and opioid requirements.[36] The role of opioid-induced hyperalgesia in developing CPSP is unknown, and future studies should be conducted to determine if it is contributory.

The decision of anesthetic modality may have an effect on the development of CPSP. In one study, the use of general anesthesia resulted in a higher prevalence of chronic posthysterectomy pain than patients who underwent spinal anesthesia. Interestingly, there was no difference in development of CPSP between patients receiving general and epidural anesthesia. Brandsbourg and colleagues[28] attributes this to the stronger blockade of central impulse traffic in spinal anesthesia. Utilization of regional anesthesia to prevent development of CPSP will be further discussed later in the article.

Acute Postoperative Pain

Many surgical procedures are associated with acute postoperative pain, as demonstrated by **Table 1**. Severe postoperative pain is frequently hypothesized to contribute to the conversion to CPSP.[37] In one study identifying risk factors for chronic pain after surgery, uncontrolled postoperative pain was found to be the sole significant risk factor.[38] Furthermore, high-intensity postoperative pain was associated with development of CPSP and functional impairment up to 6 months after surgery.[20] Acute pain has also been shown to contribute to this conversion across multiple procedures, including herniorrhaphy, surgery for breast cancer, orthopedic procedures, and cesarean deliveries.[39]

PREDICTION OF POSTOPERATIVE PAIN

Given the multiple factors associated with the development of CPSP, a concerted effort has been made to predict patient populations at risk. The use of quantitative sensory testing (QST) has shown promise, as it may predict up to 54% of the variation in response to surgical stimuli. The predictive strength of these tests is higher than any single risk factor in predicting variability of pain response in patients. QST uses mechanical, thermal, or electrical stimuli to predict pain thresholds. Electrical pain threshold testing demonstrates greater predictive power than either mechanical or thermal in prediction of postoperative pain. Preoperative psychomimetic evaluation is not as efficient as QST in predicting postoperative pain.[40]

Another metric that has been used to predict persistent postoperative pain is the Verbal Rating Scale and Numerical Pain Scale (VAS). Studies suggest that the sum of postoperative VAS for days 1 to 7 is more predictive of CPSP than maximum reported VAS. This seems to suggest that the duration of postoperative pain is related to the development of CPSP.[41]

Routine implementation of preoperative QST and psychomimetic questionnaires has not occurred yet due to time and staff constraints, but attempts have been made for simple evaluation of susceptibility to pain. Kalkman and colleagues[42] developed a multivariate prediction rule to preoperatively predict the risk of developing severe pain in the first postoperative hour. The specificity and sensitivity of the model are 61% and 74%, respectively. The investigator has since revised the model to assess both inpatient and outpatient populations and improve its content.[40]

Preoperative screening methods can be an effective tool in preventing CPSP in the future. Based on predicted risk of developing postoperative pain, these patients can be targeted with aggressive pain therapy and appropriate surgical intervention.

PROPOSED MECHANISMS OF CHRONIC POSTSURGICAL PAIN

The exact mechanism for the development of CPSP is unknown. Alternatively, the mechanism for the development of acute postsurgical pain has been extensively researched and is more clearly understood. Voscopoulos and Lema[43] claim "the transition from acute to chronic pain appears to occur in discrete pathologic and histopathological steps" (**Fig. 2**).

Following a surgically induced injury, activation of action potentials in peripheral afferent, A-∂ and C-fibers, initiate the transmission of pain signals to the central nervous system (CNS). A-∂ fibers transmit signals through mechanoreceptors and mechanothermal receptors.[44] Nonmyelinated C-fibers differ by generating action potentials more slowly via chemoreceptors in addition to mechanoreceptors. C-fibers greatly outnumber A-∂ fibers.[45]

The cell bodies for peripheral afferents reside in the dorsal root ganglion (DRG). Once thought to serve only as a metabolic "helper," it is now known that the DRG participates in signal modulation through the sensation and production of certain molecules.[46] The cell bodies of DRG neurons do not interact with one another and are separated from each other and surrounded by layers of satellite glial cells (SGCs). Following peripheral nerve injury, SGCs release multiple proinflammatory compounds, leading to neuropathic pain.[47]

Proximal to their DRG, A-∂ and C-fibers synapse with second-order neurons in laminae I and II in the dorsal horn of the spinal cord. They also synapse with wide dynamic-range neurons, given the name because they also synapse with A-ß sensory neurons. A potential for crossover stimulation may explain neuropathic pain states, such as hyperalgesia and allodynia. The laminae in the dorsal horn are chemically influenced by glutamate, and substance P as well as microglia. Projections from the dorsal horn laminae travel centrally to the thalamus, periaqueductal gray, and parabrachial area. Here they alter descending inhibitory modulation in the spinal cord and ascending third-order neuron projections to the cortex.[43]

Following intense and repeated excitation of peripheral nociceptors, *modulation* occurs. Modulation is a reversible change in cell receptor expression and protein

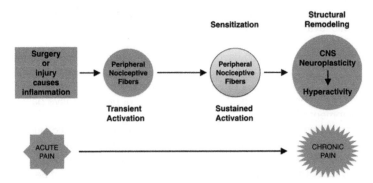

Fig. 2. Progression from acute to chronic pain. The long-term consequences of acute pain and potential for progression to chronic pain. (*Data from* Voscopoulos C, Lema M. When does acute pain become chronic? Br J Anaesth 2010;105:i69–85.)

signaling cascades in peripheral and central neurons. Nociceptor *modification* is long-lasting, often irreversible, change in neurotransmitter expression, cell receptors, and neuronal connectivity. It is likely modification that leads to CPSP.[43]

Neuroplasticity

Neuroplasticity represents the change in neuron architecture that occurs when acute pain persists, likely having evolved as a protective mechanism. With prolonged acute pain, inhibitory neurons responsible for modulation eventually undergo apoptosis, leaving spinal cord stimulation unopposed. Microglia alter the neuronal synapses to amplify the nociceptive signal and C-fibers develop more connections with the CNS. Each of these neuroplastic architectural changes contributes to central sensitization.[43]

Sensitization

Nerve injury and inflammation results in increased synthesis and release of prostanoids at the surgical site. Distal to the site of nerve injury, Schwann cell denervation and macrophage infiltration increases local tumor necrosis factor-α.[48] Upregulation of interleukin-1B (IL-1B) and COX-2 contribute to this altered milieu of neurotransmitters, ultimately responsible for activating intracellular protein kinase A (PKA) and protein kinase C (PKC).[43] These signaling pathways promote increased nociceptive sensitivity, known as peripheral sensitization, seen in **Fig. 3**. Peripheral sensitization and an increased ectopic neural activity can lead to neuropathic pain types: allodynia and hyperalgesia.

With prolonged painful stimulus, alterations in gene expression increase excitability and transmission in the DRG. Further proximally, the dorsal horn acts as the site of *central sensitization* as a result of the repetitive nociceptive stimulation (**Fig. 4**). Decreased inhibitory neurons, increased gene expression promoting excitation, and microglial activation all result in an amplification of sensory flow in the dorsal horn.[48] Additionally, the brainstem contributes to central sensitization by decreasing descending inhibitory modulation.

In the cerebral cortex, the sensation of pain is altered by sensitization as well as previous experiences and cultural factors. Preoperative fear and anxiety of eventual pain may also play a role in CPSP.[49] The limbic system influences descending projections that affect modulation of the dorsal horn.[50]

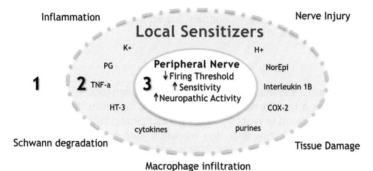

Fig. 3. Peripheral sensitization pathway. Events such as inflammation, nerve injury, tissue damage, lead to Schwann cell degradation, and macrophage infiltration of tissues (1), causing release of local sensitizers (2). These neurotransmitters are responsible for promoting increased nociceptive sensitivity (3). (*Data from* Voscopoulos C, Lema M. When does acute pain become chronic? Br J Anaesth 2010;105:i69–85.)

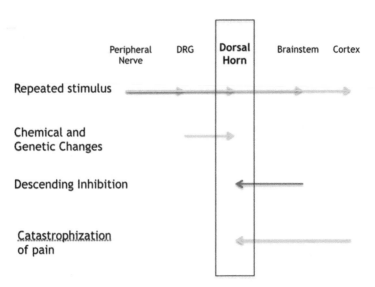

Fig. 4. Central sensitization pathway. The dorsal horn is the site of central sensitization as it receives repetitive nociceptive stimulus. Chemical and genetic changes as well as a decrease of inhibitory neurons from the brainstem contributes to central sensitization. (*Data from* Refs.[43,48–50])

N-methyl-D-aspartic acid receptors

Enhanced N-methyl-D-aspartic acid (NMDA) receptor activation plays a role in inflammatory and neuropathic pain states.[51] Repetitive stimulus from C-fibers prolongs the normal response to glutamate released by sensory fibers in the CNS. This amplified response, known as wind-up, is mediated by NMDA receptor activation. NMDA receptors are also required for descending inhibition from the brainstem.[52]

Cyclo-oxygenase-2

COX-2, located in the CNS and the periphery, is a common target of analgesics. This receptor is upregulated by IL-1B following injury to a nerve and inflammation. COX-2 expression results in increased central sensitization.[43]

Activation of COX-2 results in the expression of prostaglandin E2 (PGE2). PGE2 activates PKA and PKC, alters Na^+ channels, lowers the threshold for nociceptor excitation, and upregulates IL-1B synthesis.[53]

PREVENTION

Given the complexity and the lack of an exact mechanism for CPSP development, it is not surprising that a novel treatment has yet to be identified. Multimodal analgesic strategies are effective at preventing acute postsurgical pain but there is no evidence that they prevent CPSP; however, the evidence that severe postoperative pain is associated with a high incidence of CPSP is overwhelming.[39]

Fig. 5 demonstrates that multimodal strategies can vary greatly and must be tailored to the patient and the surgical intervention. Studies show epidural analgesia reduces postoperative pain.[54–56] Post thoracotomy pain at 6 months is reduced with epidural anesthesia.[57] Reduced chronic pain also has been observed with paravertebral blocks for patients requiring mastectomy.[58] Pectoral nerve blocks yielded promising results after breast surgery. Wahba and Kamal[59] found that patients who

measures to provide postoperative pain relief

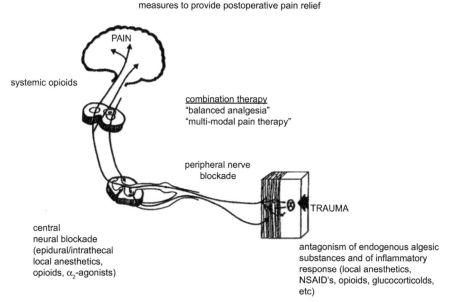

Fig. 5. Multimodal analgesic effects on the pain pathway. (*From* Kehlet H, Dahl JB. The value of "multimodal" "balanced analgesia" in postoperative pain treatment. Anesth Analg 1993;77:1048–56; with permission.)

receive a pectoral block consume less morphine in the first 24 hours after breast surgery than those who receive a paravertebral block.

The use of the alpha 2 delta ligand pregabalin resulted in a reduction in chronic neuropathic pain following total knee arthroplasty.[60] Pregabalin, like gabapentin, inhibits presynaptic Ca^{2+} influx and as a result reduces the release of excitatory neurotransmitters.[61] The evidence is not unopposed, but perioperative gabapentin and pregabalin demonstrated decreased incidence of CPSP.[62,63]

Ketamine, an NMDA receptor antagonist, has proven to be a useful adjunct. Preoperative initiation of NMDA receptor antagonists exhibits preventive effects by inhibiting central sensitization in the dorsal horn.[64] NMDA receptor antagonists limit wind-up in the CNS, activate inhibitory modulation, reduce opioid-induced hyperalgesia, and have anti-inflammatory effects.[65]

Multimodal therapy reduces postoperative pain severity. Severe postoperative pain increases one's risk of developing chronic pain.[38,66] The lack of strong evidence supporting multimodal analgesia for prevention of CPSP may be due to inadequate duration of therapy. Many of these therapies are administered intraoperatively and not continued into the postoperative, or even postdischarge period. Preventing the sensitization and the changes of neuroplasticity may require a longer therapeutic commitment.

THE "IDEAL" ACUTE TO PERSISTENT PAIN STUDY

Chronic postsurgical pain results in a significant emotional and economic burden while its prevalence is widespread over a variety of surgical procedures. To properly prevent and treat CPSP, we must develop studies to determine how acute pain develops into persistent pain. Unfortunately, most existing studies involving CPSP relied on retrospective patient surveys without a single well-validated assessment tool.[67] Such studies were helpful in determining relevant predisposing factors and assessing prevalence; however, results were clouded by the possibility of recall bias and preexisting disease. Now prospective studies must evaluate preoperative, intraoperative, and postoperative factors as well as obtain blood samples for possible future genetic testing (**Box 1**).[67]

Numerous existing studies suggest the possibility of preemptive anesthetic techniques to hinder the development of CPSP. Without prospective well-designed studies to determine the transition from acute to chronic pain, it is difficult to determine what preventive techniques will be effective. Thus, with the development of procedure-specific prospective studies using validated assessment tools throughout the preoperative, intraoperative, and postoperative periods can we better understand the development of CPSP and further techniques of prevention. Such prospective studies must extend at least 3 to 6 months postoperatively beyond the expected postsurgical inflammatory response with reevaluation for long-term outcomes.[67]

FUTURE CONSIDERATIONS/SUMMARY

Increased interest in the development of CPSP has improved our understanding of its mechanism, but there is much we do not understand about this phenomenon. We have identified multiple patient-specific and surgery-specific risk factors as well as predictive tools to allow us to identify high-risk patients. Although QST has proven predictive utility, its use in our daily practice is not currently feasible. We must continue to search for

---

Box 1
Elements of the "ideal" study design of persistent postsurgical pain

Preoperatively

Presence of preexisting pain (locally and remote)

Measurement of the functional consequences of preexisting pain

Neurophysiologic assessment

Psychosocial assessment

Analysis of pain genes

Intraoperatively

Descriptive characteristics about the incision

Descriptive characteristics about handling of nerves and muscles

Information about the disease being treated

Early postoperatively

Pain intensity and character

Pain treatment modality used

Neurophysiologic assessment

Late postoperatively

Pain intensity and character

Psychosocial consequences

Neurophysiologic assessment

From Kehlet H, Rathmell J. Persistent postsurgical pain. Anesthesiology 2010;112:514–5; with permission.

novel, easy to perform evaluations to help us accurately predict patients at risk for developing CPSP. Once reliable identification of high-risk patients is possible, an ideal surgical and analgesic plan must be designed to avoid persistent pain.

Surgical plans must be tailored so that those at risk can benefit from surgical techniques designed to minimize trauma to tissues and neural damage. From an anesthetic standpoint, intraoperative and postoperative regimens should be directed at decreasing inflammation and avoiding sensitization. Although opioids show benefit as part of a balanced analgesic technique, they have not shown effectiveness as the sole analgesic. One must consider using multiple modalities targeting different locations along the pain pathway to stop the development of persistent pain. Although our current ability to prevent CPSP is inadequate, future studies must improve our understanding of this disease process and improve management techniques.

REFERENCES

1. Kehlet H, Jensen TS, Woolf C. Persistent postsurgical pain: risk factors and prevention. Lancet 2006;367:1618–25.
2. Crombie IK, Davies HTO, Macrae WA. Cut and thrust: antecedent surgery and trauma among patients attending a chronic pain clinic. Pain 1998;76:167–71.
3. Tasmuth T, von Smitten K, Hietanen P, et al. Pain and other symptoms after different treatment modalities of breast cancer. Ann Oncol 1995;6:453–9.
4. Smith WC, Bourne D, Squair J, et al. A retrospective cohort study of post mastectomy pain syndrome. Pain 1999;83:91–5.
5. Poobalan AS, Bruce J, King PM, et al. Chronic pain and quality of life following open inguinal hernia repair. Br J Surg 2001;88(8):1122–6.
6. Katz J, Poleshuck EL, Andrus CH, et al. Risk factors for acute pain and its persistence following breast cancer surgery. Pain 2005;199:16–25.
7. Max MB, Stewart WF. The molecular epidemiology of pain: a new discipline for drug discovery. Nat Rev Drug Discov 2008;7:647–58.
8. Diatchenko L, Nackley AG, Tchivileva IE, et al. Genetic architecture of human pain perception. Trends Genet 2007;23:605–13.
9. Tegeder I, Costican M, Griffin RS, et al. GTP cyclohydrolase and tetrahydrobiopterin regulate pain sensitivity and persistence. Nat Med 2006;12:1269–77.
10. Lee YS, Kim H, Wu TX, et al. Genetically mediate interindividual variation in analgesic responses to cyclooxygenase inhibitory drugs. Clin Pharmacol Ther 2006;79:407–18.
11. Diatchenko L, Slade GD, Nackley AG, et al. Genetic basis for individual variations in pain perception and the development of chronic pain condition. Hum Mol Genet 2005;14:135–43.
12. Kambur O, Kaunisto M, Tikkanen E, et al. Effect of catechol-o-methytransferase gene variants on experimental and acute postoperative pain in 1000 women undergoing surgery for breast cancer. Anesthesiology 2013;119:1422–33.
13. Mogil JS, Wilson SG, Bon K, et al. Heritability of nociception I: responses of 11 inbred mouse strains on 12 measures of nociception. Pain 1999;80:67–82.
14. Bruce J, Drury N, Poobalan AS, et al. The prevalence of chronic chest and leg pain following cardiac surgery: a historical cohort study. Pain 2003;106:1002–12.
15. Devor M. Evidence for heritability of pain in patients with traumatic neuropathy. Pain 2004;108:200–1.
16. Becker N, Thomsen AM, Olsen AK, et al. Pain epidemiology and health related quality of life in chronic non-malignant pain patients referred to a Danish multidisciplinary pain center. Pain 1998;73:393–400.

17. Tasmuth T, Estlanderb AM, Kalso E. Effect of present pain and mood on the memory of past postoperative pain in women treated surgically for breast cancer. Pain 1996;68:343–7.
18. Joshi GP, Ogunnaike BO. Consequences of inadequate postoperative pain relief and chronic persistent postoperative pain. Anesthesiol Clin North America 2005; 23:21–36.
19. Aasvang EK, Gmaehl E, Hansen JP, et al. Predictive risk factors for persistent postherniotomy pain. Anesthesiology 2010;112:957–69.
20. Peters ML, Sommer M, de Rijke JM, et al. Somatic and psychologic predictors of long-term unfavorable outcome after surgical intervention. Ann Surg 2007;245: 487–94.
21. Hanley MA, Jensen MP, Ehde DM, et al. Psychosocial predictors of long-term adjustment to Lower-limb amputation and phantom limb pain. Disable Rehabil 2004;26:882–93.
22. Courtney CA, Duffy K, Serpell MG, et al. Outcome of patients with severe chronic pain following repair of groin hernia. Br J Surg 2002;89:1310–4.
23. Wright D, Paterson C, Scott N, et al. Five year follow-up of patients undergoing laparoscopic or open groin hernia repair: a randomized controlled trial. Ann Surg 2002;235:333–7.
24. Brummett CM, Janda AM, Schueller CM, et al. Survey criteria for fibromyalgia independently predict increased postoperative opioid consumption after lower-extremity joint arthroplasty: a prospective, observational cohort study. Anesthesiology 2013;119:1434–43.
25. Nikolajsen L, Ilkjaer S, Kroner K, et al. The influence of preamputation pain on postamputation stump and phantom pain. Pain 1997;72:393–405.
26. Keller SM, Carp NZ, Levy MN, et al. Chronic post-thoracotomy pain. J Cardiovasc Surg 1994;35(6 Suppl 1):161–4.
27. Kroner K, Knudsen UB, Lundby L, et al. Long-term phantom breast syndrome after mastectomy. Clin J Pain 1992;8:346–50.
28. Brandsborg B, Nokolasjen L, Hansen CT, et al. Risk factors for chronic pain after hysterectomy: a nationwide questionnaire and database study. Anesthesiology 2007;106:1003–12.
29. Benedetti F, Vighetti S, Ricco C, et al. Neurophysiologic assessment of nerve impairment in posterolateral and muscle sparing thoracotomy. J Thorac Cardiovasc Surg 1998;115:841–7.
30. Cerofolio RJ, Price TN, Bryant AS, et al. Intracostal sutures decrease the pain of thoracotomy. Ann Thorac Surg 2003;76:407–12.
31. Picchio M, Palimento D, Attanasio U, et al. Randomised controlled trial of preservation or elective division of ilioinguinal nerve on open inguinal hernia repair with polypropylene mesh. Arch Surg 2004;139:755–8.
32. Stiff G, Rhodes M, Kelly A, et al. Long-term pain: less common after laparoscopic than open cholecystectomy. Br J Surg 1994;81:1368–70.
33. Wallace MS, Wallace AM, Lee J, et al. Pain after breast surgery: a survey of 282 women. Pain 1996;66:195–205.
34. Poleshuck EL, Katz J, Andrus CH, et al. Risk factors for chronic pain following breast cancer surgery: a prospective study. J Pain 2006;7:626–34.
35. Fassoulaki A, Melemeni A, Paraskeva A, et al. Postoperative pain and analgesic requirements after anesthesia with sevoflurane, desflurane or propofol. Anesth Analg 2008;107:1715–9.
36. Chia YY, Liu K, Wang JJ, et al. Intraoperative high dose fentanyl induces postoperative fentanyl tolerance. Can J Anaesth 1999;46:872–7.

37. Kalso E, Perttunen K, Kaasinen S. Pain after thoracic surgery. Acta Anaesthesiol Scand 1992;36:96–100.
38. Katz J, Jackson M, Kavanagh BP, et al. Acute pain after thoracic surgery predicts long-term post-thoracotomy pain. Clin J Pain 1996;12:50–5.
39. Macrae WA. Chronic post-surgical pain: 10 years on. Br J Anaesth 2008;101:77–86.
40. Werner MU, Mjobo HN, Nielsen PR, et al. Prediction of postoperative pain: a systematic review of predictive experimental pain studies. Anesthesiology 2010;112: 1494–502.
41. Bisgaard T, Rosenberg J, Kehlet H. From acute to chronic pain after laparoscopic cholecystectomy: a prospective follow up analysis. Scand J Gastroenterol 2005; 40:1358–64.
42. Kalkman CJ, Visser K, Moen J, et al. Preoperative prediction of severe postoperative pain. Pain 2003;105:415–23.
43. Voscopoulos C, Lema M. When does acute pain become chronic? Br J Anaesth 2010;105:i69–85.
44. Gold M. Ion channels: recent advances and clinical applications. In: Flor H, Kaslo E, Dostrovsky JO, editors. Proceedings of the 11th World Congress on pain. Seattle (WA): IASP Press; 2006. p. 73–92.
45. Gold M, Gebhart G. Peripheral pain mechanisms and nociceptor sensitization. In: Fishman S, Bellantyne JC, Rathmell JP, editors. Bonica's pain management. 4th edition. Baltimore (MD): Lippincott Williams & Wilkins (LWW); 2010. p. 25–34.
46. Devor M. Unexplained peculiarities of the dorsal root ganglion. Pain Suppl 1999; 6:S27–35.
47. Krames ES. The role of the dorsal root ganglion in the development of neuropathic pain. Pain Med 2014;15:1669–85.
48. Perkins FM, Kehlet H. Chronic pain as an outcome of surgery. A review of predictive factors. Anesthesiology 2000;93:1123–33.
49. Lame IE, Peters ML, Vlaeyen JW, et al. Quality of life in chronic pain is more associated with beliefs about pain, than with pain intensity. Eur J Pain 2005;9:15–24.
50. Vera-Portocarrero LP, Zhang ET, Ossipov MH, et al. Descending facilitation from the rostral ventromedial medulla maintains nerve injury-induced central sensitization. Neuroscience 2006;140:1311–20.
51. Sindrup SH, Jensen TS. Efficacy of pharmacological treatments of neuropathic pain: an update and effect related to mechanism of drug action. Pain 1999;83: 389–400.
52. Sandkuhler J, Chen JG, Cheng G, et al. Low-frequency stimulation of afferent Adelta-fibers induces long-term depression at primary afferent synapses with substantia gelatinosa neurons in the rat. J Neurosci 1997;17:6483–91.
53. Samad TA, Moore KA, Sapirstein A, et al. Interleukin-1beta mediated induction of Cox-2 in the CNS contributes to inflammatory pain hypersensitivity. Nature 2001; 410:471.
54. Gottschalk A, Smith DS, Jobes DR, et al. Preemptive epidural analgesia and recovery from radical prostatectomy: a randomized controlled trial. JAMA 1998; 279:1076–82.
55. Moiniche S, Kehlet H, Dahl JB. A qualitative and quantitative systematic review of preemptive analgesia for postoperative relief: the role of timing of analgesia. Anesthesiology 2002;96:725–41.
56. Katz J, Cohen L, Schmid R, et al. Postoperative morphine use and hyperalgesia are reduced by preoperative but no intraoperative epidural analgesia: implications for preemptive analgesia and the prevention of central sensitization. Anesthesiology 2003;98:1449–60.

57. Obata H, Saito S, Fujita N, et al. Epidural block with mepivacaine before surgery reduces long-term postthoracotomy pain. Can J Anaesth 1999;46:1127–32.

58. Kairaluoma PM, Bachmann MS, Rosenberg PH, et al. Preincisional paravertebral block reduces the prevalence of chronic pain after breast surgery. Anesth Analg 2006;103:703–8.

59. Wahba SS, Kamal MK. Thoracic paravertebral block versus pectoral nerve block for analgesia after breast surgery. Eg Journ Anaesth 2014;30:129–35.

60. Buvanendran A, Kroin JS, Della-Valle C, et al. Perioperative oral pregabalin reduces chronic pain after total knee arthroplasty: a prospective, randomized, controlled trial. Anesth Analg 2010;110:199–207.

61. Rowbotham DJ. Gabapentin: a new drug for postoperative pain? Br J Anaesth 2006;96:152–5.

62. Clarke H, Bonin RP, Orser BA, et al. The prevention of chronic postsurgical pain using gabapentin and pregabalin: a combined systematic review and meta-analysis. Anesth Analg 2011;58:428–42.

63. Gilron I. Gabapentin and pregabalin for chronic neuropathic and early postsurgical pain: current evidence and future directions. Curr Opin Anaesthesiol 2007;20:456–72.

64. McCartney CJL, Sinha A, Katz J. A qualitative systematic review of the role of N-Methyl-D-aspartate receptor antagonists in preventive analgesia. Anesth Analg 2004;98:1385–400.

65. Hirota K, Lambert DG. Ketamine: new uses for an old drug? Br J Anaesth 2011; 107:123–6.

66. Pluijms WA, Steegers MA, Verhagen AF, et al. Chronic post-thoracotomy pain: a retrospective study. Acta Anaesthesiol Scand 2006;50:805–8.

67. Kehlet H, Rathmell J. Persistent postsurgical pain. Anesthesiology 2010;112: 514–5.

What Do We Know About the Pathophysiology of Chronic Pain?

Implications for Treatment Considerations

Gerald M. Aronoff, MD

KEYWORDS

- Nociceptive processes • Neuropathic pain • Cold hyperalgesia
- Peripheral nerve injury • Wind-up pain • Central sensitization • Pain pathophysiology

KEY POINTS

- Treatment of the specific mechanisms responsible for the pain experience should be aimed at preventing and or reducing dysfunction neuro-plasticity resulting from poorly controlled chronic pain.
- Acquiring a greater understanding of specific pain mechanisms will improve the treatment plan for chronic pain patients.
- Further study of such mechanisms is needed to reduce the probability of persistent changes that cause chronic pain.

Chronic pain has been a mystification to mankind for ages. Descartes explored the pathophysiology of chronic pain in his *Treatise of Man*, and in his writings he described the human body as a "machine" with intricate and fine-tuned systems within systems.[1] He also described a hollow pathway controlling sensory and motor perception as well as a pain pathway. The pain pathway or pathophysiology of chronic pain continued to be a perplexing factor in the field of medicine for centuries. In this article, we discuss the complex features of the pathophysiology of chronic pain and the implications for treatment.

In 1994, pain was defined by the International Association for the Study of Pain (IASP) as "An unpleasant sensory and emotional experience associated with actual or potential tissue damage, or described in terms of such damage."[2] When considering the pathophysiology of pain in context with the above-noted definition, it is important to acknowledge that chronic pain need not involve any structural pathology. This is consistent with our recognition that pain is a complex biopsychosocial experience. We now recognize that the traditional biomedical model of an acute injury with associated tissue damage does not explain the persistent pain seen in patients who

Carolina Pain Associates, PA, 1900 Randolph Road, Suite 1016, Charlotte, NC 28207, USA
E-mail address: painexpert@painexpert.com

Med Clin N Am 100 (2016) 31–42
http://dx.doi.org/10.1016/j.mcna.2015.08.004
0025-7125/16/$ – see front matter © 2016 Elsevier Inc. All rights reserved.

develop delayed recovery and chronic pain syndromes that persist long after all structural pathology has healed. It also does not explain the persistent pain of many of the patients who have chronic daily headaches. To explain these, we need to look to central nervous system (CNS), genetic, and psycho-social factors. Chronic pain has become a major public health problem in the United States and many other countries. In fact, market research from 2011 reported 1.5 billion people worldwide as suffering from chronic pain.[3] An estimated 100 million persons of our adult population in the United States suffer from chronic pain,[4] causing an estimated \$560 to \$635 billion in direct and indirect costs and is a major reason for occupational disability. Therefore, we must attempt to better understand, evaluate, and treat this multifactorial problem.

In 1999, discussing the neurobiology of normal and pathophysiological pain, Devor[5] wrote *"The role of the pain system is to process information on the intensity, location, and dynamics of strong tissue-threatening stimuli. Traditionally it is presented as a serial bottom-up system in which afferent (sensory) impulses generated by noxious stimuli are encoded in the periphery, propagated centrally, processed and perceived. While retaining this basic layout, the new synthesis adds powerful modulatory (gating) influences among the adjacent system modules. Abnormal and chronic pain states are understood in terms of the functioning of these modulatory processes as much as by variations in the primary noxious input."*

PAIN SIGNAL TRANSMISSIONS

Pathophysiological pain research studies have taught us that the pain signal initiates from the stimulation of peripheral nociceptor nerve terminals from specific receptors/ion channels. Pain circuitry activates nociceptors in response to painful stimuli. Pain is signaled to the brain via a wave of depolarization.

Such depolarization encompasses a discharge of sodium and potassium, via sodium channels. The surge of sodium is transmitted to first-order neurons ending in the brain stem within the trigeminal nucleus or dorsal horn of the spinal cord. Sensory information is then spread via small-diameter C-fibers terminating within individual regions of the dorsal horn of the spinal cord (laminae I-IV), from where the signal is transmitted to the brainstem, thalamus, and higher cortical centers.[6] Within this structure, the electrochemical signal opens voltage-gated calcium channels in the presynaptic terminal for calcium to enter and allow glutamate to release into the synaptic space. Glutamate connects with N-methyl-D-aspartate (NMDA) receptors on the second-order neurons producing depolarization. These neurons cross over the spinal cord and ascend to the thalamus, where they synapse with third-order neurons, after which they connect to the limbic system and cerebral cortex.

INHIBITORY PATHWAYS

Pathways that prevent pain signals from transmitting into the dorsal horn are referred to as inhibitory. Antinociceptive neurons start at the brain stem and stream down the spinal cord synapsing with short interneurons in the dorsal horn by releasing serotonin and norepinephrine. Interneurons modulate the synapse between first-order neuron and second-order neuron by releasing gamma amino butyric acid (GABA) an inhibitory neurotransmitter. Pain cessation is a result of synaptic inhibition between first-order and second-order synapses.

NOCICEPTIVE PAIN

Nociception is the activity in peripheral pain pathways that transmit or process information about noxious events to the brain. The process is usually associated with tissue damage. Pain itself involves the perception of nociception occurring in the brain. Nociceptive pain presents as somatic or visceral.

Somatic pain receptors are located in skin, subcutaneous tissues, fascia, other connective tissues, periosteum, endosteum, and joint capsules. Stimulation of these receptors usually produces sharp or dull localized pain. Burning sensations are uncommon if the skin or subcutaneous tissues are involved. Somatic pain is localized to the area of injury.

Visceral pain receptors are located in most viscera and the surrounding connective tissue. Visceral pain due to obstruction of a hollow organ is poorly localized, deep, and cramping and may be referred to remote cutaneous sites. Visceral pain has been known to radiate; however, generally does not radiate in a direct nerve distribution pathway. Such presentation of pain is difficult to pinpoint, at times requiring clinical acumen and often further diagnostic testing.

NEUROPATHIC PAIN

Neuropathic pain is a multifactorial acute or chronic pain state generally accompanied by tissue injury, injured nerve fibers caused by disease, injury, or a lesion of the peripheral or CNS. Nicholson[7] identified neuropathic pain as being initiated by nervous system lesions or nervous system malfunctions at times upheld by various mechanisms. This pain is a spontaneous response to noxious and innocuous stimuli triggered by lesions to the somatosensory nervous system altering its structure and function. The damaged nerve fibers begin to misfire and send the wrong pain signals to various pain centers. When one experiences neuropathic pain, its impact is not just on the nerve fiber injury, it also includes change in actual nerve function at areas around the injury.[8] These changes or alterations include ectopic generation of action potentials, enabling disinhibition of synaptic transmission and/or loss of synaptic connectivity. When synaptic connectivity is lost, it is no longer possible for new synaptic circuitries and neuro-immune interactions to form.[9]

Traditional signs of neuropathic pain are allodynia, hyperalgesia, and spontaneous pain in absence of noxious stimulation. The symptoms and signs are caused by glial activation, proinflammatory cytokine release, and differential activation of pain receptors. Inflammatory cytokines, such as interleukin-1β and tumor necrosis factor-α, are released by triggered astrocytes and microglia, enhancing glutamatergic transmission and disinhibiting GABAergic interneurons in the dorsal horn of the spinal cord; in turn, increasing spinal synaptic transmission causing neuropathic pain sensitization.[10]

Common examples of neuropathic pain include pain related to shingles[11] (acute herpes zoster) or post herpetic neuralgia, diabetes (diabetic neuropathy), back pain (lumbar radiculopathy), stroke (central pain), chronic alcohol use (alcohol neuropathy), multiple sclerosis, certain types of headaches, complex regional pain syndromes (extremity pain generally following trauma to an extremity or prolonged immobilization of an extremity with a tight fitting cast), and others.

NEUROPATHIC PAIN TRANSMISSION

Neuropathic pain studies have revealed differences in pain transmission. Neurons may increase firing if they are damaged. There is also evidence that suggests an increased number of sodium channels in damaged neurons as a result of enhanced depolarization at certain places within the fiber. This has been known to lead to spontaneous pain and pain correlated to movement. Some research suggests the impairment of inhibitory circuits at the level of the brain stem and or dorsal horn allowing impulses to travel without obstacles.[12] These research studies also suggest probable alterations in the central processing of pain in connection with the use of some medications and chronic pain. The changes in the central processing of pain are noted at the second-order and third-order neurons. The damaged neurons may cultivate a pain "memory," causing a process referred to as heightened sensitization. Risk factors for the development of chronic neuropathic pain are gender, age, and genetic polymorphisms.[13]

CHALLENGES IN CHRONIC NEUROPATHIC PAIN

1. Assessment: quality, intensity, and improvement
2. Diagnostic accuracy
3. Treatment

A combination of mechanisms can be connected to chronic neuropathic pain. Some patients present with somatic and neuropathic pain. Diagnostic tools that assist in evaluation of neuropathic pain are nerve conduction studies, functional MRI (fMRI), and PET scans. Nerve conduction studies that induce sensory capabilities help identify and quantify the extent of damage to sensory pathways. Nerve conduction studies monitor neurophysiological responses to electrical stimuli. When patients are evaluated with these studies, responses to stimuli with various intensities of electrical pulse are used to measure pain perception. Mechanical sensitivity is measured with the use of von Frey hairs, and pinpricks with weighted needles. Neuropathic pain may cause a loss of sense of vibration, as such assessment is done with the use of vibrometers. Sensitivity to hot and cold are also impacted by neuropathic pain and physicians find it helpful to evaluate thermal pain with thermodes. Other systems may be included in the impact of neuropathic pain, such as motor, sensory, and autonomic systems. Small fiber neuropathies are not often detected by electrodiagnostic testing. It is imperative that physicians consider these factors when evaluating and treating chronic neuropathic pain.

Pain and loss of function are related to the reaction of the neural damage within the nervous system; symptomatology provides insight as to where the damage has occurred. Peripheral neuropathic pain (PNP) is a result of damage from lesions to the peripheral nervous system in relation to mechanical trauma, metabolic diseases, neurotoxic chemicals, infection, or tumors. PNP involves pathophysiologic changes in both the peripheral and CNS. Pain felt in the CNS is often the result of brain or spinal cord injury, stroke, or multiple sclerosis. The classic approach to treating both CNS and PNP consists of identifying the underlying cause. However, it has been found that the etiology and neural damage causes are only the initiating factors, and proper treatment involves accurately assessing other symptoms and signs that lead to continued neuropathic pain syndrome.[14]

Cold Hyperalgesia

Patients with peripheral polyneuropathy or mononeuropathy may experience a syndrome referred to as cold hyperalgesia. Cold hyperalgesia is a mechanism of sensory disinhibition where weakened cold-specific A delta input releases cold pain input carried by C nociceptors. It presents in the symptomatic area of skin and the skin is cold to the touch.[15] It has been thought to be a result of vasospasm due to sympathetic denervation hypersensitivity. This syndrome is caused by a decrease in sympathetic efferents as part of the caliber nerve fiber. Cold hyperalgesia is normally caused by innocuous cold stimulus. It is a syndrome present in 9% of patients with a number of different neuropathies.

PERIPHERAL NERVE INJURY

Injury to peripheral nerves results in a persistent pain state encompassing hyperalgesia and allodynia mediated throughout the nerve injury. Injury to peripheral nerves results in damaged cells releasing intracellular contents. Some of the intracellular contents released may take action directly on nociceptor terminals and produce pain; other cellular structures released due to nerve damage cause sensitization to the terminals causing hypersensitivity in reaction to stimuli. Xu and Yaksh[16] reported evidence of ongoing sensations activating small afferent traffic from the distal spout of the damaged and dorsal root ganglia axons. Injured neurons may present in different ways. **Boxes 1–3** summarize the presentations of neuropathic pain based on the underlying mechanisms as adapted from research done by Griffin and Woolf.[17]

The following are the outlined spinal and peripheral mechanisms involved in peripheral nerve injury:

- Altered channel expression
- Upregulation of markers for neuronal injury
- Increased expression of neuroma and dorsal root ganglion (DRG) receptors
- Migration of non-neuronal inflammatory cells into the DRG
- Activity-induced facilitation
- Loss of inhibition
- Spinobulbospinal facilitory pathways: lead to activation through the caudal midline raphe of serotonergic projection
- Activation of non-neuronal cells
- Migration of non-neuronal inflammatory cells into dorsal horn

Proper history taking, use of interview questions, and neuropathic pain questionnaires as well as physical tests should be used to derive a proper diagnosis that encompasses all areas of concern. Proper assessment is essential to treatment as the causes of neuropathic pain vary.

WIND-UP PAIN

Wind-up is a term used to describe the frequency-dependent excitability of spinal cord neurons. Wind-up starts at the skin and travels along the peripheral nerves, resulting in hypersensitivity response from the dorsal horn and brain. These neurons are evoked by electrical stimulation of afferent C-fibers. Wind-up is produced by

---

Box 1
Injured primary sensory neurons

Peripheral and central amplification via the following:

- Changes in transmitter synthesis and signaling
- Increased membrane excitability
- Peripheral and central axon growth

Triggered by the following:

- Loss of peripheral neurotrophic factors
- Spontaneous and receptor-mediated activity
- Retrograde signaling
- Signals from immune cells and denervated Schwann cells

Data from Griffin RS, Woolf CJ. Pharmacology of analgesia. In: Golan DE, Tashjian AH, Armstrong E, et al, editors. Principles of pharmacology: the pathophysiological basis of drug therapy. 2nd edition. Baltimore (MD): Lippincott; Williams and Wilkins; 2007. p. 263–82.

Box 2
Intact primary sensory neurons

Peripheral amplification and spontaneous activity via the following:

- Altered expression and channeling of receptors and ion channels
- Change in ion channel threshold and kinetics
- Collateral axon growth

Triggered by the following:

- Neurotrophic factors
- Signals from immune cells and denervated Schwann cells

Data from Griffin RS, Woolf CJ. Pharmacology of analgesia. In: Golan DE, Tashjian AH, Armstrong E, et al, editors. Principles of pharmacology: the pathophysiological basis of drug therapy. 2nd edition. Baltimore (MD): Lippincott; Williams and Wilkins; 2007. p. 263–82.

---

glutamate (NMDA) and tachykinin neurokinin-1 (NK1) receptors, and it has been suspected that wind-up is a result of positive modulation between NMDA and tachykinin NKI receptors. Studies reveal wind-up to be an amplification system in the spinal cord of nociceptive messages received from the peripheral nociceptors connected to C-fibers. This process is the physiologic result of an intense or persistent barrage of afferent nociceptive stimuli.

Major pathways affecting wind-up are network factors, presynaptic mechanisms, and presynaptic receptors, and postsynaptic membrane properties. Herrero and colleagues[18] found network factors to play an important role in the intensity of wind-up pain. They reported Class 2 neurons profoundly located in the dorsal horn are likely to generate wind-up of greater intensity than superficially located Class 2 neurons. Class 1 and 3 neurons do not create wind-up pain. Observations of simulation reveal that the position of a neuron within a network plays a significant role in pain pathology and that build-up of excitation happens as a result of repetitive stimulation. The pain transmission observed in stimulation revealed transmission beyond sole terms of cellular mechanisms.

Box 3
Second-order sensory neurons

Central amplification and spontaneous activity via the following:

- Homosynaptic and heterosynaptic facilitation
- Disinhibition
- Altered synaptic connectivity
- Changes in central nociceptive circuits

Triggered by the following:

- Injured and uninjured primary afferents
- Descending pathways from brainstem nuclei
- Peripheral immune cells, microglia, and astrocytes

Data from Griffin RS, Woolf CJ. Pharmacology of analgesia. In: Golan DE, Tashjian AH, Armstrong E, et al, editors. Principles of pharmacology: the pathophysiological basis of drug therapy. 2nd edition. Baltimore (MD): Lippincott; Williams and Wilkins; 2007. p. 263–82.

Presynaptic Mechanisms

Increased neurotransmitter release and or the corelease of amino acids and peptides from somatic C-fiber afferents are suspected to play a significant role in the superficial dorsal horn. Wind-up in the superficial dorsal area occurs in only a few neurons and is of small magnitude. Such activity is classified as homosynaptic, whereas wind-up activity in the deep dorsal and ventral horns is classified as heterosynaptic.

Heterosynaptic mechanisms require a higher proportion of cells displaying a large level of activity within neurons located in deeper layers. These layers use other post-synaptic mechanisms involving facilitation of NMDA receptors. This increased post-synaptic activity is made possible by cumulative depolarization or the release of peptides from interneuronal bands.

CENTRAL SENSITIZATION

The state in which the CNS magnifies sensory input in multiple organ systems is defined as central sensitization (CS). Enhanced response to sensitization encompasses plasticity at neuronal levels, increasing sensitivity overall in response to future stimuli. In turn, heightened sensitivity produces allodynia (a greater than normal response to nonpainful stimuli) and or hyperalgesia (heightened response to painful stimuli). CS is the mechanistic explanation of temporal, spatial, and threshold changes in relation to pain sensibility in both acute and chronic pain settings. Visceral hypersensitivity can affect a wide range and, in some cases, all organ systems, creating extreme discomfort. These amplified sensations can range from arthralgia and myalgia to a plethora of other disease presentations.[19]

PATHOPHYSIOLOGY OF CENTRAL SENSITIZATION

CS is the result of multiple processes that alter the functional state of nociceptive neurons.

The central sensitivity phenomenon initially appears to be like peripheral sensitization; however, it differs in terms of molecular mechanisms and its manifestation. Central, unlike peripheral sensitization, designates unique inputs to nociceptive pathways encompassing pathways that do not usually transport them. For example, large low-threshold mechanoreceptor myelinated fibers impacted by CS produce Aβ fiber–mediated pain. Noninflamed tissue may become hypersensitive due to changes in the sensory response triggered by normal inputs after initial causes are no longer apparent and no peripheral pathology is present. CS is the result of changes in neuronal properties and in the superficial, deep, and ventral cord resulting in pronounced changes of their response properties. CS is a functional shift in the somatosensory system from high-threshold nociception to low-threshold hypersensitivity. This process has resulted in what many describe as a sensory illusion in which at times pain may be experienced without peripheral pathology or noxious stimuli. The processes increase membrane excitability, progression of synaptic strength, and decreased inhibitory transmission. The neurons impacted by this process show spontaneous activity. Studies of the CS process reveal reduction in activation threshold of impacted neurons as well as broadened receptive fields. This CS amplifies sensory response to normal nerve activity, such as innocuous stimuli and ordinary body activity. Sensitivity may become disjoined from intensity, duration, or the occurrence of noxious peripheral stimuli. Central sensitivity brings about changes in brain activity as detected by functional magnetic resonance, positron emission, tomographic imaging, and electrophysiologic studies.[20]

Sensitization of nociceptive pathways was once considered as a neuro-centric plasticity mechanism.[2] Findings indicate that spinal glia are the strongest modulators of the neuronal network. Increasingly, evidence supports the role of the glia in CS and pathologic pain as observed in models simulating chronic pain, peripheral inflammation, and spinal or nerve injury.

CS is a complicated process for patients with chronic pain to endure. As in neuropathic pain generally, because conventional diagnostic testing and imaging studies are often unremarkable, some patients feel their health care providers question their veracity when they complain of severe pain. They are often undertreated or may be treated with conventional analgesics (such as nonsteroidal anti-inflammatory drugs [NSAIDs] and opiates) that are often not first-line drugs in managing neuropathic pain. Often, patients do not get adequate treatment response and become frustrated and discouraged. This is why it is so important for physicians to use early and aggressive treatment before pain progresses.

Reduction of the impact of all stimuli on the CNS system is required in some patients with CS. Studies by Woolf and Chong[21] reveal that patients experiencing CS may require preemptive analgesia to withstand noxious stimuli. Such measures have been found useful in many CS chronic pain states. A double-blind placebo-controlled study revealed the use of gabapentin preoperatively for patients undergoing mastectomy and or hysterectomy as having reduced pain scores postoperatively.[22] Further studies have revealed the use of NSAIDs preoperatively as also being effective in reduction of pain in the postoperative state.[23] These findings support Woolf and Chong's[21] notation regarding preoperative and postoperative pain treatment. Postoperative treatment should include the use of "NSAIDs to reduce the activation/centralization of nociceptors, local anesthetics to block sensory inflow, and centrally acting drugs such as opiates."[21]

CENTRAL SENSITIZATION AND CLINICAL PAIN PHENOTYPE

Experimental studies reviewed by Woolf[24] revealed a patient presenting with dynamic tactile allodynia, secondary punctuate/pressure hyperalgesia, temporal summation, and sensory aftereffects and CS may be involved. Sensory experiences of large amplitude, duration, and spatial extent expected from defined peripheral input would likely boost excitability or reduce inhibition and, subsequently, reflect central amplification. This process may include "reduction in threshold, exaggerated response to noxious stimuli, pain after the end of a stimulus, and a spread of sensitivity to normal tissue."[24] Woolf[24] also noted a dilemma facing physicians currently. We are unable to measure sensory inflow. With the possibility of peripheral changes contributing to sensory amplification, like peripheral sensitization, pain hypersensitivity alone is not enough to make a definitive diagnosis of central sensitization. This factor, combined with peripheral input commonly triggers CS.

Features of patients' symptoms more likely to indicate central instead of peripheral pain pathology are as follows:

- Pain mediated by low-threshold Aβ fibers (assessed by nerve block or electrical stimulation)
- Spread of sensitivity to residual areas with no specific pathology
- After sensations
- Enhanced temporal summation
- Continued pain by low-frequency stimuli that would not normally induce long-standing pain.

Assessment of central sensitization presentation requires thorough phenotyping to re-create the changes in sensitivity and identify how, where, and why they occur. This phenotyping is normally combined with objective measures of central activity, like fMRI, so that clear diagnostic criteria are met for diagnosing CS. This would not only be useful diagnostic criteria for CS but would allow clinicians to provide pathophysiologic mechanism specific treatment (**Box 4**).

BLOCKING NERVE CONDUCTION IN PERIOPERATIVE PERIODS: PREEMPTIVE STRIKES?

Preventive measures in the development of CS include the use of nerve conduction in perioperative periods. Phantom limb syndrome (PLS) is related to the experience of spinal wind-up. Patients who receive lumbar epidural blockades with bupivacaine and morphine for 72 hours have a lessened chance of developing PLS.[24] In fact, one study revealed none of the 11 patients who received such treatment developed CS-related PLS. In contrast, 5 of 14 patients who did not receive this blockade developed PLS after surgery.[24] These measures must be taken seriously when pain results from injury or surgery, as the spinal cord may become hyperexcitable causing excessive pain response that often lasts for days, weeks, or even years.

PSYCHOLOGICAL FACTORS

One's thoughts and emotions have a great impact on the perception of pain. Many patients with chronic pain experience psychological distress, depression, and anxiety due to the lifestyle changes they undergo because of their chronic pain. At times, patients are depicted as having psychiatric disorders and are deprived of appropriate care due to misinterpretation of their actual "self-reported" pain. Oftentimes patients who are experiencing pain exacerbations report difficulty sleeping, concentrating, and completing regular activities of daily living due to the impact pain has taken on their lives. This may be misinterpreted as a primary depression rather than a frequent response to inadequately treated chronic pain. Many patients receive a psychiatric diagnosis and are started on psychiatric treatment often inappropriately.

A growing body of evidence indicates that pain itself should be considered a disease process that is self-perpetuating, causing both structural and functional changes in the CNS, and that new systems of classification are indicated based on

---

Box 4
Common clinical conditions involving central sensitization

- Rheumatoid arthritis
- Osteoarthritis
- Postsurgical pain
- Temporomandibular disorders
- Fibromyalgia
- Complex regional pain syndrome
- Central poststroke pain
- Migraines
- Neuropathic pain
- Irritable bowel syndrome (a visceral pain hypersensitivity syndrome)

this pathology.[25] In recent times, Lippe[26] suggested use of the terms Eudynia and Maldynia to distinguish normal pain from pain as a disease state. He suggests that Eudynia refers to pain as a symptom of an underlying disease process. The pain can be acute or persistent, but it is transmitted by normal physiologic pathways and generally is fairly well understood and relatively easily managed. Maldynia, on the other hand, is an abnormal pain state that serves no useful purpose to the individual and is more difficult to understand and to manage. It results from persistent untreated Eudynia or any injury of the nervous system. Dr Lippe indicates that "in clinical practice there is a continuum or spectrum in which complex pain problems are expressed as a blend of Eudynia and Maldynia."[26]

It is beyond the scope of this article to review pharmacologic pain management in detail; however, there are many research papers (some are flawed) demonstrating that one or more of the adjuvants are the medications of choice for neuropathic pain management.

Adjuvant analgesics are medications that were not primarily developed as analgesics but nonetheless have pain-relieving properties. Adjuvant therapy can enhance pain relief or diminish the side effects of traditional analgesics and can be used in conjunction with any level of analgesia. That is, the most effective treatment for the neuropathic pain process is generally one of the medication classes listed below. Drugs that act on the CNS, such as antidepressants and anticonvulsants, are commonly used medications in chronic pain. They are considered first-line drugs in the treatment of neuropathic pain and to treat concurrent psychiatric problems.[27]

Adjuvant analgesics include the following:

1. Antidepressants
2. Anticonvulsants
3. Phenothiazine tranquilizers (primarily methotrimeprazine)
4. Benzodiazepines (primarily clonazepam)
5. Topical agents
6. Local anesthetics
7. Antispasmodics
8. Antihistamines
9. Corticosteroids
10. Caffeine
11. Cannabis (federal law prohibits prescribing)
12. Psychostimulants

MEDICATION MANAGEMENT OF NEUROPATHIC PAIN, CURRENT RECOMMENDATIONS

The IASP Neuropathic Pain Special Interest Group, an international consensus process that included a diverse group of pain experts, has developed evidence-based guidelines for the pharmacologic treatment of the neuropathic pain. Other entities including the American Pain Society, the Canadian Pain Society (CPS), the Finnish Pain Society, the Latin American Federation of IASP Chapters, the Mexican Pain Society, and the European Federation of Neurologic Societies (EFNS) have either endorsed the IASP guidelines or developed their own (CPS, EFNS). The guidelines outline the following as the standard of care[28]:

First-line agents for neuropathic pain treatment:

- Tricyclic antidepressants
- Calcium channel alpha 2-delta ligands
- Selective serotonin norepinephrine reuptake inhibitors

- Topical lidocaine (for localized PNP)

Second-line or third-line agents in some instances include:

- Opioids and tramadol

Since the International consensus recommendations, studies have found that tapentadol (Nucynta) should be added to the list of opioids useful in the management of moderate to severe neuropathic pain.

SUMMARY

Pain has mystified the medical community since the age of Descartes. However, clinical investigations over the years reveal the mechanisms involved in pain pathology lead to specifically targeted treatments. Over the past 20 years, considerable strides have been made to find the cellular and molecular mechanisms responsible to make accurate diagnoses. There is still much to learn about the pathophysiology of pain. In particular, there is ongoing research attempting to better identify risk factors for developing intractable pain states and improve our specificity in treatment recommendations.

REFERENCES

1. Descartes R, Clerselier C, La Forge L, et al. L'homme et un Traitté de la ormation du Foetus du Mesme Autheur. Paris: Charles Angot; 1664.
2. Merskey H, Bogduk N. Classification of chronic pain. Seattle (WA): IASP Press; 1994.
3. Global Industry Analysts, Inc. Report, January 10, 2011. Available at: http://www.prweb.com/pdfdownload/8052240.pdf. Accessed October 16, 2015.
4. Institute of Medicine Report from the Committee on Advancing Pain Research. Care, and education: relieving pain in America, a blueprint for transforming prevention, care, education and research. Baltimore (MD): The National Academies Press; 2011.
5. Devor M. Neurobiology of normal and pathophysiological pain. In: Aronoff GM, editor. Evaluation and treatment of chronic pain. 3rd edition. Baltimore (MD): Williams &Wilkins; 1999. p. 11–25.
6. Bradesi S. Role of spinal cord glia in central processing of peripheral pain perception. Neurogastroenterol Motil 2010;22(5):499–511.
7. Available at: http://www.ajmc.com/publications/supplement/2006/2006-06-vol12-n9suppl/jun06-2326ps256-s262/1#sthash.pzGUhttp://www.painexpert.com/1Ait.dpuf. Accessed October 4, 2015.
8. Bakonja MM, Argoff CE. Neuropathic pain—definition and implications for research and therapy. J Neuropathic Pain Symptom Palliation 2005;1(2):11–7.
9. Costigan M, Scholz J, Woolf CJ. Neuropathic pain: a maladaptive response of the nervous system to damage. Annu Rev Neurosci 2009;32:1–32.
10. Silva GD, Lopes P, Fonoff ET, et al. The spinal anti-inflammatory mechanism of motor cortex stimulation: cause of success and refractoriness in neuropathic pain. J Neuroinflammation 2015;12(1):10.
11. Argoff CE. A focused review on the use of botulinum toxins for neuropathic pain. Clin J Pain 2002;18(Suppl 6):S177–81.
12. Svokos K, Goldstein LB. The pathophysiology of neuropathic pain: a discussion of the pathophysiology of neuropathic pain and an overview of the modalities used to alleviate it. Available at: http://www.practicalpainmanagement.com/pain/neuropathic/pathophysiology-neuropathic-pain?page=0,1. Accessed October 4, 2015.

13. Chen N, Zhang J, Wang P, et al. Functional alterations of pain processing pathway in migraine patients with cutaneous allodynia. Pain Med 2015;16(6): 1211–20.
14. Dworkin RH, O'Connor AB, Backonja M, et al. Pharmacologic management of neuropathic pain: evidence based recommendations. Pain 2007;132:237–51.
15. Allchorne AJ, Broom D, Woolf CJ. Detection of cold pain, cold allodynia and cold hyperalgesia in freely behaving rats. Mol Pain 2005;1:36.
16. Xu Q, Yaksh TL. A brief comparison of the pathophysiology of inflammatory versus neuropathic pain. Curr Opin Anaesthesiol 2011;24(4):400–7.
17. Griffin RS, Woolf CJ. Pharmacology of analgesia (Chapter 16). In: Golan DE, Tashjian AH, Armstrong E, et al, editors. Principles of pharmacology: the patho-physiological basis of drug therapy. 2nd edition. Baltimore (MD): Lippincott, Williams and Wilkins; 2007. p. 263–82.
18. Herrero JF, Laird JMA, Lopez-Garcia JA. Wind-up of spinal cord neurones and pain sensation: much ado about something? Prog Neurobiol 2000;61:169–203.
19. Latremoliere A, Woolf CJ. Central sensitization: a generator of pain hypersensitiv-ity by central neural plasticity. J Pain 2009;10:10895–926.
20. Aaron L, Buchwald D. A review of the evidence for overlap among unexplained clinical conditions. Ann Intern Med 2001;134(9 Pt 2):868–81.
21. Woolf CJ, Chong MS. Preemptive analgesia–treating postoperative pain by preventing the establishment of central sensitization. Anesth Analg 1993;77(2): 362–79.
22. Rorarius MG, Mennander S, Suominen P, et al. Gabapentin for the prevention of postoperative pain after vaginal hysterectomy. Pain 2004;110:175–81.
23. Rivkin A, Rivkin MA. Perioperative nonopioid agents for pain control in spinal sur-gery. Am J Health Syst Pharm 2014;71(21):1845–57.
24. Woolf CJ. Central sensitization: implications for the diagnosis and treatment of pain. Pain 2011;152(Suppl 3):S2–15.
25. Borsook D. Neurological diseases and pain. Brain 2012;135(2):320–44.
26. Lippe P. An apologia in defense of pain medicine. Clin J Pain 1998;14(3):189–90.
27. Aronoff GM, Argoff CJ. Medication management of neuropathic pain, current rec-ommendations. In: Handbook of chronic pain medication management. Trafford Victoria, Canada, in press.
28. Harden RN, Kaye AD, Kitanar T, et al. Evidence-based guidance for the manage-ment of postherpetic neuralgia in primary care. Postgrad Med 2013;125(4): 191–202.

Chronic Pain Treatment Approaches

Biopsychosocial Approach to Assessing and Managing Patients with Chronic Pain

Martin D. Cheatle, PhD

KEYWORDS

- Chronic pain • Biopsychosocial • Cognitive Behavioral Therapy • E-Health
- Primary care

KEY POINTS

- Chronic pain is a significant health care problem affecting approximately 30% of the US population.
- Chronic pain should be considered a chronic disease.
- Primary care clinicians are responsible for caring for most patients suffering from chronic pain.
- Traditional approaches to managing chronic pain have not been totally effective.
- A biopsychosocial approach to pain has been demonstrated to be efficacious and cost-effective.

INTRODUCTION

The Institute of Medicine (IOM) report, "Living Well with Chronic Illness: A Call for Public Health Action," noted that chronic illness represents approximately 75% of the $2 trillion that is spent in the United States on health care.[1] Chronic illnesses were identified that should be the focus of public health efforts to reduce disability and improve functionality and quality of life. There was an emphasis on winnable battles; in other words, illnesses with cost-cutting clinical, functional, and social implications. Nine "exemplar" disease states were identified as having significant implications for the nation's health and economy. These states included arthritis, type 2 diabetes, dementia, vision and hearing loss, posttraumatic disabling conditions, schizophrenia, cancer survivorship, depression, and, notably, chronic pain.

In spite of diagnostic and therapeutic advances in the field of medicine, the prevalence of chronic pain continues to rise. Chronic pain affects the individual suffering

Conflicts of Interest: The author does not have any conflicts of interest related to the material in this article.
Center for Studies of Addiction, Department of Psychiatry, Perelman School of Medicine, University of Pennsylvania, 3535 Market Street, 4th Floor, Philadelphia, PA 19104, USA
E-mail address: cheatle@mail.med.upenn.edu

Med Clin N Am 100 (2016) 43–53
http://dx.doi.org/10.1016/j.mcna.2015.08.007   **medical.theclinics.com**

from pain but also their families and society. One-third of adults in the United States experience chronic or recurrent pain.[2,3] The IOM report, "Relieving Pain in America: A Blueprint for Transforming Prevention, Care, Education and Research," estimated that the annual cost of chronic pain in the United States is approximately $560 to $600 billion, which includes the cost of health care and lost productivity.[4]

An individual suffering from persistent pain can develop significant concomitant conditions, including secondary physical problems due to deconditioning and weight gain (for example, hypertension, obstructive sleep apnea, diabetes), sleep disorders, substance use disorders, mood and anxiety disorders, cognitive distortions, and functional disabilities. Untreated or mismanaged pain can lead to adverse effects, such as delays in healing, changes in the central nervous system (neuroplasticity), suicidal ideation and behavior, and opioid misuse, abuse, addiction, and overdose.[5–8]

The IOM report on pain[4] challenged health care policy makers and practitioners with the following principles:

- Effective pain management is a "moral imperative"
- Pain should be considered a disease with distinct pathology
- Pain remains undertreated and underdiagnosed, particularly in disadvantaged populations
- There is a need for interdisciplinary treatment approaches

CURRENT APPROACH TO PAIN TREATMENT

The current approach to pain treatment is linear in nature, where symptoms lead to a diagnosis and then to treatment. This may be appropriate in treating an acute process, but is not efficacious for a complex pain disorder.[9] Specialty training in pain medicine has become very technical in nature, and the Accreditation Council for Graduate Medical Education (ACGME) requirements for competency in pain medicine involve primarily acquiring expertise in interventions (neural blockade, radiofrequency ablation, spinal cord stimulation, kyphoplasty, and pharmacotherapy). Although this has been the focus of pain medicine, outcome studies using these interventions on patients with chronic noncancer pain (CNCP) reveal a nominal long-term benefit. This includes the use of opioid therapy and nonopioid pharmacotherapy, injection therapy, implantable devices, and surgery, and there has been a call for changing the curriculum in pain fellowships to reflect a more balanced approach to pain care.[9,10]

Chronic pain is a complex condition with multiple medical and psychiatric comorbidities, and a more expansive and holistic approach is needed to maximize the potential for positive outcomes.

CHRONIC PAIN CARE IN THE PRIMARY CARE SETTING

More than half of all patients with chronic pain receive their pain care from primary care practitioners (PCP),[11] as there is a large discrepancy between the number of patients with chronic pain (~100,000,000) and the number of board-certified pain physicians (4000–5000). The PCP is oftentimes faced with the responsibility of fully caring for the patient with CNCP with the goal to alleviate suffering and improve their quality of life, while not causing iatrogenic complications (eg, opioid use disorders, opioid-related overdose, suicide). This clinical situation is further complicated by the reality that most PCPs do not have the time, resources, or training in pain management or addiction management to effectively and efficiently balance these important responsibilities.[12]

BIOPSYCHOSOCIAL APPROACH TO PAIN

The 2011 IOM report on pain stated that, "We believe pain arises in the nervous system but represents a complex and evolving interplay of biological, behavioral, environmental, and societal factors...."[4] According to the biopsychosocial approach to pain, physiologic stimulus (nociception, neuropathic) is filtered through the biopsychosocial context of the individual, which leads to the experience of pain. A traditional biomedical approach is ineffective in assessing psychosocial and neuro-behavioral mechanisms that can alter the manifestation and maintenance of pain (eg, kinesophobia, catastrophizing). There is evidence strongly supporting the efficacy of comprehensive pain management programs based on the biopsychosocial model of pain. These programs typically include cognitive behavioral therapy (CBT), a graded, activating exercise program, and rational pharmacotherapy with the objective to improve treatment outcomes, including return to work, pain reduction, and an increase in activity.[13–16]

INITIAL ENCOUNTER WITH PATIENT WITH CHRONIC PAIN

Patients with chronic pain typically have seen a great number of health care providers and have undergone a plethora of diagnostic evaluations, procedures, medication trials, and physical therapy. Oftentimes they do not experience appreciable improvement and seek further care.

The initial encounter with a patient with chronic pain is crucial in developing a positive physician-patient relationship, which will influence the effectiveness of and adherence to future interventions. Several steps can be followed to facilitate a collaborative and therapeutic relationship:

- *Validate:* Patients with pain can feel vilified and perceive that they are treated as if their pain is psychological. It is critical to first validate that the pain that they are experiencing is real and has compromised their life and family.
- *Educate:* Provide a framework for a biopsychosocial approach to pain emphasizing the following:
  - Pain is a chronic disease not unlike having diabetes and the goal is to manage symptoms, avoid further complications, and improve quality of life.
  - Similar to other chronic diseases, the most effective approach is a chronic disease management model.
  - Chronic disease management involves both pharmacotherapy and adopting/changing behaviors (exercise, effective communication skills, nutritional changes, stress-management techniques, pacing, making adaptations to activities of daily living).
- *Evaluate:* Conduct a thorough physical and behavioral examination establishing treatment goals and assessing the patient's expectations for treatment outcomes.
- *Treat:* Based on the comprehensive evaluation, develop a personalized treatment plan keeping in mind the patient's goals.

BIOPSYCHOSOCIAL DIAGNOSTIC EVALUATION/INTERVIEW

A comprehensive biopsychosocial pain evaluation consists of a clinical interview, mental health and substance abuse screening, physical examination, and diagnostic testing if needed.

Clinical Interview

In conducting a biopsychosocial assessment of patients with chronic pain, one should include the following:

- Pain and treatment history
  - Location
  - Onset/Duration
  - Intensity
  - Pattern/variations over time
  - What exacerbates and relieves pain
  - Impact of pain on the individual's physical, emotional, and psychosocial function
  - Patient's goals and motivation for treatment[17]
  - Past evaluations and types and efficacy of current/prior treatments
  - Timeline of functional status before the onset of pain and since the onset of pain
- Opioid medications
  - Past use
  - Current use corroborated by Prescription Drug Monitoring Program if available, urine drug testing, contacting current and previous providers, obtaining previous medical records
  - Dosage, including regimen, duration
  - Effectiveness[17]
- Nonopioid medications
  - Types (antidepressants, antiepileptics, muscle relaxants, nonsteroidal anti-inflammatory drugs)
  - Effectiveness
  - Adverse effects
- Past medical history with special attention to conditions that may be relevant to the effects of opioids (history of constipation, nausea, sleep apnea) or illnesses suggestive of a substance use disorder (hepatitis, pancreatitis, gastrointestinal disorders, cirrhosis)[18]
- History of substance use disorders, including smoking, alcohol, prescription and nonprescription drugs
- Precipitants and consequences of pain behavior (for example, family being solicitous when patient is in pain)
- Attitudes toward health care providers, family, employer if working, insurance carrier
- Current stressors, in particular changes in lifestyle/roles due to pain
- Employment, level of education
- Perform a mental status examination, assess personality traits (passive, passive-aggressive, aggressive, narcissistic)
- Level of social support
- Review of systems to include assessing for other pain complaints

Physical Examination and Diagnostic Testing

- General (vital signs, appearance, posture, gait, pain behavior)
- Musculoskeletal examination
- Neurologic examination
- Diagnostic testing (eg, MRI, computed tomography scan, electromyography) if indicated[18,19]

Mental Health/Substance Use Disorder Screening

Patients with chronic pain often present with concomitant psychiatric conditions, including mood and anxiety disorders, which can affect the expression of pain and quality of life. There are a variety of validated and reliable mental health screening tools, examples of which are outlined in **Table 1**. The Beck Depression Inventory (BDI)[20] and the Profile of Mood States (POMS)[21] are 2 measures that have been endorsed by an expert consensus group on measuring emotional functioning in chronic pain.[22] The BDI is a 21-question self-report measure of depression severity over the past week. The POMS has a full-length version (65 items) and a short-length version (35 questions), both composed of 7 scales. Three of these scales are very pertinent to the pain population (anger/hostility, depression/dejection, and tension/anxiety). The Patient Health Questionnaire (PHQ)-4[23] is a 4-item screening tool for depression and anxiety that can be easily administered in a busy primary care practice.

Likewise, many patients with chronic pain are on medications that can lead to misuse and abuse, including opioids, stimulants, and benzodiazepines. Screening for opioid misuse and substance abuse also should be part of a comprehensive biopsychosocial assessment of patients with CNCP. Examples of opioid screening tools and general substance abuse screening assessments are outlined in **Table 2**.

BIOPSYCHOSOCIAL TREATMENT PROGRAM

A comprehensive biopsychosocial treatment program includes the following:

- CBT/acceptance commitment therapy
- Rational pharmacotherapy regimen
- Graded exercise program
- Nutritional counseling/weight loss if needed
- Social support

Pharmacotherapy

A review of pharmacotherapy strategies in managing chronic pain is covered in detail by Beal and Wallace[24], but in general a practitioner must design a pharmacologic approach that targets pain, sleep, and mood and weighs benefit with risk/adverse effects.

Table 1
Examples of mental health screening tools

Tool	No. of Items	Time to Complete
Beck Depression Inventory II[20]	21	5–10 min
Beck Depression Inventory–Fast Screen for Medical Patients[25]	7	<5 min
Profile of Mood States II: Full	65	10–15 min
Short[21]	35	5–10 min
Zung Self-Rating Depression Scale[26]	20	10 min
Center for Epidemiologic Studies Depression Scale: Full	20	5–10 min
Short[27]	10	5 min
Patient Health Questionnaire[28]	9	5 min
PHQ-4[23]	4	<5 min

Table 2		
Examples of opioid misuse risk and substance use disorder screening tools		
Patients Considered for Long-Term Opioid Therapy	**Items**	**Administered**
ORT: Opioid Risk Tool[29]	5	By patient
SOAPP: Screener and Opioid Assessment for Patients with Pain[30]	24, 14, & 5	By patient
DIRE: Diagnosis, Intractability, Risk, and Efficacy Score[31]	7	By clinician
Characterize misuse once opioid treatments begins:		
PMQ: Pain Medication Questionnaire[32]	26	By patient
COMM: Current Opioid Misuse Measure[33]	17	By patient
PDUQ: Prescription Drug Use Questionnaire[34]	40	By clinician
Not specific to pain populations:		
CAGE-AID: Cut Down, Annoyed, Guilty, Eye-Opener Tool, Adjusted to Include Drugs[35]	4	By clinician
RAFFT: Relax, Alone, Friends, Family, Trouble[36]	5	By patient
DAST: Drug Abuse Screening Test[37]	28	By patient
AUDIT-C: Alcohol Use Disorders Identification Test Consumption[38]	3	By patient

Physical Therapy

Patients with chronic pain typically have had a number of previous trials of physical therapy. Oftentimes these experiences have been less than satisfactory for the patient, as they are based on a sports medicine/acute rehabilitation model of rapidly progressive and expansive exercise. This typically leads to significant pain flares in many patients with pain due to their level of deconditioning. Alternatively, physical therapy can be very passive in orientation, which would not be expected to lead to functional improvement and can reinforce the patient not being actively involved in their own recovery.

Physical therapy program goals for patients with CNCP pain should involve the following:

- *Acquiring first aid techniques for pain relief at home.* Providing the patient first aid techniques to self-manage pain flares (for example, use of transcutaneous electrical nerve stimulation, heat/cold, positioning) can help the patient avoid seeking urgent care when not necessary. This also has the benefit of engendering a sense of empowerment over their pain.
- *Establish a well-balanced, independent exercise program.* This should be done in a very graded fashion, keeping in mind that many patients with chronic pain have not been successful in traditional physical therapy due to either the level of their depression affecting their motivation, or the extent of their somatization and pain catastrophizing. Patients should be educated on the nature of chronic pain and the role of exercise in improving pain and function. Weekly goals can be established that are achievable and will not lead to an increase in pain.

Cognitive Behavioral Therapy

Patients with chronic pain can develop maladaptive thought patterns, particularly catastrophizing, and maladaptive behaviors such as kinesophobia, which will contribute to their pain and decline in function and quality of life. The objective of CBT is to guide patients in reconceptualizing their view of pain and their responsibility in promoting healing. Becoming proactive and competent rather than reactive and incompetent should be emphasized.

The process of cognitive therapy typically involves the following:

- Acquisition of specific skills, such as relaxation techniques, cognitive restructuring, effective communication, behavioral sleep hygiene, and stimulus-control techniques
- Skill consolidation and rehearsal emphasizing a generalization of the skills beyond the clinical setting
- Maintenance of new behaviors
- Relapse prevention[39]

CBT has been demonstrated as efficacious for a number of chronic pain disorders, including the following:

- Arthritis[40]
- Sickle cell disease[41]
- Chronic low back pain[42]
- Temporomandibular joint (TMJ)[43]
- Lupus[44]
- Fibromyalgia[45]

Acceptance Commitment Therapy

Acceptance commitment therapy (ACT) is a variation of CBT that is experiential in nature, based on rational frame theory. The goal of ACT is to experience life mindfully and to encourage psychological flexibility.

Core processes of ACT include the following:

- Contact with the present moment
- Self-as-context
- Diffusion
- Acceptance
- Values
- Committed action

ACT has been tested in patients with CNCP and found efficacious in improving mood and function.[46]

Barriers to Receiving Cognitive Behavioral Therapy/Acceptance Commitment Therapy

In an article by Ehde and colleagues,[47] the barriers to receiving psychological services for chronic pain were reviewed. They noted that pain is inadequately treated in primary, secondary, and tertiary care settings, and psychosocial interventions, in particular, are underutilized. Factors accounting for underutilization of psychological treatment for pain include the following:

- Financial (lack of insurance coverage for mental health care)
- Environmental (lack of transportation or lack of providers in the geographic region)
- Patient attitude–related (stigma associated with receiving psychological care)
- Health care systems barriers (no existing referral system to psychologists)

The investigators discussed the potential to use nonpsychologists to deliver CBT to patients with pain, such as dental hygienists for TMJ pain, physical therapists, and so forth. Another area that has garnered attention as an alternative to face-to-face psychological/specialist pain care is e-health.

E-Health

There has been a movement to develop alternative methods to deliver psychological services to underserved populations. This involves application of e-health technology, which refers to the use of electronic communication-based technologies to support or provide health care.

Types of e-health applications for delivering CBT and other specialty care include the following:

- *Internet-delivered interventions:* Internet-delivered CBT uses the same basic principles of face-to-face CBT but is delivered by computer and the Internet and follow a structured course. It can be either clinician guided or self-guided. This technology has been successfully applied to very refractory conditions, such as addiction[48] and chronic pain.[49]
- *Telemedicine:* Telemedicine provides face-to-face clinical care through a direct, real-time video link to a patient or group of patients or a PCP consulting with a specialist. Telemedicine has been used to deliver care to rural and other populations that have limited access to health care services. It has been effective in treating a variety of medical and mental health conditions, including chronic pain.[50,51]
- *Smartphone apps:* A significant number of smartphone applications for self-management of pain have been developed that provide a variety of tools, including self-monitoring, pain education, and goal setting. Although this is a promising endeavor, a recent analysis of available apps designed for pain management revealed that of the 279 apps that met inclusion criteria, none were comprehensive. Only 8.2% of the apps included a health care provider in their development and only one app was subjected to a scientific evaluation.[52]
- *Telecare Collaborative Pain Management:* The telecare collaborative care model is based on integrating care between the patient, the PCP, and the specialist with support from a nurse case manager using Web-based teleconferencing and telephone-based interventions. This model has been used with a stepped care approach for monitoring and managing opioid therapy in pain patients.[53,54]

FUTURE CONSIDERATIONS/SUMMARY

Chronic pain is a significant health care problem affecting more than 30% of the US population, with this number increasing yearly.

There are several models for pain care that include unimodality approaches, such as interventional pain medicine, multimodal (pain management and pharmacotherapy), multidisciplinary (care provided by several disciplines but typically not coordinated nor having shared treatment goals), and interdisciplinary (a collaborative team of health care providers that possess unique skills that are complementary). Outcome studies have revealed that biopsychosocial-based, interdisciplinary care emphasizing rational pharmacotherapy, rehabilitation, and CBT is one of the most clinically efficacious and cost-effective models in managing these complicated cases. These programs have been demonstrated to significantly improve functional status, psychological well being, reduce pain severity and opioid use and decrease health care use. Unfortunately, there are a scant few of these programs available in the United States. Most pain care is provided by PCPs who often have minimal to no training in pain medicine, and few resources or the time to effectively and efficiently manage these cases.

The 2011 IOM report on pain describes pain as "a national challenge" requiring a "cultural transformation to better prevent, assess, treat and understand pain of all types." Recently passed health care reform legislation, coupled with the development of health information technology, provides an opportunity to help meet this challenge. However, pain must be considered as complex and requiring an interdisciplinary team and systems approach. There needs to be significant changes in reimbursement policies to support this type of care model.

ACKNOWLEDGMENTS

M.D. Cheatle acknowledges the support from grant 1R01DA032776-01 from the National Institute on Drug Abuse, National Institutes of Health, in the writing of this article.

REFERENCES

1. Institute of Medicine (IOM). Living well with a chronic illness. Washington, DC: The National Academies Press; 2012.
2. Tsang A, Von Korff M, Lee S, et al. Common chronic pain conditions in developed and developing countries: gender and age differences and comorbidity with depression-anxiety disorders. J Pain 2008;9(10):883–91.
3. Johannes CB, Kim Le T, Zhou X, et al. The prevalence of chronic pain in United States adults: results of an Internet-based survey. J Pain 2010;11(11):1230–9.
4. Institute of Medicine (IOM). Relieving pain in America: a blueprint for transforming prevention, care, education, and research: a call for public action. Washington, DC: The National Academies Press; 2011.
5. Mendell JR, Sahenk Z. Painful sensory neuropathy. N Engl J Med 2003;348(13): 1243–55.
6. Cheatle MD. Depression, chronic pain, and suicide by overdose: on the edge. Pain Med 2011;12(Suppl 2):S43–8.
7. Fleming MF, Balousek SL, Klessig CL, et al. Substance use disorders in a primary care sample receiving daily opioid therapy. J Pain 2007;8(7):573–82.
8. Jones CM, Mack KA, Paulozzi LJ. Pharmaceutical overdose deaths, United States, 2010. JAMA 2013;309:657–9.
9. Peppin JF, Cheatle MD, Kirsh KL, et al. The complexity model: a novel approach to improve chronic pain care. Pain Med 2015;16(4):653–66.
10. Jamison RN. Nonspecific treatment effects in pain medicine. ISAP Pain Clinical Updates 2011;19(2):1–7.
11. Breuer B, Cruciani R, Portenoy RK. Pain management by primary care physicians, pain physicians, chiropractors, and acupuncturists: a national survey. South Med J 2010;103(8):738–47.
12. Upshur CC, Luckmann RS, Savageau JA. Primary care provider concerns about management of chronic pain in community clinic populations. J Gen Intern Med 2006;21(6):652–5.
13. Turk DC, Swanson K. Efficacy and cost-effectiveness treatment of chronic pain: an analysis and evidence-based synthesis. In: Schatman ME, Campbell A, editors. Chronic pain management: guidelines for multidisciplinary program development. New York: Informa Healthcare; 2007. p. 15–38.
14. Oslund S, Robinson RC, Clark TC, et al. Long-term effectiveness of a comprehensive pain management program: strengthening the case for interdisciplinary care. Proc (Bayl Univ Med Cent) 2009;22(3):211–4.

15. Cheatle MD, Gallagher RM. Chronic pain and comorbid mood and substance use disorders: a biopsychosocial treatment approach. Curr Psychiatry Rep 2006;8(5): 371–6.

16. McCracken LM, Turk TC. Behavioral and cognitive-behavioral treatment for chronic pain: outcome, predictors of outcome, and treatment process. Spine 2002;27(22):2564.

17. Heapy A, Kerns RD. Psychological and behavioral assessment. In: Benzon HT, Rathmel JP, Wu CL, et al, editors. Raj's practical management of pain. 4th edition. Philadelphia: Mosby/Elsevier; 2008. p. 279–95.

18. Chou R, Fanciullo GJ, Fine PG, et al. Clinical guidelines for the use of chronic opioid therapy in chronic noncancer pain. J Pain 2009;10(2):113–30.

19. Lalani I, Argoff CE. History and physical examination of the pain patient. In: Raj's practical management of pain. 4th edition. Philadelphia: Mosby/Elsevier; 2008. p. 177–88.

20. Beck A, Ward C, Mendelson M, et al. An inventory for measuring depression. Arch Gen Psychiatry 1961;4:561–71.

21. McNair D, Lorr M, Droppleman L. Profile of mood states. San Diego (CA): Educational and Industrial Testing Service; 1971.

22. Dworkin R, Turk DC, Farrar JT, et al, IMMPACT. Core outcome measures for chronic pain trials: IMMPACT recommendations. Pain 2005;113(1–2):9–19.

23. Kroenke K, Spitzer RL, Williams JB, et al. An ultrabrief screening scale for anxiety and depression: the PHQ-4. Psychosomatics 2009;50(6):613–21.

24. Beal BR, Wallace MS. An Overview of Pharmacologic Management of Chronic Pain. Med Clin N Am 2015, in press.

25. Beck A, Steer R, Brown C. Beck depression inventory-fast screen for medical patients manual. San Antonio (TX): Psychological Corporation; 2000.

26. Zung W. A self-rating depression scale. Arch Gen Psychiatry 1965;12:63–70.

27. Radloff L. The CES-D scale: a self-report depression scale for research in the general population. Appl Psychol Meas 1977;1:385–401.

28. Kroenke K, Spitzer RL, Williams JB. The PHQ-9: Validity of a brief depression severity measure. J Gen Intern Med 2001;16(9):606–13.

29. Webster LR, Webster RM. Predicting aberrant behaviors in opioid-treated patients: preliminary validation of the Opioid Risk Tool. Pain Med 2005;6:432–42.

30. Butler S, Budman S, Fernandez K, et al. Validation of a screener and opioid assessment measure for patients with chronic pain. Pain 2004;112(1–2):65–75.

31. Belgrade M, Schamber C, Lindgren B. The DIRE score: predicting outcomes of opioid prescribing for chronic pain. J Pain 2006;7(9):671–81.

32. Holmes CP, Gatchel RJ, Adams LL, et al. An opioid screening instrument: long-term evaluation of the utility of the Pain Medication Questionnaire. Pain Pract 2006;6(2):74–88.

33. Butler S, Budman SH, Fernandez KC, et al. Development and validation of the Current Opioid Misuse Measure. Pain 2007;130(1–2):144–56.

34. Compton P, Darakjian J, Miotto K. Screening for addiction in patients with chronic pain and "problematic" substance use: evaluation of a pilot assessment tool. J Pain Symptom Manage 1998;16(6):355–63.

35. Brown RL, Rounds LA. Conjoint screening questionnaires for alcohol and other drug abuse: criterion validity in a primary care practice. Wis Med J 1995;94(3): 135–40.

36. Bastiaens L, Riccardi K, Sakhrani D. The RAFFT as a screening tool for adult substance use disorders. Am J Drug Alcohol Abuse 2002;28(4):681–91.

37. Skinner HA. The drug abuse screening test. Addict Behav 1982;7(4):363–71.

38. Bush K, Kivlahan DR, McDonell MB, et al. The AUDIT alcohol consumption questions (AUDIT-C): an effective brief screening test for problem drinking. Ambulatory Care Quality Improvement Project (ACQUIP). Alcohol Use Disorders Identification Test. Arch Intern Med 1998;158(16):1789–95.
39. Turk DC, Flor H. Etiological theories and treatments for chronic back pain. II. Psychological models and interventions. Pain 1984;19(3):209–33.
40. Keefe FJ, Caldwell DS. Cognitive behavioral control of arthritis pain. Med Clin North Am 1997;81:277–90.
41. Chen E, Cole SW, Kato PM. A review of empirically supported psychosocial interventions for pain and adherence outcomes in sickle cell disease. J Pediatr Psychol 2004;29:1997–2009.
42. Glombiewski JA, Hartwich-Tersek J, Rief W. Two psychological interventions are effective in severely disabled, chronic back pain patients: a randomized controlled trial. Int J Behav Med 2010;17(2):97–107.
43. Turner JA, Manci L, Aaron LA. Short- and long-term efficacy of brief cognitive-behavioral therapy for patients with chronic temporomandibular disorder pain: a randomized, controlled trial. Pain 2006;121(3):181–94.
44. Greco CM, Rudy TE, Manzi S. Effects of a stress-reduction program on psychological function, pain, and physical function of systemic lupus erythematosus patients: a randomized controlled trial. Arthritis Rheum 2004;51(4):625–34.
45. Thieme K, Flor H, Turk D. Psychological pain treatment in fibromyalgia syndrome: efficacy of operant behavioral and cognitive behavioral treatments. Arthritis Res Ther 2006;8(4):R121.
46. McCracken LM, Eccleston C, Vowles KE. Acceptance-based treatment for persons with complex, long standing chronic pain: a preliminary analysis of treatment outcome in comparison to a waiting phase. Behav Res Ther 2005;43:1335–46.
47. Ehde DM, Dillworth TM, Turner JA. Cognitive-behavioral therapy for individuals with chronic pain: efficacy, innovations, and directions for research. Am Psychol 2014;69(2):153–66.
48. Carroll KM, Kiluk BD, Nich C, et al. Computer-assisted delivery of cognitive-behavioral therapy: efficacy and durability of CBT4CBT among cocaine-dependent individuals maintained on methadone. Am J Psychiatry 2014;171(4):436–44.
49. Dear BF, Titov N, Perry KN, et al. The pain course: a randomized controlled trial of a clinician-guided Internet-delivered cognitive behaviour therapy program for managing chronic pain and emotional well-being. Pain 2013;154(6):942–50.
50. Keogh E, Rosser BA, Eccleston C. E-health and chronic pain management: current status and developments. Pain 2010;151(1):18–21.
51. Sato AF, Clifford LM, Silverman AH, et al. Cognitive-behavioral interventions via telehealth: applications to pediatric functional abdominal pain. Child Health Care 2009;38(1):1–22.
52. Lalloo C, Jibb LA, Rivera J, et al. "There's a pain app for that": review of patient-targeted smartphone applications for pain management. Clin J Pain 2015;31(6):557–63.
53. Kroenke K, Krebs EE, Wu J, et al. Telecare collaborative management of chronic pain in primary care: a randomized clinical trial. JAMA 2014;312(3):240–8.
54. Cahana A, Dansie EJ, Theodore BR, et al. Redesigning delivery of opioids to optimize pain management, improve outcomes, and contain costs. Pain Med 2013;14(1):36–42.

Multimodal Treatment of Chronic Pain

Rebecca Dale, DO[a,*], Brett Stacey, MD[b]

KEYWORDS

- Multimodal • Combination therapy • Chronic pain treatment
- Multidisciplinary chronic pain treatment • Interdisciplinary pain treatment

KEY POINTS

- Most patients with chronic pain receive multimodal treatment.
- Combination pharmacotherapy should be carefully selected to avoid additive side effects and drugs with similar mechanisms of action or other interactions while still providing benefit.
- Structured interdisciplinary programs that include psychological treatments, rehabilitation, and medical management are beneficial yet costly, and may be applicable to only a minority of patients.
- Interventions including surgery and injections should rarely be first-line treatments and should be combined with other domains—rehabilitation, pharmacotherapy, attention to mental health, and coping.
- Complementary and alternative medicine as an addition to conventional pain treatment is a safe yet largely understudied area.

INTRODUCTION

Chronic pain of all sorts is not only responsible for considerable personal suffering worldwide, it also contributes to substantial costs to society. Although suffering cannot be quantified, the economic burden of pain in the United States alone is estimated at $650 billion per year in health care and lost productivity.[1] Although there are many treatment options available, none are universally endorsed, and many come with counterproductive side effects, or in the case of interventions, may lead to further complications.

The authors have nothing to disclose.
[a] Harborview Medical Center, Anesthesiology and Pain Medicine, Box 359724, 325 Ninth Ave, Seattle, WA 98104, USA; [b] Anesthesiology and Pain Medicine, UW Center for Pain Relief, University of Washington, 4225 Roosevelt Way Northeast, Box 354693, Seattle, WA 98105, USA
* Corresponding author.
E-mail address: rdale@uw.edu

Med Clin N Am 100 (2016) 55–64
http://dx.doi.org/10.1016/j.mcna.2015.08.012   medical.theclinics.com

When treating chronic pain, a common goal is to provide a lasting and meaningful reduction in suffering with concomitant improvements in overall functioning and health-related quality of life. Additional considerations are to minimize side effects and adverse events, and to deliver the care in a cost-effective manner. Ongoing pain is multidimensional with physical, cognitive, psychological, and behavioral aspects. Given the complex nature of chronic pain and the goals for treating it, it is not surprising that any 1 treatment by itself is rarely adequate to achieve these objectives. Rather, chronic pain lends itself to a multimodal treatment approach (**Fig. 1**). Treatment often includes medication(s), physical rehabilitation, lifestyle changes, psychology, advanced pain interventions, surgery, and complementary and alternative medicine in various combinations. Combination, multimodal therapy can be on an ad hoc basis, come about as an evolution in patient care owing to partial or incomplete treatment response, or take place in a more formalized setting such as a structured rehabilitation program. Although combination therapy is commonplace in clinical practice, such approaches are very little studied. In this article, we review multimodal, combination therapy for chronic pain.

PHARMACOLOGIC TREATMENT

With ongoing chronic pain, it is unusual for a single medication to result in satisfactory pain relief in a unimodal, stand-alone fashion. Therefore, combination pharmacologic treatment is an important aspect of multimodal chronic pain management. A key component of treating pain with medications is finding the balance between effective treatment and acceptable side effects (**Fig. 2**).

"Effective treatment" is difficult to define, because it will almost never mean a complete remission of pain. An analysis from a collection of industry-sponsored chronic pain trials suggest that a reduction of pain by 30% is clinically meaningful, because it is at this this level that patient ratings demonstrate a "much improved" pain experience.[2]

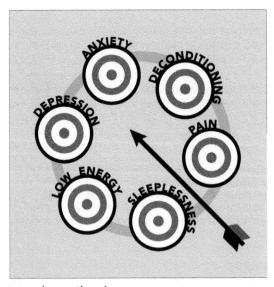

Fig. 1. Many targets need more than 1 arrow.

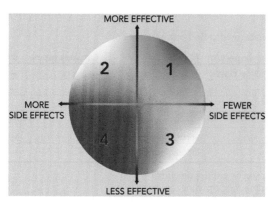

Fig. 2. The potential outcomes of combination pharmacotherapy. (*1*) Better pain control through a synergistic effect of the medications with minimal or improved side effect profile. (*2*) Better pain control, but worsened side effects. (*3*) No change in pain control with the addition of the second drug with improved side effect profile owing to antagonistic side effects (stimulant vs depressant). (*4*) No change or worsening pain control and worsened side effect profile.

Many of the pharmacologic agents used to treat chronic pain are central nervous system depressants and may impair the patient's energy, mobility, memory, and ability to exercise, all of which are crucial for successful rehabilitation. Although the mechanisms behind chronic pain vary and are poorly understood, it is generally characterized by a heightened sensitivity and hyperexcitability of the nervous system, which may be amenable to treatment with anticonvulsants and antidepressants, as well as opioids. To minimize sedation caused by a single pharmacologic agent, a reduction in dose is often desired, but this dose reduction may come at the cost of lessened analgesic effects. Ideally, the addition of a second agent would have an additive analgesic effect, but not a cumulative side effect profile, allowing the practitioner to use the lowest dose possible without losing analgesia and minimizing side effects. The use of combination pharmacotherapy has a wide evidence base in acute pain and so the rational that it may work for chronic pain as well is not unfounded.[3]

THEORY BEHIND COMBINED PHARMACOLOGIC TREATMENT

Studies have shown that, at best, most medications give a positive response in only a small percentage of people.[4] So until new more effective medications are developed, there is a need to identify medications that work well in combination. Another rationale for combination drug therapy (CDT) is to target the different pain mechanisms that contribute to the patient's overall pain syndrome. For example, a patient with chronic neck pain may have both a neuropathic as well as inflammatory component to their pain and may benefit from a combination therapy that targets each of these components. In clinical practices, this in fact seems to be a common perception. Recent studies show that more than one-third to one-half of chronic pain patients are taking more than 1 analgesic.[5–7] Unfortunately, some studies show that certain combinations of medications cannot only worsen the side effect profile, but have no synergistic analgesic effect at all.[8,9] There is a glaring need for further research to identify first-line combination pharmacotherapy for specific chronic pain conditions to guide practitioners in a rational approach to the medical treatment of patients with chronic pain (**Table 1**).

Table 1 Potentially problematic medication combinations	Gabapentin	TCAs[a]	Carbamazepine	Duloxetine
Pregabalin	Same class	—	—	—
Cyclobenzaprine	—	Same class	—	—
Topiramate	—	—	Same class	—
Venlafaxine	—	Serotonin syndrome	—	Same class
Tramadol	—	Serotonin syndrome	—	Serotonin syndrome
Methadone	—	QT prolongation	—	—

Abbreviation: TCAs, tricyclic antidepressants.
[a] Doxepin, imipramine, nortriptyline, amitriptyline.

STUDIED COMBINATIONS OF ANALGESIC MEDICATIONS IN COMMON PAIN CONDITIONS

There are a number of ways to approach the available information on CDT for chronic pain. We have organized this section by type of pain.

Neuropathic Pain

The International Association for the Study of Pain defines neuropathic pain as, "Pain caused by a lesion or disease of the somatosensory system." This includes central disorders (eg, spinal cord injury pain, multiple sclerosis pain, poststroke thalamic pain) as well as peripheral disorders (eg, diabetic neuropathy, postherpatic neuralgia, and tic douloureux) A number of studies explore CDT for neuropathic pain. One such successful combination is a gabapentenoid together with a tricyclic antidepressant. Both tricyclic antidepressants and gabapentinoids are proposed as first-line agents for neuropathic pain.[10] These medications have completely different mechanisms of actions (gabapentinoids are alpha-2-delta calcium channel modulators and tricyclic antidepressants have multiple mechanisms of action, including norepinephrine and serotonin reuptake inhibition), and so are logical candidates for combination therapy. This CDT has been studied in the treatment of diabetic peripheral neuropathy and postherpetic neuralgia and was found to be more effective than either drug given alone.[11] Opioids and gabapentinoids were also studied for neuropathic pain and the combination was found to be positive.[12–14] However, a 2012 Cochrane review looked at the combination pharmacotherapy for neuropathic pain[15] and concluded that many 2-drug combination therapies demonstrate superior efficacy than either drug alone, but that limited trial size and the short duration of the studies precluded them from making recommendations for any 1 specific recommendation for neuropathic pain.

Arthritis

Rheumatologic conditions associated with ongoing pain have a strong peripheral nociceptive component, although recent data suggest a component of central sensitization in many patients, as evidenced by limited correlation between pain complaints and disease severity.[16] There have been a number of studies evaluating successful CDT in arthritis. Tramadol mixed with acetaminophen and/or a nonsteroidal anti-inflammatory drug is 1 example that was found to be efficacious.[17,18] Again, however, a Cochrane review was preformed in 2011 for inflammatory arthritis, and they found the studies available for review had inadequate study design, were industry funded, or were dated before the advent of disease-modifying antirheumatic drug therapy. Because of this, they were unable to make any recommendations.[19]

Back Pain

Back pain is among the most common (if not the most common) chronic pain conditions, but despite this, a recent systemic review of CDT for this condition only found 6 studies eligible for review.[20] Chronic low back pain has been shown to be secondary to both neuropathic as well as nociceptive pain mechanisms.[21] This mixed pain picture lends itself to multimodal pharmacologic treatment. Studies examining the combination of an opioid and acetaminophen[22–24] found the combination to be beneficial. However, one must proceed with caution when prescribing opioids for chronic low back pain, because opioids are associated with significant risk and no long-term studies support their use. A 2013 Cochrane Review looked at opioid use in chronic back pain and found very low to moderate quality of evidence in their short-term use for pain and function.[25] One of the examined trials found no difference when comparing tramadol with a nonsteroidal anti-inflammatory drug.[26] Another trial examined in the review compared nortriptyline with morphine to the combination of the 2 to an active placebo and found that none of the treatments were effective.[8]

Fibromyalgia

Because of the physiologic, behavioral, and social issues that often surround patients with fibromyalgia, it is a complicated condition to treat. Our current understanding of fibromyalgia leads us to believe that it is mainly a centralized pain disorder with widespread pain as its defining feature. It is often accompanied by fatigue, sleep disturbance, and memory and mood difficulties. With successful treatment, several of these symptoms will typically improve.[27] When treating a polygenic chronic illness such as this, how does one decide on an appropriate CDT without exacerbating the central nervous system depressant components of the disease? Studies looking into CDT for fibromyalgia are limited. Positive CDT trials include the combination of tramadol and acetaminophen,[28] cyclobenzaprine plus fluoxetine,[29] pregabalin added to either quetiapine or trazodone,[30] and fluoxetine and amitriptyline.[31] However, the study evaluating tramadol and acetaminophen was industry sponsored and short term (13 weeks). It also did not include a group evaluating tramadol or acetaminophen alone. Since that study was published, other studies have found chronic opioids to be of little benefit, if not detrimental, to overall functioning in patients with fibromyalgia.[32,33] The study evaluating fluoxetine paired with amitriptyline was also short, with a limited number of study participants and the effects were modest. Clearly, there is a need for further trials.

That being said, when presented with a patient suffering from fibromyalgia, who has received only partial benefit from monotherapy, it may be prudent to try CDT. Calandre and colleagues[34] suggests starting with the US Food and Drug Administration–approved drugs pregabalin, duloxetine, and milnacipran. Begin by carefully evaluating the patient's symptoms and matching the CDT with the desired effects. Addition of a third drug, or a drug that is, not US Food and Drug Administration approved such as trazodone or quetiapine, may be desired. As always, careful titration and avoidance of drugs with similar mechanisms or dangerous synergistic side effects is important.

PSYCHOLOGICAL APPROACHES

Ongoing pain is commonly complicated by sleep interference, mood disturbances, maladaptive behaviors, and ineffective coping strategies, making psychological interventions a logical treatment component. However, many studies examining cognitive–behavioral therapy (CBT) and other mental health approaches as stand-alone treatment demonstrate only modest impact on pain, mood, or function.[35] Currently CBT is the first-line psychological treatment for chronic pain.[35] CBT focuses on the reduction of disability by emphasizing patient coping, adaption, and self-management. It teaches the patient skills such as relaxation, activity pacing, and identification and elimination of negative appraisals, fear avoidance, and catastrophizing. CBT has been shown to be helpful for pain, depression, anxiety, and insomnia. Similar to other pain management modalities, treatment effects of CBT have been shown to be only modest.[36] Again, this highlights the need for a multimodal approach.

One likely combination is CBT paired with pharmacologic management. Calderon Pdos and colleagues[37] did a small pilot study on the combination of amitriptyline with CBT in patients with temporomandibular joint pain and found no differences between groups. However, the authors thought that this was owing to a number of weaknesses in the study design. Monticone and colleagues[38] performed a study comparing CBT combined with exercise versus exercise alone in patients with low back pain and found that the combination group had longer lasting improvement in fear avoidance, reduced disability, and pain.

INTERVENTIONS

Often, radicular pain leads to a referral to an interventionalist, be it a surgeon or a pain specialist. This often leads to an epidural steroid injection, facet procedures, other injections, or surgical intervention. Nonsurgical interventional techniques are among the major modalities contributing to the increasing costs of treating chronic pain patients in the United States.[1] In fact, epidural steroid injections are the most commonly performed procedure in the United States, yet evidence is controversial and inconclusive as to their long-term effectiveness.[39,40] Similarly, most randomized studies evaluating the effectiveness of neurosurgical interventions for neuropathic pain have found minimal long-term benefits.[39] These results are perhaps because we have not been able to match patients with the correct treatment, or because patients with ongoing pain often have multiple components to their pain and suffering that do not lend themselves to a single treatment modality. Perhaps a combination of treatments, tailored to a particular patient's need, would be more beneficial. For example, surgery might play a greater role in a patient with serious neurologic symptoms, whereas epidural steroid injections may work better for patients with ongoing inflammatory pathology, and patients with ectopic nerve impulses stemming from central sensitization or chronic nerve injury may respond better to pharmacotherapy.

Recently, Cohen and colleagues[39] performed a randomized study comparing the effectiveness of epidural steroid injections, conservative treatment, or combination treatment in patients with cervical radicular pain. They found that patients in the conservative group receiving gabapentin or nortriptyline or both along with physical therapy fared the same as patients in the epidural steroid injection group. The patients in the combination group fared slightly better on some outcome measures, but most differences were not significant. Until further studies have elucidated patient selection criteria, the take home message with regard to interventions is that owing to the risk/benefit ratio, interventional and operative techniques should not be first-line treatments. This sage advice goes for many common interventional procedures, including sacroiliac joint injections, medial branch blocks, and radiofrequency ablative procedures.

INTERDISCIPLINARY PAIN REHABILITATION PROGRAMS

Research trends indicating that chronic pain is best understood as a combination of physical, psychological, and social interactions has led us to the current "bio-psychosocial" treatment paradigm. Interdisciplinary pain rehabilitation programs that target all of these aspects of a patient's pain have been developed to address this need and are the ultimate in multimodal pain treatments. Interdisciplinary pain rehabilitation programs do not have a standardized format, but as a whole, offer co-ordinated care between physicians, psychologists, physical therapists, and other health care providers in either an inpatient or outpatient setting. Often, rehabilitation programs are a last ditch attempt after all other alternatives have been proven insuf-ficient. There have been a number of positive studies to assess the efficacy of multi-component therapy in this population often regarded as "treatment resistant."

Fibromyalgia

Both the American Pain Society and the German guidelines for the management of fi-bromyalgia give strong recommendations to multicomponent therapy. A 2009 metaa-nalysis for multicomponent treatment in fibromyalgia found that, although there is limited evidence for long-term effects, there is strong evidence for reduction of symp-toms in key areas of fibromyalgia syndrome such as pain, fatigue, depression, and physical fitness.[41]

Chronic Low Back Pain

A 2014 Cochran Review analyzed multidisciplinary biopychosocial rehabilitation pro-grams for low back pain and found moderate quality evidence that multidisciplinary biopychosocial rehabilitation treatment results in modest improvements (1 point out of 10) for pain when compared with usual care or physical therapy alone, and that it doubled the likelihood that people were able to return to work in the next 6 to 12 months.[42] They emphasized the need to weigh the cost–benefit ratio as well as the time–benefit ratio when considering enrolling a patient in such a program.

COMPLEMENTARY AND ALTERNATIVE MEDICINE AND SELF-MANAGEMENT

For no lack of effort, conventional treatment of chronic pain is lacking in many aspects. Intolerable side effects, serious risks, and lack of efficacy have led many patients to seek complimentary and alternative medicine and self-management strategies such as acupuncture, relaxation, yoga, message therapy, and biofeedback.[43] A recent re-view of the literature behind such treatments was able to find evidence in favor of use of yoga, tai chi, and music therapy for self-management of pain, but was unable to find quality evidence to support any other common complementary and alternative med-icine modalities.[44] This was mainly owing to the fact that there is a dearth of quality randomized control studies available, and not because the evidence points away from these modalities as being effective. In 2014, Lee and colleagues[43] performed a review looking at multimodal integrative therapies for chronic pain, and came to a similar conclusion. There is not enough high-quality research to make a recommenda-tion regarding multimodal integrative therapies for chronic pain.

SUMMARY

Combination therapy for the treatment of chronic pain remains an important and com-mon, yet understudied, approach. The development of refined clinical strategies to predict positive outcomes and to optimize individualized combination therapy is the goal for future improvements. Until more information becomes available, a prudent and rational approach with careful attention to the potential risks and monitoring for patient improvement is vital.

REFERENCES

1. Gaskin DJ, Richard P. The economic costs of pain in the United States. J Pain 2012;13(8):715–24.
2. Farrar JT, Young JP Jr, LaMoreaux L, et al. Clinical importance of changes in chronic pain intensity measured on an 11-point numerical pain rating scale. Pain 2001;94(2):149–58.
3. Elvir-Lazo OL, White PF. The role of multimodal analgesia in pain management after ambulatory surgery. Curr Opin Anaesthesiol 2010;23(6):697–703.
4. Moore RA, Derry S, McQuay HJ, et al. Clinical effectiveness: an approach to clinical trial design more relevant to clinical practice, acknowledging the importance of individual differences. Pain 2010;149(2):173–6.
5. Gore M, Tai KS, Sadosky A, et al. Clinical comorbidities, treatment patterns, and direct medical costs of patients with osteoarthritis in usual care: a retrospective claims database analysis. J Med Econ 2011;14(4):497–507.
6. Gore M, Sadosky A, Stacey BR, et al. The burden of chronic low back pain: clinical comorbidities, treatment patterns, and health care costs in usual care settings. Spine 2012;37(11):E668–77.
7. Berger A, Sadosky A, Dukes E, et al. Clinical characteristics and patterns of healthcare utilization in patients with painful neuropathic disorders in UK general practice: a retrospective cohort study. BMC Neurol 2012;12:8.
8. Khoromi S, Cui L, Nackers L, et al. Morphine, nortriptyline and their combination vs. placebo in patients with chronic lumbar root pain. Pain 2007;130(1–2):66–75.
9. Graff-Radford SB, Shaw LR, Naliboff BN. Amitriptyline and fluphenazine in the treatment of postherpetic neuralgia. Clin J Pain 2000;16(3):188–92.
10. Dworkin RH, O'Connor AB, Audette J, et al. Recommendations for the pharmacological management of neuropathic pain: an overview and literature update. Mayo Clin Proc 2010;85(3 Suppl):S3–14.
11. Gilron I, Bailey JM, Tu D, et al. Nortriptyline and gabapentin, alone and in combination for neuropathic pain: a double-blind, randomised controlled crossover trial. Lancet 2009;374(9697):1252–61.
12. Gatti A, Sabato AF, Occhioni R, et al. Controlled-release oxycodone and pregabalin in the treatment of neuropathic pain: results of a multicenter Italian study. Eur Neurol 2009;61(3):129–37.
13. Gilron I, Bailey JM, Tu D, et al. Morphine, gabapentin, or their combination for neuropathic pain. N Engl J Med 2005;352(13):1324–34.
14. Hanna M, O'Brien C, Wilson MC. Prolonged-release oxycodone enhances the effects of existing gabapentin therapy in painful diabetic neuropathy patients. Eur J Pain 2008;12(6):804–13.
15. Chaparro LE, Wiffen PJ, Moore RA, et al. Combination pharmacotherapy for the treatment of neuropathic pain in adults. Cochrane Database Syst Rev 2012;(7):CD008943.
16. Meeus M, Vervisch S, De Clerck LS, et al. Central sensitization in patients with rheumatoid arthritis: a systematic literature review. Semin Arthritis Rheum 2012; 41(4):556–67.
17. Lee EY, Lee EB, Park BJ, et al. Tramadol 37.5-mg/acetaminophen 325-mg combination tablets added to regular therapy for rheumatoid arthritis pain: a 1-week,

randomized, double-blind, placebo-controlled trial. Clin Ther 2006;28(12): 2052–60.

18. Wilder-Smith CH, Hill L, Spargo K, et al. Treatment of severe pain from osteoar-thritis with slow-release tramadol or dihydrocodeine in combination with NSAID's: a randomised study comparing analgesia, antinociception and gastrointestinal effects. Pain 2001;91(1–2):23–31.

19. Ramiro S, Radner H, van der Heijde D, et al. Combination therapy for pain management in inflammatory arthritis (rheumatoid arthritis, ankylosing spondy-litis, psoriatic arthritis, other spondyloarthritis). Cochrane Database Syst Rev 2011;(10):CD008886.

20. Romano CL, Romano D, Lacerenza M. Antineuropathic and antinociceptive drugs combination in patients with chronic low back pain: a systematic review. Pain Res Treat 2012;2012:154781.

21. Baron R, Binder A. How neuropathic is sciatica? The mixed pain concept. Ortho-pade 2004;33(5):568–75 [in German].

22. Gatti A, Sabato AF, Carucci A, et al. Adequacy assessment of oxycodone/para-cetamol (acetaminophen) in multimodal chronic pain : a prospective observa-tional study. Clin Drug Investig 2009;29(Suppl 1):31–40.

23. Ruoff GE, Rosenthal N, Jordan D, et al. Tramadol/acetaminophen combination tablets for the treatment of chronic lower back pain: a multicenter, randomized, double-blind, placebo-controlled outpatient study. Clin Ther 2003;25(4):1123–41.

24. Peloso PM, Fortin L, Beaulieu A, et al. Analgesic efficacy and safety of tramadol/ acetaminophen combination tablets (Ultracet) in treatment of chronic low back pain: a multicenter, outpatient, randomized, double blind, placebo controlled trial. J Rheumatol 2004;31(12):2454–63.

25. Chaparro LE, Furlan AD, Deshpande A, et al. Opioids compared to placebo or other treatments for chronic low-back pain. Cochrane Database Syst Rev 2013;(8):CD004959.

26. O'Donnell JB, Ekman EF, Spalding WM, et al. The effectiveness of a weak opioid medication versus a cyclo-oxygenase-2 (COX-2) selective non-steroidal anti-in-flammatory drug in treating flare-up of chronic low-back pain: results from two randomized, double-blind, 6-week studies. J Int Med Res 2009;37(6):1789–802.

27. Ablin J, Fitzcharles MA, Buskila D, et al. Treatment of fibromyalgia syndrome: rec-ommendations of recent evidence-based interdisciplinary guidelines with special emphasis on complementary and alternative therapies. Evid Based Complement Alternat Med 2013;2013:485272.

28. Bennett RM, Kamin M, Karim R, et al. Tramadol and acetaminophen combination tablets in the treatment of fibromyalgia pain: a double-blind, randomized, placebo-controlled study. Am J Med 2003;114(7):537–45.

29. Cantini F, Bellandi F, Niccoli L, et al. Fluoxetine combined with cyclobenzaprine in the treatment of fibromyalgia. Minerva Med 1994;85(3):97–100 [in Italian].

30. Calandre EP, Morillas-Arques P, Molina-Barea R, et al. Trazodone plus pregabalin combination in the treatment of fibromyalgia: a two-phase, 24-week, open-label uncontrolled study. BMC Musculoskelet Disord 2011;12:95.

31. Goldenberg D, Mayskiy M, Mossey C, et al. A randomized, double-blind cross-over trial of fluoxetine and amitriptyline in the treatment of fibromyalgia. Arthritis Rheum 1996;39(11):1852–9.

32. Brummett CM, Janda AM, Schueller CM, et al. Survey criteria for fibromyalgia independently predict increased postoperative opioid consumption after lower-extremity joint arthroplasty: a prospective, observational cohort study. Anesthesi-ology 2013;119(6):1434–43.

33. Fitzcharles MA, Faregh N, Ste-Marie PA, et al. Opioid use in fibromyalgia is associated with negative health related measures in a prospective cohort study. Pain Res Treat 2013;2013:898493.

34. Calandre EP, Rico-Villademoros F, Rodriguez-Lopez CM. Monotherapy or combination therapy for fibromyalgia treatment? Curr Rheumatol Rep 2012;14(6): 568–75.

35. Ehde DM, Dillworth TM, Turner JA. Cognitive-behavioral therapy for individuals with chronic pain: efficacy, innovations, and directions for research. Am Psychol 2014;69(2):153–66.

36. Williams AC, Eccleston C, Morley S. Psychological therapies for the management of chronic pain (excluding headache) in adults. Cochrane Database Syst Rev 2012;(11):CD007407.

37. Calderon Pdos S, Tabaquim Mde L, Oliveira LC, et al. Effectiveness of cognitive-behavioral therapy and amitriptyline in patients with chronic temporomandibular disorders: a pilot study. Braz Dent J 2011;22(5):415–21.

38. Monticone M, Ferrante S, Rocca B, et al. Effect of a long-lasting multidisciplinary program on disability and fear-avoidance behaviors in patients with chronic low back pain: results of a randomized controlled trial. Clin J Pain 2013;29(11): 929–38.

39. Cohen SP, Hayek S, Semenov Y, et al. Epidural steroid injections, conservative treatment, or combination treatment for cervical radicular pain: a multicenter, randomized, comparative-effectiveness study. Anesthesiology 2014;121(5): 1045–55.

40. Cohen SP, Deyo RA. A call to arms: the credibility gap in interventional pain medicine and recommendations for future research. Pain Med 2013;14(9):1280–3.

41. Hauser W, Bernardy K, Arnold B, et al. Efficacy of multicomponent treatment in fibromyalgia syndrome: a meta-analysis of randomized controlled clinical trials. Arthritis Rheum 2009;61(2):216–24.

42. Kamper SJ, Apeldoorn AT, Chiarotto A, et al. Multidisciplinary biopsychosocial rehabilitation for chronic low back pain. Cochrane Database Syst Rev 2014;(9):CD000963.

43. Lee C, Crawford C, Swann S, Active Self-Care Therapies for Pain Working Group. Multimodal, integrative therapies for the self-management of chronic pain symptoms. Pain Med 2014;15(Suppl 1):S76–85.

44. Crawford C, Lee C, Buckenmaier C 3rd, et al. The current state of the science for active self-care complementary and integrative medicine therapies in the management of chronic pain symptoms: lessons learned, directions for the future. Pain Med 2014;15(Suppl 1):S104–13.

An Overview of Pharmacologic Management of Chronic Pain

Benjamin R. Beal, MD, Mark S. Wallace, MD*

KEYWORDS

- Chronic pain • Pharmacologic management • Neuropathic pain
- Intrathecal drug delivery • Nonopiate pain medication • Evidence based

KEY POINTS

- The need to adequately treat chronic pain is widely accepted.
- Proper patient selection is essential for initiation of long-term opiate therapy.
- Multiple alternatives to opioids for treating chronic pain are effective and widely available.
- Intrathecal drug delivery systems can be used both for cancer-related and non–cancer-related pain.

OVERVIEW OF THE PHARMACOLOGIC MANAGEMENT OF CHRONIC PAIN

The treatment of patients with chronic painful conditions can at times be difficult at best. Historically, the opiates were the primary class of medications used to treat patients with both acute and chronic pain. More recently, multiple studies have been published revealing the adverse consequences of chronic opiate therapy in the non-cancer population and questioning its safety.[1] This has resulted in an increased interest in nonopiate pain medications currently available for the management of chronic pain.

Pain can be broadly categorized in several ways. However, for the purpose of this article, pain will be broadly categorized into 2 major subtypes: nociceptive pain and neuropathic pain. Nociceptive pain is due to normal activity in neural pathways resulting from actual tissue damage or potential tissue damage as seen with postoperative pain, osteoarthritis-related pain, or mechanical low back pain.[2] Neuropathic pain is pain that results from damage to the nervous system itself, as is seen, for example, in painful diabetic peripheral neuropathy, central poststroke pain, and postherpetic neuralgia.[3] Although many of the therapies mentioned in this article have been shown

Division of Pain Medicine, Department of Anesthesiology, University of California, San Diego, San Diego, CA, USA
* Corresponding author. 9300 Campus Point Drive, MC 7651, La Jolla, CA 92037-1300.
E-mail address: mswallace@ucsd.edu

Med Clin N Am 100 (2016) 65–79
http://dx.doi.org/10.1016/j.mcna.2015.08.006
0025-7125/16/$ – see front matter

to have some degree of efficacy in treating nociceptive pain, the primary focus of this article is on medications used for the treatment of chronic neuropathic pain.

The types of medications used to manage both chronic and acute pain can be broadly classified into 8 major categories: opiates, nonopioid analgesics (primarily nonsteroidal anti-inflammatories), antidepressants, anticonvulsants, cannabinoids, botulinum toxin, topical agents, and intrathecal drugs. The focus of this review is on the more common oral preparations used in the treatment of chronic pain.

CLASSES OF MEDICATIONS
Nonsteroidal Anti-inflammatory Drugs

Nonsteroidal anti-inflammatory drugs (NSAIDs) affect varying degrees of pain modulation through the inhibition of prostaglandin (PG) synthesis. Prostaglandins are synthesized from arachidonic acid via cyclooxygenase (COX) and have both proinflammatory effects as well as homeostatic effects, which are necessary for the proper maintenance of kidney, gut mucosa, and smooth muscle function.[4] The COX-2 isoform is responsible for synthesizing the proinflammatory prostaglandins and is the target of the newer NSAIDs known collectively as COX-2 inhibitors.[5] The remainder of the NSAIDs nonselectively inhibit both COX-1 and COX-2 to varying degrees.

NSAIDs have been shown to be effective in the treatment of chronic low back pain as well as chronic pain due to osteoarthritis.[5,6] There is also some evidence that NSAIDs are modestly effective in treating lumbar radiculopathy; however, in general, NSAIDs are considered minimally effective in treating other types of neuropathic pain states.[7] Additionally, multiple studies as well as a recent meta-analysis have consistently shown that the addition of an NSAID to a pain management regimen can have an opioid-sparing effect of between 20% and 35%.[8,9]

OPIOIDS

The opioids as a class are medications whose clinical effects are similar in that they cause analgesia, respiratory depression, sedation, and constipation primarily through their action as agonists of the mu opioid receptor. In addition to the mu receptor, the kappa and delta opioid receptors also contribute to the clinical effects, such as respiratory depression and sedation to lesser degrees.[10] The opioid receptors are located centrally throughout the brain and spinal cord, more specifically on primary afferent dorsal horn neurons. High densities of mu receptors are found throughout the periaqueductal gray (PAG) of the midbrain. Agonism of the mu receptor in the PAG is thought to remove a tonic inhibitory gamma aminobutyric acid (GABA)-ergic tone, allowing the PAG to exert its inhibitory effect at the level of the spinal cord.[11] Opioids acting on the dorsal horn neurons inhibit glutamine release, thereby decreasing the transmission of nociceptive information from A-delta and C nerve fibers.[10]

Over the past decade, an increased awareness of the undertreatment of chronic pain has paralleled a significant increase in opioid prescribing.[12] Between 1991 and 2011, opioid prescriptions dispensed by retail pharmacies increased from 76 million to 219 million. With this increase in opioid use by people experiencing chronic pain, the number of drug overdose deaths involving opiate analgesics increased fourfold and the number of admissions for the treatment of opioid dependence has increased to an almost identical degree.[12]

Recent studies have called into question both the efficacy and safety of chronic opiate therapy in the non–cancer-related pain population. Although there is a rather large volume of strong evidence supporting the short-term use of opiates in managing pain, the evidence supporting the long-term use of non-cancer pain is not as strong.[13,14] Unwanted adverse effects, such as opioid tolerance, dependence, constipation, respiratory depression, impaired cognitive ability, immune suppression, and opioid-related endocrinopathies, are only some of the known physical alterations associated with the chronic use of opiate medications.[15,16]

Current recommendations for initiating chronic opiate therapy are intended to better identify patients at risk for abusing and/or misusing opiate medications or from suffering their adverse physical effects (**Fig. 1**).[12,13] This includes a detailed medical history, psychiatric history, and substance use history as well as establishing a physical diagnosis and the medical necessity for chronic opiate therapy.[17] Urine drug screening as well as establishing an agreement between the provider and patient in which the goals and expectations of the therapy are clearly stated reduces misuse, abuse, or diversion of opiate medications.[13]

ANTIDEPRESSANTS

The effectiveness for antidepressants in the treatment of chronic pain disorders with a strong neuropathic component has long been established in the literature.[14] Tricyclic antidepressants (TCA), which include the tertiary amines amitriptyline and imipramine as well as the secondary amines nortriptyline and desipramine, have been shown to be effective in treating a variety of painful neuropathic conditions, such as painful diabetic peripheral neuropathy (DPN), postherpetic neuralgia (PHN), painful polyneuropathy, postmastectomy pain, and central poststroke pain.[14,18] The analgesic effect of TCAs occurs at a lower dose than doses expected for the treatment of depression and with a more rapid onset. Furthermore, studies have shown that the analgesic effects are independent of the presence of any changes in depression or mood state.[19,20]

TCAs as a class have multiple mechanisms of action that contribute to analgesia to varying degrees. Their primary mechanism of action is through reuptake inhibition of norepinephrine and serotonin, which increases the activation of descending inhibitory pathways in the midbrain and spinal cord.[14,21] Other mechanisms that contribute both to antinociception and the adverse effects of the drugs include interactions with

Mark each box that applies	Female	Male	
1. Family Hx of substance abuse			
Alcohol	❑ 1	❑ 3	
Illegal drugs	❑ 2	❑ 3	**Administer**
Rx drugs	❑ 4	❑ 4	• On initial visit
2. Personal Hx of substance abuse			• Prior to opioid
Alcohol	❑ 3	❑ 3	therapy
Illegal drugs	❑ 4	❑ 4	
Rx drugs	❑ 5	❑ 5	**Scoring (risk)**
3. Age between 16–45 yrs	❑ 1	❑ 1	• 0–3: low
4. Hx of preadolescent sexual abuse	❑ 3	❑ 0	• 4–7: moderate
5. Psychologic disease			• ≥8: high
ADD, OCD, bipolar, schizophrenia	❑ 2	❑ 2	
Depression	❑ 1	❑ 1	
Scoring totals:			

Fig. 1. Opioid risk tool. ADD, attention-deficit disorder; Hx, history; OCD, obsessive-compulsive disorder; Rx, prescription. (*From* Webster LR, Webster RM. Predicting aberrant behaviors in opioid-treated patients: preliminary validation of the opioid risk tool. Pain Med 2005;6(6):433; with permission.)

histamine, cholinergic, and N-methyl-D-aspartate receptors, as well as direct blockade of membrane ion channels (reducing neuronal influx of Ca^{2+} or Na^+).[21,22] The side-effect profiles of the TCAs are not insignificant and oftentimes lead to an individual's inability to tolerate the medication. The most common side effects include postural hypotension, dry mouth, and sedation for which reason these medications are typically taken at bedtime. Additionally, these side effects can be of particular concern in the elderly population, which may increase the risk for falls. Other disadvantages of TCAs are the risk of serotonin syndrome, when used in conjunction with other serotonin reuptake inhibitors, cardiac conduction abnormalities, and lethal overdose.[23]

In addition to the TCAs, the serotonin and norepinephrine reuptake inhibitor agents, duloxetine and venlafaxine, have shown efficacy in treating peripheral neuropathic pain and other chronic pain conditions. Duloxetine has been approved by the Food and Drug Administration (FDA) in the treatment of painful DPN, fibromyalgia, and chronic musculoskeletal pain but venlafaxine has not received FDA approval for pain treatment.[24] The mechanism of action is thought to be due to activation of descending inhibitory pathways via serotonin and norepinephrine reuptake inhibition. However, it is likely that the mood-elevating effects of the medications also have a significant contribution to the reported decreases in pain scores. A recent placebo-controlled trial of duloxetine in patients with depression and moderate-to-severe pain of an unclear etiology found a significant benefit from duloxetine for both pain and depression symptoms.[25]

ANTICONVULSANTS

The first anticonvulsant used in clinical trials to treat a neuropathic pain disorder (trigeminal neuralgia) was carbamazepine; in fact, it was first FDA approved for trigeminal neuralgia, NOT seizure treatment.[26] Carbamazepine acts to stabilize the inactivated state of voltage-gated sodium channels thereby decreasing the excitability of frequency-dependent neuronal activity of A-delta and C-fibers, suppressing spontaneous activity.[27] Common side effects include somnolence, dizziness, and gait disturbance. More serious adverse reactions that have been reported include Stevens-Johnson syndrome, toxic epidermal necrolysis, and blood dyscrasias (severe blood dyscrasias estimated at 7.2 per 10,000 treated patients).[28,29]

Carbamazepine has continued to be used for the treatment of trigeminal neuralgia but has not been shown to be as effective in treating other neuropathic pain disorders.[14] Valproic acid, oxcarbazepine, topiramate, and lamotrigine have also been studied for efficacy in treating various neuropathic pain disorders showing inconsistent evidence of efficacy.[14]

Gabapentin is a structural analog of GABA, but does not bind to the $GABA_A$ or $GABA_B$ receptor to achieve its effect. Instead, it binds to the α_2-δ site of voltage-dependent calcium channels and modulates the influx of calcium with a resulting reduction in excitatory neurotransmitter release and a decrease in pain signaling.[30] Pregabalin has a similar mechanism of action but has greater bioavailability (absolute bioavailability of >90%) and displays linear pharmacokinetics over the range of recommended dosages. Gabapentin, however, does not display linear pharmacokinetics and, as a result, the absolute bioavailability decreases from 60% to 33% with increased dosing from 900 to 3600 mg per day.[31] The linear versus nonlinear pharmacokinetics may explain the lower incidence of unwanted side effects in individuals taking pregabalin. Whereas the site of action of pregabalin is thought to be modulation of N-type calcium channels in the dorsal horn, recent animal studies suggest that the site of action of gabapentin may be supraspinal at the locus coeruleus.[32]

The most common side effects reported for both drugs are dizziness, somnolence, and ataxia. In the case of gabapentin, these side effects may become apparent at doses below those that are considered therapeutic (1800 mg per day).[30] In addition, peripheral edema has been reported as a side effect of both drugs with a possibly higher incidence in pregabalin.[33]

Gabapentin and pregabalin have been shown to be effective when compared with placebo in treating painful DPN, PHN, painful polyneuropathy, neuropathic cancer pain, central poststroke pain, and spinal cord injury pain.[14] Given the high safety profile and the relative effectiveness in treating neuropathic pain, gabapentin and pregabalin are considered first-line therapy by the International Association for the Study of Pain Neuropathic Pain Special Interest Group.

TOPICAL AGENTS

Topical lidocaine, either in the form of the lidocaine patch 5% or in the form of lidocaine gel 5%, has been shown to be effective in treating patients' peripheral neuropathic pain conditions with allodynia as well as PHN with allodynia for which it has FDA approval.[18,34] Lidocaine works by blocking abnormal activity in sodium channels located on peripheral neurons in the painful regions. When used appropriately, there are no clinically significant drug plasma levels, so the treatment is achieved via blocking the abnormal peripheral neuronal conduction. The lidocaine patch also acts as a physical barrier between the painful area and the environment.

Topical NSAIDs were developed to achieve the localized anti-inflammatory effects of these medications while avoiding the adverse effects associated with systemic administration of the same drugs.[35] The most widely studied topical NSAIDs include diclofenac, ibuprofen, and ketoprofen.[36] A review of these studies concluded that topical NSAIDs can be recommended for short-term pain relief in the treatment of soft tissue injuries and chronic joint-related pain.[36]

Topical high-dose capsaicin (8%) has been shown to be effective in providing rapid and sustained pain relief in patients with PHN and painful human immunodeficiency virus (HIV)-associated neuropathies.[37,38] Capsaicin is a TRPV-1 receptor agonist, which are receptors located on cutaneous nociceptors. When high-dose capsaicin is applied topically, TRPV-1 activation results in a large and sustained influx of intracellular calcium causing a breakdown in the cytoskeletal components of the neuronal fibers. This breakdown results in a "defunctionalization" of the spontaneously firing nociceptor, providing pain relief for up to 12 weeks.[38,39] Transient treatment-related pain and localized erythema is to be expected and can best be managed by pretreatment with a short-acting opioid.

CANNABINOIDS

There are 2 cannabinoid receptors: CB1 and CB2. CB1 receptors are located in the brain, spinal cord, and on primary sensory nerve terminals. CB2 is found on microglia, monocytes, macrophages, and B/T lymphocytes. Activation of CB1 receptors reduces pain transmission at multiple levels of the nervous system both peripherally and centrally. Activation of CB2 receptors on peripheral inflammatory cells has been shown to decrease inflammatory cell mediator release, plasma extravasation, and the sensitization of afferent terminal.[40,41]

The term cannabinoid refers to a variety of compounds that are (1) derived from cannabis plants (phytocannabinoids), (2) endogenous cannabinoids (referred to as endocannabinoids), and (3) synthetic cannabinoids.[42] The most abundant and main psychoactive compound in cannabis is delta-9-tetrahydrocannabinol (THC). Cannabidiol (CBD) is the second most abundant compound in the plant. CBD is less psychoactive than THC and appears to enhance the effects of THC. In addition, CBD has analgesic, antiseizure and anti-inflammatory effects.[43,44] Although cannabis remains a schedule I drug, at the time of this writing 23 states plus the District of Columbia have legalized medicinal marijuana. Nonetheless, there have been many placebo-controlled randomized studies showing efficacy in neuropathic pain.[45–49] Exactly how it should be integrated into medical practice is still up for debate, given the lack of quality control over marijuana products.

Cannabis-based extract (CBME) is derived by extracting compounds directly from the marijuana plant. There are currently 2 CBMEs that have undergone clinical trials, Cannador and Sativex, both with a combination of THC and CBD.[50,51] Sativex is approved in Canada for the treatment of spasticity related to multiple sclerosis. Although Sativex was positive in relieving cancer pain in a phase II trial, the phase III trial failed to reach the primary end point.[52]

There are 2 synthetic cannabinoids on the market: Dronabinol and Nabilone. Dronabinol is an oral synthetic THC that has been on the market since 1985 to treat nausea associated with chemotherapy and as an appetite stimulant in HIV/AIDS. Nabilone is a semisynthetic analog of THC that is approximately 10 times more potent with a longer duration and is FDA approved to treat chemotherapy-induced nausea. Neither has been studied in neuropathic pain and both have mixed results in treating acute pain, most likely due to the erratic and unpredictable absorption from the gastrointestinal tract.[53,54]

Some states provide guidelines for recommending medicinal marijuana (see California Medical Board Web site www.mbc.ca.gov/Licensees/Prescribing/medical_marijuana_cma-recommend.pdf). Because it is a drug of abuse, chronic opioid therapy guidelines can be applied. Clinicians should educate patients on marijuana safety and efficacy, counsel patients on their responsibilities, and follow-up with patients to assess efficacy and side effects. Not allowing the coadministration of marijuana and an opioid should be strongly considered.

BOTULINUM TOXIN

The botulinum toxins are derived from the anaerobic bacterium *Clostridium botulinum*. Of the 7 different toxins, only botulinum toxin types A and B are available for clinical use. The toxin acts to inhibit the presynaptic release of acetylcholine from cholinergic nerve terminals. However, this does not completely explain the analgesic effect of the toxins. It is likely that the inhibition of the release of glutamate, substance P, and calcitonin gene-related peptide resulting in a decreased afferent nociceptive transmission is also involved, independent of the inhibition of acetylcholine release.[55] Although the unwanted side effects of botulinum toxin administration are few, there is a black box warning for the use of botulinum toxin. This warning indicates that the use of botulinum toxin may result in the unwanted spread of the medication from its intended site to distant parts of the body, resulting in botulismlike symptoms. Although most of these events were associated with high-dose botulinum toxin injections in children with cerebral palsy–associated spasticity, similar cases have been reported in adults.[56]

Botulinum toxin has been shown to be effective in decreasing the number and severity of headaches in chronic migraine, and one preparation, onabotulinum toxin A (Botox), has FDA approval for this indication.[57] Multiple studies have also looked at the effect that botulinum toxin has on tension-type headache, cluster headache, and chronic daily headache with mixed results.

Each of the 4 FDA-approved botulinum toxins are considered first-line therapy for the treatment of cervical dystonia (**Table 1**). This syndrome is the result of abnormal, involuntary contractions of the cervical and shoulder muscles resulting in significant musculoskeletal pain. Botulinum toxin injections can improve head positioning, pain, and disability in up to 90% of individuals with this condition.[57] Two recent studies found that there was insufficient evidence to support its use in myofascial and musculoskeletal pain.[58,59]

INTRATHECAL DRUG THERAPY

Intrathecal drug delivery (IDD) consists initially of an intrathecal trial of the medication to be used. After a successful trial, the patient is taken to the operating room for permanent implant of an intrathecal catheter and pump. IDD is considered both an invasive and labor-intensive therapy and therefore proper patient selection is crucial to its success.

Indications for IDD include (1) individuals with cancer pain whose life expectancy is longer than 3 months and has had inadequate pain relief or intolerable side effects from systemic agents, and (2) noncancer pain with objective evidence of pathology, lack of drug-seeking behavior, and inadequate pain relief or intolerable side effects from systemic agents.[60]

It has been shown that patients without major psychological or psychiatric illness have more favorable outcomes than those who do. Appropriate screening should exclude individuals with any of the following: (1) active psychosis, (2) active suicidality, (3) active homicidality, (4) major uncontrolled depression or other mood disorders, (5) somatization or other somatoform disorders, (6) alcohol or drug dependency, (7) compensation or litigation resolution, (8) lack of appropriate social support, and (9) neurobehavioral or cognitive deficits.[61–63]

Of the medications used in IDD, only morphine, ziconotide, and baclofen are FDA approved for intrathecal therapy. However, other medications commonly used in IDD include local anesthetics and clonidine. All of the intrathecal medications are commonly used in combination, but opioids, baclofen, and ziconotide can be used as monotherapy.[64]

Morphine, when delivered at its site of action in the dorsal horn of the spinal cord, allows for decreased dosing and decreased side effects when compared with systemic dosing. Morphine, hydromorphone, fentanyl, and sufentanil are all commonly used opioids and can still result in side effects, such as respiratory depression with overdose, nausea, urinary retention, pruritus, and peripheral edema.[65] Furthermore, highly concentrated opiates can result in the formation of catheter tip granulomas and may cause spinal cord compression with associated neurologic findings.[66]

The mechanism of action of ziconotide is via presynaptic N-type calcium channel blockade resulting in decreased neurotransmitter release. Two studies, 1 for cancer-related pain and 1 for non–cancer-related pain, showed a 53.1% versus 18.1% and 31.2% versus 6.0% reduction in pain (ziconotide vs placebo), respectively.[67,68] Dizziness, somnolence, confusion, and abnormal gait are some of the most common side effects seen with rapid titration of this medication due to a narrow therapeutic window.[68]

Local anesthetics are typically used in combination with other medications. Their mechanism of action is via blockade of both presynaptic and postsynaptic sodium channels. When used in low doses, minimal sensory or motor deficits are noted and tachyphylaxis is avoided.[60]

Table 1
Prescribing recommendations for first-line medications and for opioid agonists

Medication Class	Starting Dosage	Titration	Maximum Dosage	Duration of Adequate Trial	Major Side Effects	Precautions	Other Benefits
Antidepressant medications							
Secondary amine TCAs							
Nortriptyline[a] Desipramine[a]	25 mg at bedtime	Increase by 25 mg daily every 3–7 d, as tolerated, until pain relief	150 mg daily; if blood level of active drug and its metabolite is <100 ng/mL (mg/mL), continue titration with caution	6–8 wk with ≥2 wk at maximum tolerated dosage	Sedation, dry mouth, blurred vision, weight gain, urinary retention	Cardiac disease, glaucoma, suicide risk, seizure disorder, concomitant use of tramadol	Improvement of depression, improvement of insomnia, low cost
SSNRIs							
Duloxetine	30 mg once daily	Increase to 60 mg once daily after 1 wk	60 mg twice daily	4 wk	Nausea	Hepatic dysfunction, renal insufficiency, alcohol abuse, concomitant use of tramadol	Improvement of depression
Venlafaxine	37.5 mg once or twice daily	Increase by 75 mg each week, as tolerated until pain relief	225 mg daily	4–6 wk	Nausea	Concomitant use of tramadol, cardiac disease, withdrawal syndrome with abrupt discontinuation	Improvement of depression

Calcium channel $\alpha_{2-\delta}$ ligands

Drug	Starting dose	Titration	Maximum dose	Duration of trial	Adverse effects	Precautions	Benefits
Gabapentin[a]	100–300 mg at bedtime or 100–300 mg 3 times daily	Increase by 100–300 mg 3 times daily every 1–7 d, as tolerated, until pain relief	3600 mg daily (1200 mg 3 times daily); reduce if impaired renal function	3–8 wk for titration + 2 wk at maximum dose	Sedation, dizziness, peripheral edema	Renal insufficiency	Improvement of sleep disturbance, no clinically significant drug interactions
Pregabalin[a]	50 mg 3 times daily or 75 mg twice daily	Increase to 300 mg daily after 3–7 d, then by 150 mg/d every 3–7 d, as tolerated, until pain relief	600 mg daily (200 mg 3 times daily or 300 mg twice daily); reduce if impaired renal function	4 wk	Sedation, dizziness, peripheral edema	Renal insufficiency	Improvement of sleep disturbance, improvement of anxiety, no clinically significant drug interactions

Topical lidocaine

Drug	Starting dose	Titration	Maximum dose	Duration of trial	Adverse effects	Precautions	Benefits
5% lidocaine patch	Maximum of 3 patches daily for a maximum of 12 h	None needed	Maximum of 3 patches daily for a maximum of 12–18 h	3 wk	Local erythema, rash	None	No systemic side effects

Opioid agonists[b]

Drug	Starting dose	Titration	Maximum dose	Duration of trial	Adverse effects	Precautions	Benefits
Morphine, oxycodone, methadone, levorphanol[a]	10–15 mg morphine every 4 h or as needed (equianalgesic dosages should be used for other opioid analgesics)	After 1–2 wk, convert total daily dosage to long-acting opioid analgesic and continue short-acting medication as needed	No maximum dosage with careful titration; consider evaluation by pain specialist at relatively high dosages (eg, 120–180 mg morphine daily; equianalgesic dosages should be used for other opioid analgesics)	4–6 wk	Nausea/vomiting, constipation, drowsiness, dizziness	History of substance abuse, suicide risk, driving impairment during treatment initiation	Rapid onset of analgesic Benefit

(continued on next page)

Table 1
(continued)

Medication Class	Starting Dosage	Titration	Maximum Dosage	Duration of Adequate Trial	Major Side Effects	Precautions	Other Benefits
Tramadol[c]	50 mg once or twice daily	Increase by 50–100 mg daily in divided doses every 3–7 d, as tolerated, until pain relief	400 mg daily (100 mg 4 times daily); in patients aged >75 y, 300 mg daily	4 wk	Nausea/vomiting, constipation, drowsiness, dizziness, seizures	History of substance abuse, suicide risk, driving impairment during treatment initiation, seizure disorder, concomitant use of SSRI, SSNRI, or TCA	Rapid onset of analgesic benefit

Opioid agonists generally considered second-line drugs but can be used for first-line treatment in select clinical circumstances.

Abbreviations: SSNRI, selective serotonin and norepinephrine reuptake inhibitors; SSRI, selective serotonin reuptake inhibitor; TCA, tricyclic antidepressant (use tertiary amine TCA only if a secondary amine TCA is not available).

[a] Consider lower starting dosages and slower titration in geriatric patients.

[b] First-line only in certain circumstances; see text.

[c] Consider lower starting dosages and slower titration in geriatric patients; dosages given are for short-acting formulation.

From O'Connor AB, Dworkin RH. Treatment of neuropathic pain: an overview of recent guidelines. Am J Med 2009;122(10A):S27–8; with permission.

Baclofen is a $GABA_B$ agonist used for its antispasmodic effects through decreasing the release of excitatory neurotransmitters from afferents in the spinal cord. It does have analgesic properties as well, but at doses that result in significant motor weakness.[60]

Clonidine is another agent typically used in combination with other medications. It acts via agonism of presynaptic and postsynaptic adrenergic α2 receptors, reducing the release of presynaptic neurotransmitters. Its side effects can include sedation, hypotension, and bradycardia.[60]

The most common complications seen with IDD systems are due to catheter malfunction, such as obstruction, as is seen with catheter tip granuloma formation, or catheter fracture. Other less common complications include pump rotor stall, pump pocket fill, filling errors, concentration errors, and pump programming errors. All of these complications may result in either an underinfusion of drug precipitating withdrawal, or overinfusion leading to medication overdose. Either of these clinical scenarios can be life-threatening and one must have a knowledge of the medications used in the pump and a high index of suspicion if a patient presents with symptoms consistent with drug withdrawal or overdose.[69]

SUMMARY

The treatment of patients with chronic pain can present a significant challenge to medical providers. Medications such as NSAIDs, tricyclic antidepressants, SSRI/SNRI antidepressants, anticonvulsants, and topical agents have shown to be effective in treating chronic pain with a good safety profile. There is some evidence for the use of opiate medications in the treatment of chronic non-cancer pain. However, practitioners must be vigilant in selecting appropriate patients for this therapy due to concerns for abuse or misuse of these medications. There has been a surge of interest in the use of cannabinoids for treating chronic pain. Many placebo-controlled, randomized studies have shown efficacy in treating neuropathic pain, however cannabis remains a schedule 1 drug but some states have legalized medical marijuana. Lastly, botulinum toxin is being used to effectively treat chronic pain conditions not related to muscle dystonia, such as migraine headache, and intrathecal preparations of systemic medications can be used in order to decrease the common side effects of systemic administration and decrease the overall dose of these medications.

REFERENCES

1. Rosenblum A, Marsch L. Opioids and the treatment of chronic pain: controversies, current status, and future directions. Exp Clin Psychopharmacol 2008; 16(5):405–16.
2. Management of chronic pain syndromes: issues and interventions. Pain Med 2005;6:S1–21.
3. IASP Taxonomy - IASP. Philadelphia: Lippincott Williams & Wilkins Publishers. Available at: http://www.iasp-pain.org/Taxonomy. Accessed January 24, 2015.
4. Loeser JD, Butler SH, Chapman CR, et al. Bonica's management of pain. 3rd edition. 2001.
5. Van Tulder MW, Scholten RJ, Koes BW, et al. Nonsteroidal anti-inflammatory drugs for low back pain. Spine (Phila Pa 1976) 2000;25(1):2501–13.
6. Myers J, Wielage RC, Han B, et al. The efficacy of duloxetine, non-steroidal anti-inflammatory drugs, and opioids in osteoarthritis: a systematic literature review and meta-analysis. BMC Musculoskelet Disord 2014;15(1):76.

7. Dreiser R, Le Parc J, Velicitat P, et al. Oral meloxicam is effective in acute sciatica: two randomised, double-blind trials versus placebo or diclofenac. Inflamm Res 2001;50:17–23.

8. Rømsing J, Møiniche S, Mathiesen O, et al. Reduction of opioid-related adverse events using opioid-sparing analgesia with COX-2 inhibitors lacks documentation: a systematic review. Acta Anaesthesiol Scand 2005;49:133–42.

9. Kehlet H, Callesen T. Postoperative opioid analgesia: time for reconsideration? J Clin Anesth 1996;3180(96):441–5.

10. McDonald J, McDonald J, Lambert DG, et al. Opioid receptors. Cont Educ Anaesth Crit Care Pain 2005;5(1):22–5.

11. Kukuda K. Opioids. In: Miller's anesthesia. Philadelphia: Churchill Livingstone Elsevier; 2010. p. 769–824.

12. Centers for Disease Control and Prevention. Prescription drug abuse overdose public health perspective. 2012. Available at: http://www.cdc.gov/primarycare/materials/opoidabuse/docs/pda-phperspective-508.pdf. Accessed October 2, 2015.

13. Manchikanti L, Abdi S, Atluri S, et al. American Society of Interventional Pain Physicians (ASIPP) guidelines for responsible opioid prescribing in chronic non-cancer pain: part I–evidence assessment. Pain Physician 2012;15:S1–65. Available at: http://www.ncbi.nlm.nih.gov/pubmed/22786448.

14. O'Connor AB, Dworkin RH. Treatment of neuropathic pain: an overview of recent guidelines. Am J Med 2009;122(10 Suppl):S22–32.

15. Benyamin R, Trescot AM, Datta S, et al. Opioid complications and side effects. Pain Physician 2008;11:S105–20.

16. Daniell HW. Hypogonadism in men consuming sustained-action oral opioids. J Pain 2015;3(5):377–84.

17. Webster LR, Webster RM. Predicting aberrant behaviors in opioid-treated patients: preliminary validation of the opioid risk tool. Pain Med 2005;6(6):432–42.

18. Dworkin RH, O'Connor AB, Backonja M, et al. Pharmacologic management of neuropathic pain: evidence-based recommendations. Pain 2007;132:237–51.

19. Woolf C, Mannion RJ. Neuropathic pain: aetiology, symptoms, mechanisms, and management. Lancet 1999;353(9168):1959–64.

20. Park HJ, Moon DE. Pharmacologic management of chronic pain. Korean J Pain 2010;23:99–108.

21. Vranken J. Mechanisms and treatment of neuropathic pain. Cent Nerv Syst Agents Med Chem 2009;9(1):71–8.

22. Gillman PK. Tricyclic antidepressant pharmacology and therapeutic drug interactions updated. Br J Pharmacol 2007;151(6):737–48.

23. Pacher P, Kecskemeti V. Cardiovascular side effects of new antidepressants and antipsychotics: new drugs, old concerns? Curr Pharm Des 2004;10(20):2463–75.

24. FDA drug label. 1–31. 2010. Available at: http://www.accessdata.fda.gov/drugsatfda_docs/label/2010/022516lbl.pdf. Accessed February 24, 2015.

25. Brecht S, Courtecuisse C, Debieuvre C, et al. Efficacy and safety of duloxetine 60 mg once daily in the treatment of pain in patients with major depressive disorder and at least moderate pain of unknown etiology: a randomized controlled trial. J Clin Psychiatry 2007;68:1707–16.

26. Backonja M. Use of anticonvulsants for the treatment of neuropathic pain. Neurology 2002;59(5 Suppl 2):S14.

27. Ambrósio AF, Silva AP, Malva JO, et al. Carbamazepine inhibits L-type Ca2+ channels in cultured rat hippocampal neurons stimulated with glutamate receptor agonists. Neuropharmacology 1999;38:1349–59.

28. Chung WH, Hung SI, Chen YT. Genetic predisposition of life-threatening antiepileptic-induced skin reactions. Expert Opin Drug Saf 2010;9:15–21.

29. Blackburn SC, Oliart AD, García Rodríguez LA, et al. Antiepileptics and blood dyscrasias: a cohort study. Pharmacotherapy 1994;18:1277–83.

30. Beal B, Moeller-Bertram T, Schilling JM, et al. Gabapentin for once-daily treatment of post-herpetic neuralgia: a review. Clin Interv Aging 2012;7:249–55.

31. Bockbrader HN, Wesche D, Miller R, et al. A comparison of the pharmacokinetics and pharmacodynamics of pregabalin and gabapentin. Clin Pharmacokinet 2010;49(10):661–9.

32. Yoshizumi M, Parker RA, Eisenach JC, et al. Gabapentin inhibits γ-amino butyric acid release in the locus coeruleus but not in the spinal dorsal horn after peripheral nerve injury in rats. Anesthesiology 2012;116(6):1347–53.

33. Ifuku M, Iseki M, Hidaka I, et al. Replacement of gabapentin with pregabalin in postherpetic neuralgia therapy. Pain Med 2011;12:1112–6.

34. Finnerup NB, Otto M, McQuay HJ, et al. Algorithm for neuropathic pain treatment: an evidence based proposal. Pain 2005;118:289–305.

35. Green S, Buchbinder R, Barnsley L, et al. Non-steroidal anti-inflammatory drugs (NSAIDs) for treating lateral elbow pain in adults. Cochrane Database Syst Rev 2002;(4):CD003686.

36. Argoff CE. Topical analgesics in the management of acute and chronic pain. Mayo Clin Proc 2013;88(2):195–205.

37. Backonja M, Wallace MS, Blonsky ER, et al. NGX-4010, a high-concentration capsaicin patch, for the treatment of postherpetic neuralgia: a randomised, double-blind study. Lancet Neurol 2008;7(12):1106–12.

38. Simpson D, Brown S, Tobias J, NGX-4010 C107 Study Group. Controlled trial of high-concentration capsaicin patch for treatment of painful HIV neuropathy. Neurology 2008;70:2305–13.

39. Anand P, Bley K. Topical capsaicin for pain management: therapeutic potential and mechanisms of action of the new high-concentration capsaicin 8 patch. Br J Anaesth 2011;107(4):490–502.

40. Burstein S, Tepper M. In vitro metabolism and metabolic effects of ajulemic acid, a synthetic cannabinoid agonist. Pharmacol Res Perspect 2013;1:1–9.

41. Pacher P, Batkai S, Kunos G. The endocannabinoid system as an emerging target of pharmacotherapy. Pharmacol Rev 2006;53:389–462.

42. Pertwee R. Pharmacological actions of cannabinoids. Handb Exp Pharmacol 2005;168:1–51.

43. Pertwee RG. The diverse CB1 and CB2 receptor pharmacology of three plant cannabinoids: delta9-tetrahydrocannabinol, cannabidiol and delta9-tetrahydro-cannabivarin. Br J Pharmacol 2008;153(2):199–215.

44. Hayakawa K, Mishima K, Hazekawa M, et al. Cannabidiol potentiates pharmacological effects of Delta(9)-tetrahydrocannabinol via CB1 receptor-dependent mechanism. Brain Res 2008;1188(1):157–64.

45. Abrams DI, Jay CA, Shade SB, et al. Cannabis in painful HIV-associated sensory neuropathy: a randomized placebo-controlled trial. Neurology 2007;68(7):515–21.

46. Ellis RJ, Toperoff W, Vaida F, et al. Smoked medicinal cannabis for neuropathic pain in HIV: a randomized, crossover clinical trial. Neuropsychopharmacology 2009;34(3):672–80.

47. Wilsey B, Marcotte T, Tsodikov A, et al. A randomized, placebo-controlled, crossover trial of cannabis cigarettes in neuropathic pain. J Pain 2008;9(6): 506–21.

48. Wilsey B, Marcotte T, Deutsch R, et al. Low-dose vaporized cannabis significantly improves neuropathic pain. J Pain 2013;14(2):136–48.

49. Ware MA, Wang T, Shapiro S, et al. Smoked cannabis for chronic neuropathic pain: a randomized controlled trial. CMAJ 2010;182(14):E694–701.

50. Zajicek J, Fox P, Sanders H, et al. Cannabinoids for treatment of spasticity and other symptoms related to multiple sclerosis (CAMS study): multicentre randomised placebo-controlled trial. Lancet 2003;362(9395):1517–26.

51. Zajicek JP, Sanders HP, Wright DE, et al. Cannabinoids in multiple sclerosis (CAMS) study: safety and efficacy data for 12 months follow up. J Neurol Neurosurg Psychiatry 2005;76(12):1664–9.

52. Portenoy RK, Ganae-Motan ED, Allende S, et al. Nabiximols for opioid-treated cancer patients with poorly-controlled chronic pain: a randomized, placebo-controlled, graded-dose trial. J Pain 2012;13(5):438–49.

53. Beaulieu P. Effects of nabilone, a synthetic cannabinoid, on postoperative pain. Can J Anaesth 2006;53:769–75.

54. Buggy DJ, Toogood L, Maric S, et al. Lack of analgesic efficacy of oral delta-9-tetrahydrocannabinol in postoperative pain. Pain 2003;106(1–2):169–72.

55. Cui M, Li Z, You S, et al. Mechanisms of the antinociceptive effect of subcutaneous Botox: inhibition of peripheral and central nociceptive processing. Arch Pharmacol 2002;365:R17.

56. Kuehn B. FDA requires black box warnings on labeling for botulinum toxin products. JAMA 2009;301(22):4462.

57. Lew M. Review of the FDA-approved uses of botulinum toxins, including data suggesting efficacy in pain reduction. Clin J Pain 2002;18:S142–6.

58. Soares A, Andriolo RB, Atallah AN, et al. Botulinum toxin for myofascial pain syndromes in adults. J Pain Palliat Care Pharmacother 2012;26(7):283.

59. Singh JA. Use of botulinum toxin in musculoskeletal pain. F1000Res 2013; 2:52.

60. Wallace M, Yaksh T. Long-term spinal analgesic delivery: a review of the preclinical and clinical literature. Reg Anesth Pain Med 2000;25(2):117–57.

61. Brandwin M, Kewman D. MMPI indicators of treatment response to spinal epidural stimulation in patients with chronic pain and patients with movement disorders. Psychol Rep 1982;51:1059–64.

62. Prager J, Jacobs M, Ph D, et al. Evaluation of patients for implantable pain modalities: medical and behavioral assessment. Clin J Pain 2001;17:206–14.

63. Schocket KG, Gatchel RJ, Stowell AW, et al. A demonstration of a presurgical behavioral medicine evaluation for categorizing patients for implantable therapies: a preliminary study. Neuromodulation 2008;11(4):237–48.

64. Deer TR, Prager J, Levy R, et al. Polyanalgesic consensus conference-2012: recommendations on trialing for intrathecal (intraspinal) drug delivery: report of an interdisciplinary expert panel. Neuromodulation 2012;15:420–35.

65. Paice JA, Penn RD, Shott S. Intraspinal morphine for chronic pain: a retrospective, multicenter study. J Pain Symptom Manage 1996;11(2):71–80.

66. Ver Donck A, Vranken JH, Puylaert M, et al. Intrathecal drug administration in chronic pain syndromes. Pain Pract 2014;14(5):461–76.

67. Staats PS, Presley RW, Wallace MS, et al. Intrathecal ziconotide in the treatment of refractory pain in patients with cancer or AIDS: a randomized controlled trial. JAMA 2004;291(1):63–70.

68. Wallace MS, Charapata SG, Fisher R, et al. Intrathecal ziconotide in the treatment of chronic nonmalignant pain: a randomized, double-blind, placebo-controlled clinical trial. Neuromodulation 2006;9(2):75–86.
69. Deer TR, Levy R, Prager J, et al. Polyanalgesic consensus conference-2012: recommendations to reduce morbidity and mortality in intrathecal drug delivery in the treatment of chronic pain. Neuromodulation 2012;15:467–82.

Exploring the Use of Chronic Opioid Therapy for Chronic Pain: When, How, and for Whom?

Abigail Brooks, PharmD, BCPS[a], Courtney Kominek, PharmD, BCPS, CPE[b], Thien C. Pham, BS, PharmD[c], Jeffrey Fudin, BS, PharmD[d,e,f,g,*]

KEYWORDS

- Chronic opioid therapy • Chronic noncancer pain • Pain management
- Opioid risk management • Opioid induced respiratory depression

KEY POINTS

- Chronic opioid therapy (COT) for the treatment of chronic noncancer pain (CNCP) should be individualized based on a comprehensive evaluation and assessment.
- COT should be initiated on a trial basis; phases of the trial include initiation, titration, and maintenance.
- Prescribers of COT must ensure that appropriate monitoring (eg, urine drug tests, prescription drug monitoring programs) and follow-up is done at regular intervals.
- COT, if deemed appropriate, is just one piece of a complete treatment plan for patients with CNCP.

Conflicts of Interest: This commentary is the sole opinion of the authors and does not reflect the opinion of employers, employee affiliates, and/or pharmaceutical companies mentioned or specific drugs discussed. It was not prepared as part of official government duties for authors Brooks, Kominek, Pham, or Fudin. Dr J. Fudin is an expert legal advisor and on the speakers' bureau for Millennium Laboratories, Inc. He is on speakers' bureaus for Kaléo Pharma and Astra Zeneca. He is a consultant to Zogenix, Astra Zeneca, Millennium Health LLC, and to Practical Pain Management in the development of the online Opioid Calculator. He is founder and owner of Remitigate LLC. Dr J. Fudin's participation does not reflect the opinion of employers, employee affiliates, and/or pharmaceutical companies listed.
[a] Pain Management, Minneapolis VA Health Care System, Minneapolis, MN, USA; [b] Pain Management, Harry S. Truman Memorial Veterans' Hospital, Columbia, MO, USA; [c] Pain & Palliative Care, Stratton VA Medical Center, Albany, NY, USA; [d] Pain Management, PGY2 Pain & Palliative Care Pharmacy Residency, Stratton VA Medical Center, Albany, NY, USA; [e] Western New England University College of Pharmacy, Springfield, MA, USA; [f] Albany College of Pharmacy & Health Sciences, Albany, NY, USA; [g] University of Connecticut School of Pharmacy, Storrs, CT, USA
* Corresponding author. PO Box 214, Delmar, NY 12054-0214.
E-mail address: jeff@paindr.com

INTRODUCTION

Prescribed chronic opioid therapy (COT) has dramatically increased over the past decade with resultant startling increased mortality.[1] No doubt, a large portion of associated morbidity and mortality arise from inadequate education, lack of specialty providers, and ineffective support systems for excellent opioid pharmacotherapeutic management. Nevertheless, at the expense of legitimate patient access, media sensationalism has run amok collaterally with various political agendas[2,3] irrespective of potential harm to patients requiring opioids.[4,5]

A 2014 Agency for Healthcare Research and Quality report identified 16,917 fatal prescription opioid overdoses occurred in 2011.[6] Risks increase with higher daily opioid doses, concomitant benzodiazepine or sedative hypnotics, and in patients with mental health comorbidities. Patients receiving 100 or more morphine equivalents per day (MED) are at a 9-fold higher risk for opioid overdose. Moreover, the combination of prescription opioids and benzodiazepines is the most common cause of polysubstance overdose deaths nationwide.[7–10] Nevertheless, correlation of MED to opioid risk should be interpreted carefully because there are no universally accepted morphine equivalents.[11] Long-term efficacy data related to functional improvement on COT has come under great scrutiny with multiple review articles and position statements published in the last 12 months.[12]

INITIAL EVALUATION AND ASSESSMENT

Appropriate treatment considerations for chronic noncancer pain (CNCP) start with a comprehensive physical examination and assessment to determine which treatment modalities are most suitable.[13] Before starting any medication, it is important to obtain the patient's medical and psychiatric history and a family history, including various risk factors for substance abuse disorder, and to perform a psychosocial assessment. All of these elements are components of risk stratification that become critical in determining whether or not COT is appropriate.

Components of a comprehensive assessment are similar to those identified as the "universal precautions" in pain management related to diagnosis and treatment selection: (1) make a diagnosis with appropriate differential, (2) psychological assessment including risk of addictive disorders, and (3) periodically review pain diagnosis and comorbid conditions, including addictive disorders.[14] It is suggested to triage patients based on results and findings in the initial assessment into one of several treatment level categories: primary care patients (those with the lowest risk; no past/current history of substance abuse and absence of major mental health comorbidity), primary care patients with specialist support (moderate risk patients; may have past or remote history of substance use or significant family history but are not actively addicted), and specialty pain management (those with the highest risk; active substance abuse or addiction and/or presence of major mental health comorbidities).[14] Validated risk tools as outlined in **Tables 1** and **2** are available for assessing opioid abuse and misuse; at least one from each category should be used before initiating COT.

Pharmacologic Strategies: Opioid Trial

Before considering COT, appropriate nonopioid medications should be trialed after initial and ongoing attempts of lifestyle changes, diet and exercise, stretching, physical therapy, behavior modification, yoga, and/or other nonmedical modalities, particularly where there is supportive evidence.[15]

Opioids may be considered when a patient has moderate to severe pain that is affecting their function or quality of life, documented failure of alternative therapies,

Table 1
Comparison of risk stratification tools

Risk Tool	Indication	Question Format	Scoring	Advantages	Disadvantages
DIRE	Risk of opioid abuse and suitability of candidate for long-term opioid therapy	7 via patient interview	Numeric, simple to interpret	2 min to complete Correlates well with patient's compliance and efficacy of long-term opioids therapy	Prospective validation needed
ORT	Categorizes patients as low, medium, high risk	5	Numeric, simple to interpret	<1 min to complete Simple scoring High sensitivity and specificity for stratifying patients Validated	1 question based on patient's knowledge of family history of substance abuse
PDUQ	Assess for presence of addiction in chronic pain patients	42 items via patient interview	Numeric, simple to interpret	3 items correctly predicted addiction or no addiction in 92% of patients	20 min to administer
SOAPP-R	Primary care	24	Numeric, simple to interpret	5 min to complete Cross-validated Easy to interpret results	

Abbreviations: DIRE, Diagnosis; Intractability, Risk; Efficacy Score; ORT, opioid risk tool; PDUQ, prescription drug use questionnaire; SOAPP-R, Screener and Opioid Assessment for Patients with Pain-Revised.

Adapted from Fudin J. Opioid risk stratification tools summarized. Available at: http://paindr.com/wp-content/uploads/2012/05/Risk-stratification-tools-summarized_tables.pdf. Accessed May 5, 2015, with permission; and *Data from* Compton P, Darakjian J, Miotto K. Screening for addiction in patients with chronic pain and "problematic" substance use: evaluation of a pilot assessment tool. J Pain Symptom Manage 1998;16(6):355–63.

Table 2
Comparison of opioid misuse assessment tools

Tool	Indication	Question Format	Scoring	Advantages	Disadvantages
ABC	Ongoing assessment of patients on COT	20	≥3 indicates possible inappropriate opioid	Concise Easy to score Studied at VA	Need validation outside VA
COMM	Assess aberrant medications related behaviors in chronic pain	17	Numeric	10 min to complete Useful for adherence assessment	Unknown reliability long term
PADT	Streamline assessment of chronic pain outcomes using the 4 As	N/A	N/A	5 min to complete Documents progress Complements	Not intended to predict drug-seeking behavior or positive/ negative outcomes

Abbreviations: ABC, Addiction Behaviors Checklist; COMM, Current Opioid Misuses Measure; PADT, Pain Assessment and Documentation Tool.

Adapted from Fudin J. Opioid risk stratification tools summarized. Available at: http://paindr.com/wp-content/uploads/2012/05/Risk-stratification-tools-summarized_tables.pdf. Accessed May 5, 2015; with permission.

and when the benefits of therapy are expected to outweigh the potential risks. Implementing opioids should be considered a therapeutic trial of short-term duration to determine suitability for continued use based on assessment of risks versus benefits. When discussing an opioid trial with the patient and significant others, it is important to establish realistic therapeutic goals with the patient that will help to determine whether the trial was successful. These goals should be individualized to the patient and include components of reduction in pain, improvements in functioning and/or quality of life, and minimization of side effects or risk. Opioids should be just one piece of a patient's pain management plan.[16–18]

Informed consent and opioid treatment agreements

Before COT is initiated, it is essential to obtain informed consent, which is intended to ensure that the patient has all the necessary information to make a knowledgeable and informed decision commensurate with personal goals and preferences. Acknowledgment of benefits, risks, and alternatives to opioid therapy are essential components. Common and serious risks should be reviewed carefully with the patient and caregiver.[16,18] Throughout therapy, there should be ongoing reevaluation of patient risks and benefits of therapy to ensure COT remains appropriate.[16,18] Patients should understand the differences between addiction, tolerance, and physical dependence (**Table 3**).[19]

Multiple guidelines advocate for the use of opioid treatment agreements in patients on COT. These may be implemented before initiating opioids and continually revisited throughout therapy.[16–18] Generally, opioid treatment agreements (**Box 1**) are used to foster the exchange of information, improve adherence, and develop treatment goals.[20] Opioid treatment agreements outline the responsibilities of both the patient

Table 3
Definitions of addiction, tolerance, and physical dependence

Term	Addiction
Addiction (Association 2013)	"A problematic pattern of opioid use leading to clinically significant impairment or distress."
Tolerance (VA/DoD 2010)	"A form of neuroadaptation to the effects of chronically administered opioids, which is manifested by the need for increasing or more frequent doses of the medication to achieve the initial effects of the drug."
Physical dependence (VA/DoD 2010)	"A physiologic state in which abrupt cessation of the opioid, rapid tapering, or administration of an opioid antagonist, results in a withdrawal syndrome."

Data from American Psychiatric Association. Diagnostic and statistical manual of mental disorders. 5th edition. Washington, DC: Author; 2013; and VA/DoD. Clinical practice guidelines for management of opioid therapy for chronic pain. Available at: http://www.healthquality.va.gov/guidelines/Pain/cot/COT_312_Full-er.pdf. Accessed December 17, 2014.

and provider and the conditions for continuation or discontinuation of COT.[20] See other important practice considerations outlined in **Box 1**.

Adverse effects and risks associated with opioids

Common adverse opioid effects include constipation, nausea/vomiting, dizziness, sedation, respiratory depression, and pruritus. Tolerance often develops to these side effects in time with the exception of constipation. To mitigate opioid-induced constipation, patients are often started on prophylactic bowel regimens including a stool softener and stimulant laxative(s). More recently we have seen an introduction of

Box 1
Characteristics of an opioid treatment agreement

- Goals of therapy
- Discussion of risks and benefits
- Expectations about prescribing and taking opioids
  - Considered a trial
  - Use of one prescriber and one pharmacy
  - Avoiding abruptly stopping opioids
  - No early refills
  - No replacement of lost, stolen, or destroyed medication
  - Patients must inform providers of all medications being taken
- Avoidance of alcohol and illicit substances while on opioids
- Prohibition of sharing, selling, or providing others access to opioids
- Follow-up and monitoring parameters
  - Office visits
  - Urine drug screening[a]
  - Prescription drug monitoring programs
  - Pill counts[b]
- Reasons for continuing or discontinuing opioids
- Secure storage of medications

[a] Discussed in further detail elsewhere in this article.
[b] Pill counts are flawed because patients can borrow or rent medications from others.
Data from Refs.[16,18,20]

peripherally acting mu receptor opioid antagonists as an alternative to traditional therapies for opioid-induced constipation. Slow dose titration, opioid dose reduction, opioid rotation, extended release formulations, and symptom treatment are ways to prevent and manage opioid adverse effects.[17] To date, there are no established consensus guidelines for the treatment of opioid-induced constipation.

Despite the use of opioids with the intent to reduce pain, high-dose opioids may lead to increased pain by what some believe to be opioid-induced hyperalgesia. Recently, Eisenberg and colleagues[21] provided a comprehensive overview of opioid-induced hyperalgesia, which demonstrates limited evidence supporting opioid-induced hyperalgesia.

A major concern with opioid therapy is diminished respiration. Opioids contribute to sleep-disordered breathing. Opioid-induced respiratory depression may contribute to overdose and death. Opioid-induced respiratory depression is dose related and increased when combined with central nervous system depressants like alcohol, benzodiazepines, and/or other sedative–hypnotics such as carisoprodol.[12,16–18,22] Opioid overdose risk increases 4-fold at 50 to 100 mg (MED).[12,22]

Endocrine and immune system effects can occur with COT. By interacting with the hypothalamic–pituitary axis, opioids have been shown to decrease testosterone levels, leading to hypogonadism, sexual dysfunction, infertility, and a host of other medical anomalies associated with hypotestosteronemia.[12,16–18,22,23] Other associated morbidities include falls and fractures, neonatal abstinence syndrome, cardiovascular effects including increased risk for myocardial infarction and QT prolongation (methadone), depression, and increased motor vehicle accidents.[12,22]

Contraindications to opioids

Absolute contraindications to opioid therapy are listed in **Box 2**. Opioid allergies are often incorrectly assigned and are specifically owing to histamine release, which is the most common cause of opioid-induced pruritus, but not a true allergy. Even anaphylaxis to one opioid does not preclude use of opioids from other structural classes. **Table 4** outlines the chemistries of these various agents with relative cross-sensitivities.

Box 2
Contraindications to opioids

- Respiratory instability

- Acute psychiatric instability

- Uncontrolled suicide risk

- Active, untreated alcohol or substance use disorder

- True opioid allergy

- Concomitant medications with potential to cause life-limiting drug interactions

- Prolonged QTc ($\geq$500 ms) with methadone

- Active diversion

Data from Manchikanti L, Abdi S, Atluri S, et al. American Society of Interventional Pain Physicians (ASIPP) guidelines for responsible opioid prescribing in chronic non-cancer pain: Part 2–guidance. Pain Physician 2012;15(Suppl 3):S67–116; and VA/DoD. Clinical Practice Guidelines for Management of Opioid Therapy for Chronic Pain. Available at: http://www.healthquality.va.gov/guidelines/Pain/cot/COT_312_Full-er.pdf. Accessed August 25, 2015.

Table 4
Chemical classes of opioids

Phenanthrenes	Benzomorphans	Phenylpiperidines	Diphenylheptanes	Phenylpropyl Amines
Morphine	Pentazocine	Meperidine	Methadone	Tramadol
Buprenorphine[a]	Diphenoxylate	Alfentanil	Methadone	Tapentadol
Butorphanol[a]	Loperamide	Fentanyl	Propoxyphene	Tramadol
Codiene	Pentazocine	Meperidine		
Heroin (diacetyl-morphine)		Remifentanil		
Hydrocodone[a]		Sufentanil		
Hydromorphone[a]				
Levorphanol[a]				
Morphine				
Nalbuphine				
Naloxone[a]				
Oxycodone[a]				
Oxymorphone[a]				
Cross-sensitivity risk				
Probable	Possible	Low risk	Low risk	Low risk

[a] Agents lacking the 6-OH group of morphine, possibly decreases cross-sensitivity within the phenanthrene group.
Adapted from Fudin J. Chemical classes of opioids. Available at: http://paindr.com/wp-content/uploads/2012/05/Opioid-Chemistry-09-2011.pdf. Accessed May 5, 2015; with permission.

Codeine is contraindicated for use in pediatric patients undergoing tonsillectomy or adenoidectomy. A Black Box Warning has been issued for this indication owing to potential mortality among pediatric patients, including nursing infants. Several deaths occurred in children who were found to be ultrarapid metabolizers of the CYP2D6 enzyme, which is the enzyme that converts codeine into morphine.[24]

TREATMENT INITIATION, TITRATION, AND MAINTENANCE
Initiation

An opioid trial consists of initiation, titration, and maintenance phases.[17] The initial selection of an opioid medication and dose is patient individualized. For opioid-naïve patients, low doses should be initiated to ensure safety and tolerability. Patient preference, health status, dosing schedule, route of administration, patient's prior experience, and tolerance level (**Box 3**) should be considered.[25,26] Most guidelines prefer long-acting opioids in chronic pain for more consistent pain relief and uninterrupted sleep, adherence, and a possible lesser risk of addiction or abuse; however, this is not evidence based.[18]

Titration

The titration phase involves gradual dose increases to achieve the lowest effective dose that meets patient goals. Caution must be exercised to slowly titrate doses, because rapid escalation may lead to unintentional overdose. Opioid doses should not be adjusted until steady state has been reached, which is typically 5 half-lives (**Table 5**). During this phase, patients should be monitored closely with follow-up every 2 to 4 weeks until stable.[17]

Breakthrough Pain

Breakthrough pain is defined as a period of increased pain in patients with cancer-related pain with otherwise stable well-controlled pain; however, many have expanded the concept to include non–cancer-related pain. Different types of breakthrough pain include spontaneous, incidental, and end-of-dose failure.[27] Ultimately, the use of breakthrough pain medications should be minimized in chronic pain patients through titration of the baseline opioid dose or use of adjunctive agents.[17] A reasonable dose for breakthrough pain medication is 10% to 15% of the total daily opioid dose.[27]

Box 3
Criteria for opioid tolerance

Patients receiving opioids on a daily basis for at least 1 week of

- 60 mg oral morphine/d
- 25 µg transdermal fentanyl/h
- 30 mg oral oxycodone/d
- 8 mg oral hydromorphone/d
- 25 mg oral oxymorphone/d
- Or an equianalgesic dose of any other opioid combination

From FDA. FDA blueprint for prescriber education for extended release and long-acting opioid analgesics. Available at: http://www.fda.gov/downloads/Drugs/DrugSafety/InformationbyDrug Class/UCM277916.pdf. Accessed August 24, 2015.

Table 5
Comparison of extended-release (ER) opioid analgesics (or immediate release with $*T_{1/2} > 12$ h)

Opioid	Brand	Extended-Release Technology	FDA-Approved Abuse Deterrent Technology	Initial Dose	Opioid Tolerant Only Doses/Dosage Forms	Half-life (h)
Buprenorphine[a]	Butrans	Matrix	No	5 µg/h patch Q7days	≥5 µg/h patch	26
Fentanyl	Duragesic	Matrix	No	12 µg/h patch Q72H	≥25 µg/h patch	20–27 after removal
Hydrocodone	Hysingla ER	Film-coated	Yes	20 mg PO Q24H	Single dose ≥80 mg daily dose	7–9
	Zohydro ER	Beadtek	Yes (not yet available)	10 mg PO Q12H	Single dose ≥40 mg or ≥80 mg daily dose	8
Hydromorphone	Exalgo	OROS	Yes	8 mg PO Q24H	All tablets	10–11
Levorphanol*	—	—	—	2 mg PO Q8H	—	11–16
Methadone*	Dolophine	—	—	5 mg PO Q8H	—	8–60
Morphine	Avinza	SODAS	No	30 mg PO Q24H	90, 120 mg capsules	24
	Embeda	Pellets	Yes	30 mg PO Q24H	100/4 mg capsules	29
	Kadian	Polymer-coated pellets	No	10 mg PO Q24H	100, 130, 150, 200 mg capsules	11–13
	MS Contin	Film coated	No	15 mg PO Q12H	100, 200 mg tablets	Not listed
Oxycodone	Oxycontin	Film coated	Yes	10 mg PO Q12H	Single dose ≥40 mg or ≥80 mg daily dose	4.5
	Targiniq ER	Film coated	No	10 mg/5 mg PO Q12H	Single dose ≥40/20 mg or ≥80/40 mg daily dose	3.9–5.3
	Xartemis XR	PolyOx	No	(2) 7.5–325 mg PO Q12H	None	4.5
Oxymorphone	Opana ER	INTAC	No	5 mg PO Q12H	None	9.4–11.3
Tapentadol[b]	Nucynta ER	Film-coated	No	50 mg PO Q12H	None	5

Abbreviation: FDA, US Food and Drug Administration.
[a] Buprenorphine is a partial mu opioid agonist, kappa-opioid antagonist, delta-opioid receptor agonist, and a partial ORL-1 (nociceptin) agonist.
[b] Tapentadol is a centrally-acting synthetic analgesic with mu-opioid receptor agonist and norepinephrine reuptake inhibitor activity.
Data from Refs.[57–72]

Opioid Rotation

When patients fail to achieve analgesic and functional benefits with escalating doses of opioids, the potential cause for this must be evaluated, for example, adherence, drug–drug interactions, polymorphism, or worsening of the condition. If there is no identifiable reason, rotation to another opioid may be considered.[16–18] Opioid rotation can be defined as a therapeutic strategy that involves switching from 1 opioid to another in an effort to improve patient outcomes. Opioid rotations may be within the same opioid chemical class or between opioid chemical classes. Opioid alternatives could be considered in the cases of poor tolerability owing to side effects. Other considerations for opioid rotation include changes in patient status (consider buprenorphine transdermal once weekly), as well as availability, cost, and patient preference. Conversion tables are available but are not standardized. These tables list the doses of different opioids that presumably result in similar analgesic benefits. **Table 6** provides one example.[27]

Frequently, a 25% to 50% decrease in dose is used in opioid rotations to account for incomplete cross-tolerance.[16–18] Conversions may be completed via 2 strategies: stepwise or single step. In single-step rotations, the previous opioid is discontinued and the new opioid is initiated. When switching between large doses of opioids, the authors recommend a stepwise conversion be used. This involves reducing the initial opioid MED by 25% to 50% and converting that to an equianalgesic dose of an alternate opioid.[17]

Equianalgesic charts are subject to several flaws. Limited equianalgesic dosing data are available from the chronic pain population. Conversion tables are notoriously flawed and none consider patient specific factors like age, weight, body surface area, pharmacogenetics, drug interactions, organ dysfunction, or comorbid conditions. When using equianalgesic dosing tables or online calculators, it is often assumed the data are bidirectional when they may only be unidirectional and conservative only in one direction.[27] Given all of these concerns, equianalgesic dosing tables are only guides and patient-specific factors should be incorporated into the ultimate dose with a monitoring plan to ensure safety and efficacy.[28]

REASSESSMENT AND FOLLOW-UP

When pain regimens are reviewed for appropriateness, the popularized 4 As—analgesia, adverse effects, activities, and adherence—should be evaluated.[16,17,29] It is

Table 6 Equianalgesic opioid dosing		
Opioid	Parenteral (mg)	Oral (mg)
Buprenorphine	0.3	0.4 (SL)
Codeine	100	200
Fentanyl	0.1	N/A
Hydrocodone	N/A	30
Hydromorphone	1.5	7.5
Methadone	Multiple strategies*	N/A
Morphine	10	30
Oxycodone	10	20
Oxymorphone	1	10

Abbreviation: N/A, not applicable.

  * Methadone dosing is highly variable and conversion to/from other opioids is NOT linear.

  Data from McPherson ML. Demystifiying opioid conversion calculations: a guide for effective dosing. Bethesda (MD): American Society of Health-System Pharmacists; 2010.

prudent to follow-up with patients within 2 to 4 weeks depending on stratified risk level, concomitant therapy, and comorbid conditions. High-risk patients should be seen more frequently and include patients with a history of substance use disorder, older patients, patients with comorbid physical or psychological conditions, and those with an unstable or dysfunctional social milieu.[17,18] For patients with an increased risk of substance abuse or misuse, if they can be safely and reasonably maintained on opioids with strict compliance monitoring and have limited other therapeutic options, abuse deterrent formulations may be considered. Long-acting opioids with US Food and Drug Administration (FDA)–approved indications are listed in **Table 5**. And finally, stable lower risk patients may be seen in clinic every 3 to 6 months.[18]

MONITORING PARAMETERS

Appropriate and timely COT monitoring is vital in the management of chronic pain. Urine drug tests (UDT) generally by immunoassay (IA), prescription drug monitoring programs, behavioral assessments, and "pill counts" have been used in the monitoring of COT.[16] In the authors' experience, the latter is a futile exercise serving only to promulgate inconvenience and hardship for legitimate patients, because it is quite easy for substance abusers to borrow medications from others. Patients on methadone should have baseline electrocardiograms and be monitored closely for electrolyte abnormalities (eg, hypokalemia and hypomagnesemia) and liver function impairment.[30] Guidelines for methadone electrocardiogram monitoring are summarized in **Table 7**.[30]

Table 7 Guidelines for methadone electrocardiogram (ECG) monitoring		
Frequency	**Recommendations**	**Considerations**
Baseline	Before initiation of methadone: Risk factors for QTc interval prolongation[a] Any record of previous ECG with QTc >450 ms Past medical history of ventricular arrhythmia An ECG with a QTc <450 ms within the past 3 mo with no new risk factors is acceptable	Any patient with no known risk factors for QTc interval prolongation An ECG within the past year with QTc <450 ms with no new risk factors QTc interval prolongation
Follow-up	Pending baseline ECG results, methadone dose changes, and risk factors for QTc prolongation: Performed 2–4 wk after initiation of methadone therapy After significant dose increases in patients with risk factors for QTc interval prolongation Any prior ECG demonstrating a QTc > 450 ms Have a history of syncope	For all patients: Methadone doses titrated up to 30–40 mg/d Methadone doses titrated up to 100 mg/d New risk factors for QTc interval prolongation Signs or symptoms signifying arrhythmia

Abbreviations: ECG, electrocardiogram; QTc, corrected QT interval.
  [a] Risk factors for QTc interval prolongation: electrolyte abnormalities (eg, hypokalemia, hypomagnesemia), impaired liver function, structural heart disease (eg, congenital heart disease, history of endocarditis, congestive heart failure), genetic predisposition, QTc-prolonging drugs.
  Data from Chou R, Cruciani RA, Fiellin DA, et al. Methadone safety: a clinical practice guideline from the American Pain Society and College on Problems of Drug Dependence, in collaboration with the Heart Rhythm Society. J Pain 2014;15(4):321–37.

Urine Drug Tests

UDTs have become a standard of care tool to monitor patients for treatment adherence, detecting nonprescribed drugs, and use of illicit substances. The use of IA UDT poses several advantages in providing clinicians at the point of care with objective, noninvasive, low-cost results to assess patient adherence and possible diversion.[31] Notwithstanding, IA UDT comes with a high risk of false negatives and positives. However, IA UDT could be performed initially and as clinically indicated as part of the COT monitoring.[14,16–18,32] The typical IA UDT primarily screens for morphine, but will detect semisynthetic and synthetic opioids at high doses.[33–35] The detection time on a UDT varies based on the type of opioid, dose, frequency of use, and time of collected specimen in relation to the last dose.[32] **Table 8** provides window of detection times. Nonphenanthrene opioids such as methadone and fentanyl will not be detected on an IA UDT screen, and therefore require a specific qualitative IA test or separate definitive test by chromatography.[36] Published data indicate deficiencies in clinicians' abilities to accurately interpret UDT results, because accurate interpretation requires an understanding of IA limitations, clinical chemistry, and opioid metabolism.[31,33,35,36]

Prescription Drug Monitoring Program

State prescription drug monitoring programs are vital tools developed to assist with combatting prescription drug abuse, doctor shopping, and diversion. Unfortunately, prescribers have encountered several barriers with using these programs, which has prompted states to consider implementing legal mandates to access and use of these programs.[37–39] These can provide a powerful tool for clinicians and should be routinely used in practice.

HIGH-RISK PATIENTS AND SPECIAL POPULATIONS
High-Dose Opioids and the Morphine-Equivalent Dose

According to the American Pain Society and the International Association for the Study of Pain, chronic pain is defined as "daily or near-daily use of opioids for at least 90 days, often indefinitely" and "pain that persists beyond normal tissue healing time, which is assumed to be 3 months."[18,40] High-dose opioid therapy is defined as more than 200 mg of oral morphine or opioid equivalent per day.[17,18] In addition, a 120-mg dose threshold and greater was recommended by the Centers for Disease Control and Prevention to seek pain specialty consultation owing to the increased risk of opioid-related overdoses.[1]

Extended-Release or Long-Acting Opioids

"Improper use of any opioid can result in serious side effects including overdose and death, and this risk can be greater with ER/LA opioid analgesics."[41] The FDA recommends that extended-release/long-acting opioid analgesics should only be prescribed by clinicians who are experienced in the use of opioids for the management of pain and it is their responsibility to ensure safe and effective use of these potent drug products (see **Table 5**).[41] Clinicians should be aware that by FDA guidelines, extended-release/long-acting opioid analgesic formulations and doses are only "indicated for the management of pain severe enough to require daily, around-the-clock, long-term opioid treatment and for which alternative treatment options are inadequate," as defined in the product labeling.[41]

Table 8
Opioid metabolism and detection times

Opioid	Metabolism	PGT Impact from Phenotype for CYP450	Active Metabolites	Inactive Metabolites	Detection Time (h)
Buprenorphine TM	CYP3A4	Y	Norbuprenorphine	Buprenorphine-3-glucuronide	9–76
Buprenorphine TD	CYP3A4				—
Codeine	CYP2D6	Y	Morphine Hydrocodone	Norcodeine	48
Fentanyl TD	CYP3A4	Y	None	Norfentanyl	—
Heroin (diacetyl morphine)	Glucuronidation via UGT2B7	Y	Morphine 6-Monoacetylmorphine	Normorphine	24–72
Hydrocodone	CYP2D6	Y	Hydromorphone	Norhydrocodone	20–25
Hydromorphone	Glucuronidation via UGT2B7	N	Hydromorphone-3-glucuronide	Minor metabolites	48–96
Levorphanol	Glucuronidation via UGT2B7	N	Levorphanol-3-glucuronide	None	—
Meperidine	CYP3A4 CYP2B6 CYP2C19	Y	Normeperidine	Meperidinic acid	15–20
Methadone	CYP3A4 CYP2B6 CYP2D6 CYP2C19 CYP2C9	Y	None	2-Ethylidene-1,5-dimethyl-3,3-diphenylpyrrolidine 2-Ethyl-5-methyl-3,3-diphenylpyrroline	72
Morphine	Glucuronidation via UGT2B7	N	Hydromorphone Morphine-3-G glucuronide Morphine-6-G glucuronide	Normorphine	48–72
Oxycodone	CYP3A4 CYP2D6	Y	Noroxycodone Oxymorphone	None	48–96
Oxymorphone	Glucuronidation via UGT2B7	N	6-Hydroxy-oxymorphone	Oxymorphone-3-glucuronide	—

Abbreviations: CYP, cytochrome P450; PGT, pharmacogenetics; TD, transdermal; TM, transmucosal; UGT2B7, uridine diphosphate glucuronosyltransferase 2B7.
Data from Refs.[33–35,46,57–75]

Neuropathy

Opioids such as methadone, levorphanol, tapentadol, and tramadol may offer superiority for neuropathic pain syndromes.[42] However, when using these unique opioids in conjunction with antiretroviral therapy, methadone and tramadol may be especially problematic with respect to its CYP450 drug interactions that can result in decreased efficacy and increased toxicity.[42,43] Careful consideration for patients actively being treated for hepatitis C is in order owing to potential dangerous drug interaction risks associated with p-glycoprotein inhibitors like telaprevir or boceprevir used concomitantly with methadone or morphine.[44] For this reason, levorphanol or tapentadol may be the best options because both avoid CYP450 metabolisms and neither has proven problematic with p-glycoprotein.[45]

Pharmacogenetics in Pain Management

Genetic variability to opioid analgesics in chronic pain management can be complex and involves various genes and phenotypes.[46] Several studied genes have been identified that can alter the perception of pain, affect analgesic activity and drug metabolism, and increase risk for toxicity when polymorphisms occur. These important variations and their applicability are outlined in **Table 9**.

Discontinuation of Therapy

Whenever opioid risks outweigh benefits and functional improvement is limited, adjustments to the treatment plan must be made and may include discontinuation of

Table 9
Pharmacogenetics in pain management

Site of Activity	Genes of Interest	Function
Cytochrome P450 (CYP)	CYP2D6	Involved in the metabolism of several opioids analgesics such as codeine to morphine, oxycodone to oxymorphone, tramadol to O-desmethyltramadol, and hydrocodone to hydromorphone
P-glycoprotein (P-gp)	ABCB1/MDR1	Decreased P-gp expression and activity can affect opioid concentrations and increase patient's risk for toxicity
Catechol-O-methyltransferase (COMT) enzyme	COMT Val158Met variant	May produce an increase of dopaminergic stimulation owing to dysfunctional COMT activity, upregulating expression of MORs, resulting in increased morphine efficacy
Mu opioid receptor (MOR)	OPRM1	Codes for the expression of MOR higher binding affinity of β-endorphin to the opioid-μ receptor
Kappa opioid receptor (KOR)	melanocortin 1 receptor (MC1R)	Associated with sex-specific increased analgesic response via the KOR

Abbreviations: ABCB1, ATP-binding cassette, sub-family B, member 1; MDR1, multidrug resistance protein 1.
Data from Refs.[46,74,76,77]

Table 10
Naloxone

Route	Dose and Administration	Time to "Response"	Advantages	Disadvantages	Approved for In-home Use?
IN naloxone	Spray 1 mg in 1 mL in each nostril using atomizer device (each syringe contains 2 mg in 2 mL). May repeat dose in 3–5 min if no response. Dose may be repeated if apnea or hypopnea recurs.	Mean 4.2 ± 2.7 min; median 3 min. Range 2–13 min.	Decreases risk of bloodborne virus transmission. Decreases risk of needlestick injuries. Obviates need for needle disposal. Easy access to nares. May be preferred by people with an aversion to needles or injections.	May have lower bioavailability vs IM route. Similar or slower onset vs IM route. Similar or slightly lower responder rates vs IM naloxone. May be more likely to require supplemental doses of naloxone. Not manufactured in a formulation for this route (the injectable form is aerosolized). Nasal abnormalities and prior intranasal drug use may reduce effectiveness. Involves more steps to assemble. Inconvenience and bulkiness of carrying the product and necessary supplies.	Yes
IM naloxone	Inject 0.4 mg in 1 mL IM (using vials), through clothing if necessary. May repeat dose in 3–5 min if no response. Dose may be repeated if apnea or hypopnea recurs.	Mean 6–8 min.	Formulation manufactured for this route. Similar responder rates vs IV naloxone in prehospital settings. Fewer steps to assemble. Simpler for some people (eg, those familiar with using injections).	Risk of bloodborne virus transmission (eg, HIV, HBV, HCV). Risk of needlestick injuries. Risk of injury from improper injection technique. Proper use requires training. Requires adequate muscle mass. Inconvenience and bulkiness of carrying the product and necessary supplies.	Yes

(continued on next page)

Table 10
(continued)

Route	Dose and Administration	Time to "Response"	Advantages	Disadvantages	Approved for In-home Use?
Autoinjector naloxone	Administer 0.4 mg in 0.4 mL into the anterolateral aspect of the thigh, through clothing if necessary. May repeat doses every 2–3 min (each carton contains 2 doses).	Mean 6–8 min (IM). Mean 9.6 ± 4.6 min (subcutaneous or SC).	Pocket-size; convenient; portable. Shown to be relatively easy to use even without prior training (adults took on average about 60 s [range, 30–160]) to administer simulated injections. Retractable needle may reduce accidental needle sticks and risk of bloodborne virus transmission. The needle is not seen before, during, or after the injection; this may be a desirable feature for persons who have an aversion to the sight of needles. Discourages reuse of the device by injection drug users. The autoinjector cannot be opened by hand and modified; opening it by using a tool is difficult and renders it nonfunctional.	If the voice instructions fail, persons with poor vision may have difficulty reading the label instructions because of the small font size. Restriction to IM or SC route of administration. Needle length in children <1 y old; the skin should be pinched to prevent the needle from contacting bone. If the needle strikes bone, the needle may be broken or damaged and delivery of drug may be obstructed. Lack of field testing by OEND programs.	Yes

| IV naloxone | Within 2 min. | May be diluted for IV infusion in 0.9% sodium chloride injection or 5% dextrose injection (2 mg naloxone in 500 mL solution provides concentration of 0.004 mg/mL). Initial dose of 0.4 mg to 2 mg and may be repeated at 2–3 min intervals. If no response after administration of 10 mg of naloxone, diagnosis should be questioned. | Rate of administration can be titrated to the patient's response. More rapid onset of action compared with IM or SC routes. May be more effective in the setting of ER or LA opioid formulations. | Administered in a hospital setting. Requires IV access. Mixture should be used within 24 h. | No |

Abbreviations: ER, extended release; HBV, hepatitis B virus; HCV, hepatitis C virus; HIV, human immunodeficiency virus; IM, intramuscular; IN, intranasal; LA, long acting; OEND, Overdose Education and Naloxone Distribution; SC, subcutaneous.

Note: Naloxone administration in the home using a rescue kit does not preclude the need to activate the emergency response system (calling "911") or perform the "ABCs" (airway, breathing, circulation) of emergency response while waiting for help to arrive.

Data from Naloxone Kits and Naloxone Autoinjectors: recommendations for Issuing Naloxone Kits and Naloxone Autoinjectors for the VA Overdose Education and Naloxone Distribution (OEND) Program. Washington, DC: Veterans Affairs Pharmacy Benefits Management, Medical Advisory Panel and VISN Pharmacist Executives in collaboration with the VA OEND National Support and Development Work Group, Veterans Health Administration, Department of Veterans Affairs; 2015; and Naloxone [package insert]. Lake Forest, IL: Hospira, Inc; 2007.

opioid therapy. Patient individualized goals are established at the outset of the opioid trial, throughout therapy, and progress toward all of these goals requires close and ongoing monitoring. When patients fail to achieve the desired outcomes, opioid therapy should be discontinued. In situations where there are severe, unmanageable adverse effects, misuse or abuse of opioids, or significant nonadherence to the treatment plan, the risks of continuing opioid therapy outweigh the benefits.[17]

If opioids are being tapered owing to aberrant behaviors or safety concerns, a more rapid opioid taper schedule is indicated. For less urgent reasons, a taper can be completed over the course of weeks to months. Typically, the goal in designing a taper is to minimize the potential for opioid withdrawal and maximize the patient's comfort during the taper. The Veteran's Administration/Department of Defense (VA/DoD) Clinical Practice Guidelines for COT recommend tapering by 20% to 50% per week of the original dose for nonaddicted patients.[17] Other suggestions for opioid taper include reduction by 10% each day, reduction by 20% every 3 to 5 days, or reduction by 25% each week.[47] The VA/DoD practice guidelines indicate that 20% of the previous day's dose is required to prevent withdrawal symptoms.[17]

Opioid Reversal: Naloxone

Risks for opioid overdose exist outside of the substance abuse population, some of which include high-daily MED, age, gender, concomitant use of benzodiazepines and/or alcohol with or without other sedative–hypnotics, chronic lung disease, chronic kidney and/or liver impairment, sleep apnea, and accidental exposure to young children in the home.[48–50] Patients on lower doses of opioids (eg, 20 MED/d)[6] and even those on COT for several years remain at risk for opioid overdose as their coprescribed medications and medical status changes.

During an opioid overdose, basic life support is provided and naloxone, a mu-opioid receptor antagonist, is administered to reverse opioid-induced respiratory depression. Possible routes of administration include subcutaneous, intramuscular (traditional or by autoinjector), intravenous, or intranasally. Naloxone administration, routes of administration, advantages, and disadvantages are outlined in **Table 10**.

Use in Obstetrics, Gynecology, and Neonatology

The use of buprenorphine versus methadone during gestation, delivery, post partum, and in the neonate has historic and emerging new evidence suggesting that buprenorphine is the safer, more practical alternative for opioid-dependent mothers and neonatal abstinence syndrome treatment.[51–56] This exciting therapeutic area requires more evidence-based research, requires experienced clinical teams, and is beyond the scope of this article.

SUMMARY

COT is a viable analgesic option for the management of chronic pain in select patient populations to help improve function and overall quality of life. Clinicians should optimize nonpharmacologic and nonopioid modalities for pain management where possible before considering COT. The risks and benefits must be discussed thoroughly and documented with the patient, including a realistic understanding of expectations for functional improvement and ongoing level of pain. This is a conversation that should be revisited periodically while patients are prescribed COT and the risks versus benefits should be continuously evaluated by the treating clinician and treatment team. Universal precautions should be observed in accordance with current published clinical practice guidelines, including regular and intermittent examination with urine testing. It is crucial that clinicians stress the importance of communication, routine monitoring for efficacy and safety, appropriate and timely follow-up, and patient engagement with the treatment plan and goals while receiving COT.

REFERENCES

1. Centers for Disease Control and Prevention. CDC's issue brief: unintentional drug poisoning in the United States. 2010.
2. Fudin J. 2015. Available at: http://paindr.com/massachusetts-politics-surrounding-zohydro-reaches-biblical-proportions/. Accessed April 14, 2015.
3. Kean N. PROP Versus PROMPT: FDA Speaks Practical Pain Management 2013. 2013. Available at: http://www.practicalpainmanagement.com/treatments/pharmacological/opioids/prop-versus-prompt-fda-speaks. Accessed April 14, 2015.
4. Rich BA. Pain: a political history pain: a political history. Keith Wailoo. Baltimore Johns Hopkins University Press 2014, Hardcover 284 pages, List price: $29.95. ISBN 1-4214-1365-5 Also available as an e-book. J Pain Palliat Care Pharmacother 2015;29(1):75–8.
5. Atkinson TJ, Schatman ME, Fudin J. The Damage done by the war on opioids: the pendulum has swung too far. J Pain Res 2014;7:265–8.
6. Chou R DR, Devine B, Hansen R, et al. The effectiveness and risks of long-term opioid treatment of chronic pain. evidence report/technology assessment No. 218. (Prepared by the pacific northwest evidence-based practice center under contract no. 290-2012-00014-I.). AHRQ Publication No 14-E005-EF. Rockville, MD: Agency for Healthcare Research and Quality. September 2014. www.effectivehealthcare.ahrq.gov/reports/final.cfm.
7. Calcaterra S, Glanz J, Binswanger IA. National trends in pharmaceutical opioid related overdose deaths compared to other substance related overdose deaths: 1999-2009. Drug Alcohol Depend 2013;131(3):263–70.
8. Dunn KM, Saunders KW, Rutter CM, et al. Opioid prescriptions for chronic pain and overdose: a cohort study. Ann Intern Med 2010;152(2):85–92.
9. Kobus AM, Smith DH, Morasco BJ, et al. Correlates of higher-dose opioid medication use for low back pain in primary care. J Pain 2012;13(11):1131–8.
10. Turner BJ, Liang Y. Drug overdose in a retrospective cohort with non-cancer pain treated with opioids, antidepressants, and/or sedative-hypnotics: interactions with mental health disorders. J Gen Intern Med 2015;30(8):1081–96.
11. Rennick A, Atkinson TJ, Cimino NM, et al. Variability in Opioid Equivalence Calculations. Pain Medicine 2015, in press. Available at: http://authorservices.wiley.com/bauthor/onlineLibraryTPS.asp?DOI=10.1111/pme.12920&ArticleID=4251185. Accessed September 25, 2015.
12. Chou R, Turner JA, Devine EB, et al. The effectiveness and risks of long-term opioid therapy for chronic pain: a systematic review for a National Institutes of Health Pathways to Prevention Workshop. Ann Intern Med 2015;162(4):276–86.
13. Gatchel RJ, Peng YB, Peters ML, et al. The biopsychosocial approach to chronic pain: scientific advances and future directions. Psychol Bull 2007;133(4):581–624.
14. Gourlay DL, Heit HA, Almahrezi A. Universal precautions in pain medicine: a rational approach to the treatment of chronic pain. Pain Med 2005;6(2):107–12.
15. Cunningham NR, Kashikar-Zuck S. Nonpharmacological treatment of pain in rheumatic diseases and other musculoskeletal pain conditions. Curr Rheumatol Rep 2013;15(2):306.

16. Manchikanti L, Abdi S, Atluri S, et al. American Society of Interventional Pain Physicians (ASIPP) guidelines for responsible opioid prescribing in chronic noncancer pain: Part 2–guidance. Pain Physician 2012;15(Suppl 3):S67–116.

17. Veterans' Administration/Department of Defense. Clinical practice guidelines for management of opioid therapy for chronic pain [Internet]. 2010. Available at: www.healthquality.va.gov/guidelines/Pain/cot/COT_312_Full-er.pdf. Accessed December 17, 2014.

18. Chou R, Fanciullo GJ, Fine PG, et al. Clinical guidelines for the use of chronic opioid therapy in chronic noncancer pain. J Pain 2009;10(2):113–30.

19. American Psychiatric Association. Diagnostic and statistical manual of mental disorders. 5th edition. Washington, DC: American Psychiatric Association; 2013.

20. Cheatle MD, Savage SR. Informed consent in opioid therapy: a potential obligation and opportunity. J Pain Symptom Manage 2012;44(1):105–16.

21. Eisenberg E, Suzan E, Pud D. Opioid-induced hyperalgesia (OIH): a real clinical problem or just an experimental phenomenon? J Pain Symptom Manag 2015; 49(3):632–6.

22. Franklin GM. Opioids for chronic noncancer pain: a position paper of the American Academy of Neurology. Neurology 2014;83(14):1277–84.

23. Deyo RA, Von Korff M, Duhrkoop D. Opioids for low back pain. BMJ (Clinical research ed) 2015;350:g6380.

24. FDA. FDA news release: FDA warning on codeine use by nursing mothers, may increase chance of serious side effects in infants. 2007. Available at: http://www.fda. gov/NewsEvents/Newsroom/PressAnnouncements/2007/ucm108968. Accessed April 15, 2015.

25. Webster LR, Fine PG. Overdose deaths demand a new paradigm for opioid rotation. Pain Med 2012;13(4):571–4.

26. Webster LR, Fine PG. Review and critique of opioid rotation practices and associated risks of toxicity. Pain Med 2012;13(4):562–70.

27. McPherson ML. Demystifiying opioid conversion calculations: a guide for effective dosing. Bethesda (MD): American Society of Health-System Pharmacists; 2010.

28. Shaw K, Fudin J. Evaluation and comparison of online equianalgesic opioid dose conversion calculators. Pract Pain Manage 2013;13(7):61–6.

29. Federation of State Medical Boards (FSMB). Model policy on the use of opioid analgesics in the treatment of chronic pain [Internet]. 2013. Available at: www.fsmb.org/Media/Default/PDF/FSMB/Advocacy/pain_policy_july2013.pdf. Accessed December 17, 2014.

30. Chou R, Cruciani RA, Fiellin DA, et al. Methadone safety: a clinical practice guideline from the American Pain Society and College on Problems of Drug Dependence, in collaboration with the Heart Rhythm Society. J Pain 2014; 15(4):321–37.

31. Pesce A, West C, Egan-City K, et al. Diagnostic accuracy and interpretation of urine drug testing for pain patients: an evidence-based approach. In: Bill Acree, editor. Toxicity and drug testing. InTech; 2012. Available at: http://www.intechopen.com/ books/toxicity-and-drug-testing/urine-drug-testing-in-pain-patients.

32. Peppin JF, Passik SD, Couto JE, et al. Recommendations for urine drug monitoring as a component of opioid therapy in the treatment of chronic pain. Pain Med 2012;13(7):886–96.

33. Gourlay D, Heit HA. The art and science of urine drug testing. Clin J Pain 2010; 26(4):358.

34. Moeller KE, Lee KC, Kissack JC. Urine drug screening: practical guide for clinicians. Mayo Clin Proc 2008;83(1):66–76.
35. Hammett-Stabler C, Webster L. A clinical guide to urine drug testing: augmenting pain management and Enhancing patient care. University of Medicine and Dentistry of New Jersey - Center for Continuing and Outreach Education; 2008.
36. Reisfield GM, Salazar E, Bertholf RL. Rational use and interpretation of urine drug testing in chronic opioid therapy. Ann Clin Lab Sci 2007;37(4):301–14.
37. Haffajee RL, Jena AB, Weiner SG. Mandatory use of prescription drug monitoring programs. JAMA 2015;313(9):891–2.
38. Rutkow L, Turner L, Lucas E, et al. Most primary care physicians are aware of prescription drug monitoring programs, but many find the data difficult to access. Health Aff (Project Hope) 2015;34(3):484–92.
39. Laws NAfMSD. States that require prescribers and/or dispensers to access PMP database in certain circumstances. Available at: www.namsdl.org/library/2155A1A5-BAEF-E751-709EAA09D57E8FDD/. Accessed April 4, 2015.
40. Classification of chronic pain. Descriptions of chronic pain syndromes and definitions of pain terms. Prepared by the International Association for the Study of Pain, Subcommittee on Taxonomy. Pain Suppl 1986;3:S1–226.
41. US Food and Drug Administration (FDA). FDA blueprint for prescriber education for extended release and long-acting opioid analgesics. Atlanta (GA): FDA; 2014.
42. Zorn KE, Fudin J. Treatment of neuropathic pain: the role of unique opioid agents. Pract Pain Manage 2011;11(4):26–33.
43. Crana S, Fudin J. Drug interactions among HIV patients receiving concurrent antiretroviral and pain therapy. Pract Pain Manage 2011;11(8):20–4.
44. Fudin J, Fontenelle DV, Fudin HR, et al. Potential P-glycoprotein pharmacokinetic interaction of telaprevir with morphine or methadone. J Pain Palliat Care Pharmacother 2013;27(3):261–7.
45. Pham TC, Fudin J, Raffa RB. Is levorphanol a better option than methadone? Pain Med 2015;16(9):1673–9.
46. Kapur BM, Lala PK, Shaw JL. Pharmacogenetics of chronic pain management. Clin Biochem 2014;47(13–14):1169–87.
47. Kral LA. Safely discontinuing opioid analgesics. Pain Treatment Topics 2006.
48. Evzio [package insert]. Richmond, VA: Kaleo, Inc; 2014.
49. Opioid Overdose Risk Assessment Checklist. Kaleo, Inc. 2014. Available at: www.evzio.com/pdfs/Evzio-Opioid-Overdose-Risk-Assessment-Checklist.pdf. Accessed April 14, 2015.
50. Substance Abuse and Mental Health Services Administration. SAMHSA opioid overdose prevention toolkit. Rockville (MD): Substance Abuse and Mental Health Services Administration; 2014. p. 2014. HHS Publication No. (SMA) 14-4742.
51. Kraft WK, Dysart K, Greenspan JS, et al. Revised dose schema of sublingual buprenorphine in the treatment of the neonatal opioid abstinence syndrome. Addiction (Abingdon, England) 2011;106(3):574–80.
52. Kraft WK, Gibson E, Dysart K, et al. Sublingual buprenorphine for treatment of neonatal abstinence syndrome: a randomized trial. Pediatrics 2008;122(3):e601–7.
53. Hoflich AS, Langer M, Jagsch R, et al. Peripartum pain management in opioid dependent women. Eur J Pain 2012;16(4):574–84.
54. Meyer M, Paranya G, Keefer Norris A, et al. Intrapartum and postpartum analgesia for women maintained on buprenorphine during pregnancy. Eur J Pain 2010;14(9):939–43.

55. Meyer MC, Johnston AM, Crocker AM, et al. Methadone and buprenorphine for opioid dependence during pregnancy: a retrospective cohort study. J Addict Med 2015;9(2):81–6.
56. Jones HE, Heil SH, Baewert A, et al. Buprenorphine treatment of opioid-dependent pregnant women: a comprehensive review. Addiction 2012;107(Suppl 1):5–27.
57. MS Contin (morphine sulfate) [prescribing information]. Stamford, CT: Purdue Pharma; 2014.
58. Kadian (morphine sulfate) [prescribing information]. Parsippany, NJ: Actavis Pharma Inc; 2014.
59. Avinza (morphine sulfate) [prescribing information]. Gainesville, GA: Alkermes Gainesville; 2014.
60. Embeda (morphine/naltrexone) [prescribing information]. New York: Pfizer; 2014.
61. Hysingla ER (hydrocodone bitartrate) [prescribing information]. Stamford, CT: Purdue Pharma L.P; 2014.
62. Zohydro ER (hydrocodone) [prescribing information]. San Diego, CA: Zogenix Inc; 2015.
63. Exalgo (hydroxymorphone) [prescribing information]. Hazelwood, MO: Mallinckrodt Brand Pharma; 2014.
64. OxyContin (oxycodone) [prescribing information]. Stamford, CT: Purdue Pharma; 2014.
65. Targiniq ER (oxycodone and naloxone) [prescribing information]. Stamford, CT: Purdue Pharma; 2014.
66. Xartemis XR (oxycodone/acetaminophen) [prescribing information]. Hazelwood, MO: Mallinckrodt Brand Pharmaceuticals, Inc; 2015.
67. Opana ER (oxymorphone) [prescribing information]. Chadds Ford, PA: Endo Pharmaceuticals Inc; 2014.
68. Duragesic (fentanyl transdermal system) [prescribing information]. Titusville, NJ: Janssen; 2014.
69. Butrans (buprenorphine) [prescribing information]. Stamford, CT: Purdue Pharma; 2014.
70. Nucynta ER (tapentadol) [prescribing information]. Titusville, NJ: Janssen Pharmaceuticals; 2014.
71. Dolophine (methadone hydrochloride) [package insert]. Roxane Laboratories, Inc. Columbus, OH; 2014.
72. Levorphanol tartrate [package insert]. Roxane Laboratories, Inc. Columbus, OH; 2011.
73. Kronstrand R, Nystrom I, Andersson M, et al. Urinary detection times and metabolite/parent compound ratios after a single dose of buprenorphine. J Anal Toxicol 2008;32(8):586–93.
74. Smith HS. Opioid metabolism. Mayo Clin Proc 2009;84(7):613–24.
75. Christo PJ, Manchikanti L, Ruan X, et al. Urine drug testing in chronic pain. Pain Physician 2011;14(2):123–43.
76. Janicki PK. Pharmacogenomics of pain management. Comprehensive treatment of chronic pain by medical, interventional, and integrative approaches. New York: American Academy of Pain Medicine; 2013.
77. Nielsen LM, Olesen AE, Branford R, et al. Association between human pain-related genotypes and variability in opioid analgesia: an updated review. Pain Pract 2015;15(6):580–94.

The Role of Invasive Pain Management Modalities in the Treatment of Chronic Pain

Heather Smith, BA[a], Youngwon Youn, BA[a], Ryan C. Guay, DO, MBA[b], Andras Laufer, MD[b], Julie G. Pilitsis, MD, PhD[a],*

KEYWORDS

- Chronic pain • Neuropathic pain • Interventional pain management

KEY POINTS

- Because of the easy, safe, and cost-effective nature of spinal epidural steroid injections, this therapy is an appropriate starting point for certain patients.
- Spinal nerve root blocks can be both diagnostic in localization of pain sources and therapeutic for chronic pain.
- Radiofrequency ablation is backed by moderate evidence for the treatment of chronic neck and back pain, and offers an effective alternative for patients who do not qualify for surgery, such as elderly patients.
- Intrathecal drug delivery and stimulation therapies provide alternatives to pain management for selected chronic pain patients.
- Patients should undergo thorough multidisciplinary evaluation and screening before being considered for invasive pain management treatments.

INTRODUCTION

Low back pain (LBP) is estimated to affect 37% of the general adult population, with a 60% to 80% lifetime prevalence.[1] In the United States alone, the annual cost of LBP management is estimated to be between $12.2 billion and $90.6 billion.[1] Medical management is unable to relieve many people of their chronic pain and in the last few decades the use of invasive procedural therapies has increased. These invasive therapies include spinal injections, nerve root blocks (NRBs), radiofrequency ablation (RFA), neurostimulation, and intrathecal drug delivery (IDD) (**Box 1**).

The risk/benefit ratio of stopping anticoagulation must always be considered.[2] To assess risk the physician prescribing the medication should be contacted and a

[a] Department of Neurosurgery, Albany Medical Center, 47 New Scotland Avenue, MC 10, Albany, NY 12208, USA; [b] Department of Anesthesiology, Albany Medical Center, 47 New Scotland Avenue, MC 10, Albany, NY 12208, USA
* Corresponding author.
E-mail address: jpilitsis@yahoo.com

Med Clin N Am 100 (2016) 103–115
http://dx.doi.org/10.1016/j.mcna.2015.08.011   medical.theclinics.com
0025-7125/16/$ – see front matter © 2016 Elsevier Inc. All rights reserved.

> **Box 1**
> **General recommendations**
>
> *Contraindications*
>
> - Absolute contraindications include coagulopathy, and systemic or site infections.[2,3] Local malignancy and acute spinal cord compression are contraindications for epidural steroid injections (ESIs).[3]
> - Relative contraindications include allergies to injected materials, steroid psychosis, pregnancy, hyperglycemia, adrenal suppression, immunocompromised state, or congestive heart failure.[2]
> - Fluoroscopy is contraindicated with pregnancy.[3]
> - The risks and benefits of temporary discontinuation of anticoagulation therapy should be considered individually. Refer to **Table 1**.
>
> *Patient preparation*
>
> - Injection sites are adequately sterilized to avoid infection and patients are physiologically monitored.[2]
> - Sedation is often given to prevent procedure-related pain and anxiety, but is limited or short-acting to prevent systemic analgesic effects.[2]
>
> *Postprocedure care*
>
> - Patients are asked to rate their pain on a numeric rating scale of 1 to 10. Significant pain relief lasting the expected duration of the anesthetic suggests a positive response to the injection.[2]
> - Monitor for any adverse reaction to the injectants.
> - There is small risk of intradural injection during an intended epidural injection; approximately 5%, even with experienced providers.[4]
>   - Although puncturing the dura is not particularly dangerous, it can cause a spinal headache.[3] Effects can be reduced with lying flat, hydration, administering caffeine, or giving a blood patch.[5]
>
> *Complications (strategies to reduce these are discussed in **Table 2**)*
>
> - Physicians should be attentive for any adverse side effects after the procedure, including:
>   - Infections: cellulitis, epidural abscess meningitis, and sepsis.[4]
>   - Bleeding: epidural and subdural hematomas.[2]
>   - Spinal cord trauma: weakness, pain, numbness, bowel, bladder, and sexual dysfunction.
>   - Irritation and inflammation: arachnoiditis.[3]
>   - Cardiovascular: dysrhythmias, hypotension, bradycardia, vasovagal reactions, and congestive heart failure.
>   - Systemic side effects of corticosteroid therapy: suppression of pituitary-adrenal axis, hyperadrenocorticism, Cushing syndrome, osteoporosis, avascular necrosis of bone, steroid myopathy, lipomatosis, weight gain, fluid retention, and hyperglycemia.[3,4]

suitable plan, including bridging with short-acting medication, should be considered (see **Box 1**).

PROCEDURE 1: CORTICOSTEROID INJECTIONS
Facet Joint Injections

Indications
Between 15% and 45% of patients with chronic LBP experience lumbar facet joint pain.[6,7] There is moderate evidence for short-term and long-term improvement in LBP symptoms when using intra-articular injections of local anesthetics and steroids.[8]

Facet injections (FI) for LBP without radiculopathy remain debated.[4] Facet pain may be induced by palpation and may be diagnosed with a thorough history and physical.[4]

Approach
Injections can be used for both diagnostic and therapeutic purposes, and may facilitate the effectiveness of other concurrent therapies, such as physical therapy. For patients with severe limitation of function, these injections may be offered before more conservative therapies, such as physical therapy (**Box 2**).[2]

PROCEDURE 2: EPIDURAL STEROID INJECTIONS
Lumbar Epidural Injection

Indications
Epidural steroid injections (ESIs) are primarily implicated for radicular pain from a herniated disc.[4,11] ESI may also be used for patients with spinal stenosis; however, the success rates tend to be lower with a shorter duration of pain relief.[12]

Approach
There are 3 approaches for entry (caudal, interlaminar, and transforaminal), with transforaminal being most supported in the literature.[3] All three approaches use fluoroscopic guidance (**Box 3**).

Cervical Injections

Indications
Cervical ESI can be used to treat cervical radicular pain symptoms (eg, shooting pain down the arm).[2] In contrast, cervical facet joint injections are used primarily for diagnostic purposes, and only in patients who have failed conservative treatments such as nonsteroidal antiinflammatory drugs and oral corticosteroids.[2]

Approach
As per our practice, we always perform a physical examination to ensure the patient does not have signs of myelopathy and recommend an MRI before cervical injections to confirm the absence of stenosis.

Postprocedural care
One special consideration for cervical injections remains the risk for vasovagal syncope, the risk of which is much higher with cervical injections (8%) compared with lumbar ESI (1%–2%). These symptoms are self-limiting (**Box 4**).[3]

PROCEDURE 3: NERVE ROOT BLOCKS
Indications

NRBs are percutaneous injections of analgesics into a specific location. The main purpose of nerves blocks is localization of pain for diagnosis or treatment.[19]

Box 2	
Outcomes and evidence for facet joint injection	
Boswell et al,[8] 2007	Systematic review of randomized and nonrandomized trials found moderate evidence for FI for short-term and long-term pain relief
Fuchs et al,[9] 2005	Randomized, controlled, blind-observer clinical study with 60 patients with lumbar facet pain. Found improved quality of life and improved function at 3-mo and 6-mo follow-up with both glucocorticoid and control hyaluronidase injections
Civelek et al,[10] 2012	Compared FI with RFA. Found RFA to be more effective

Box 3
Outcomes and evidence for ESIs

Chou et al,[13] 2009 Depalma et al,[14] 2005 Roberts et al,[15] 2009	ESI provides short-term relief for radicular pain. The evidence for long-term relief, disability, and axial pain is more variable
Valet & Rozenberg,[4] 2007	228 patients with sciatica; ESI significantly improved Oswestry Disability Index and leg pain score after 3 wk, but not after 6 wk
Benny & Azari,[16] 2011	Review of 10 randomized trials, 4 retrospective studies, and 8 prospective studies found strong evidence for ESI for radiculopathy

Approach

NRBs are most commonly ordered by surgeons trying to assess whether an operation to relieve pressure on the nerve root will be beneficial. In cases of multilevel disease, this procedure may be used similarly to an electromyogram to isolate the nerve involved.

Postprocedural Care

As shown in **Table 1**, immediately following the procedure the patient should be instructed to be careful walking because the nerve root will remain anesthetized for hours (**Box 5**).[20]

PROCEDURE 4: SYMPATHETIC NERVE BLOCKS
Lumbar Sympathetic Block

Indications
Indicated pain syndromes that can be treated with this modality include phantom limb, complex regional pain syndromes, and peripheral neuropathies, as well as painful vascular diseases (eg, vascular insufficiency, frostbite, Buerger disease) of the lower extremities.

Approach
Local anesthetic or neurolytic agent is deposited with fluoroscopy guidance ventral to the psoas muscle along the lumbar sympathetic chain.

Reducing complications
The most common complication associated with lumbar sympatholysis is genitofemoral neuralgia.[22] Intravascular injection should be negligible if fluoroscopy is used throughout the injection (**Box 6**).[23]

Box 4
Outcomes and evidence for cervical injections

Boswell et al,[8] 2007	Systematic review examining randomized and nonrandomized trials concluded that the evidence is limited for short-term and long-term pain relief following cervical FI
Abdi et al,[17] 2007	Moderate level of evidence to support ESI for short-term neck pain relief
Carragee et al,[18] 2008	Recommend only for patients with severe radicular symptoms

Table 1
Recommended holding times for common anticoagulant medications before spinal procedures

Medication	Recommended Amount of Time to Hold Before Procedure
Aspirin and aspirin-containing medication	7 d
Nonsteroidal antiinflammatory drugs	3 d
Warfarin	6 d
Ticlopidine	14 d
Clopidogrel	10 d
Cilostazol and pentoxifylline	2 d
Dipyridamole dipyridamole/aspirin	7 d
Herbal medications containing ginger, ginkgo biloba, or feverfew	7 d
Danaparoid	5 d
Heparin	4 h
Enoxaparin, tinzaparin, dalteparin, ardeparin (BID)	12 h
Vitamin E (>400 IU)	7 d

Abbreviation: BID, twice a day.
Adapted from Pauza KJ. Education Guidelines for Interventional Spine Procedures. American Academy of Physical Medicine and Rehabilitation. Available at: http://www.aapmr.org/practice/guidelines/Documents/edguidelines.pdf. Accessed August 25, 2015.

Box 5
Outcomes and evidence for nerve blocks

Boswell et al,[8] 2007	Review of randomized and nonrandomized trials showed moderate evidence for medial nerve branch blocks for short-term and long-term pain relief
Ko et al,[21] 2015	Prospective, randomized, double-blind trial with 252 patients found concurrent injection of hyaluronidase to reduce rebound pain 2–4 wk following NRB

Box 6
Outcomes and evidence for lumbar sympathetic block

Cameron et al,[24] 1994	A prospective study on 29 patients with reflex sympathetic dystrophy following total knee replacement found 45% of patients showed complete relief after 1.8 lumbar sympathetic blocks
Meier et al,[25] 2009	A double-blinded, placebo-controlled trial of children with complex regional pain syndrome comparing lumbar sympathetic block with intravenous lidocaine. The patients who received the lumbar plexus block had a significant reduction in pain intensity compared with pretreatment scores for variables measured

STELLATE GANGLION BLOCK
Indications

Indications include complex regional pain syndromes or vascular syndromes (eg, Raynaud syndrome) of the upper extremity, and also pain syndromes of the head and neck.

Approach

Local anesthetic is deposited to infiltrate the inferior cervical ganglion, which is fused with the first thoracic sympathetic ganglion forming the larger stellate ganglion at the anterolateral surface of the C7 vertebral body. This procedure is performed from an anterior approach with blind technique or ultrasonography or with fluoroscopy localization.

Reducing Complications

Proper visualization and contrast media are used to prevent intravascular and neuroaxial injection, which could result in severe, life-threatening complications. Further potential complications include pneumothorax, potential blockade of recurrent laryngeal nerve with resulting hoarseness and dysphagia, as well as blockade of the superior cervical ganglion causing an ipsilateral Horner syndrome. The optimal method for checking needle location and then solution spread uses fluoroscopy or computed tomography (CT) (**Box 7**).[26]

CELIAC PLEXUS BLOCK
Indications

The areas of blockade include the visceral organs from the stomach to mid–transverse colon, including the gallbladder and pancreas. Many case reports and randomized controlled trials have proved the effectiveness of neurolytic celiac plexus blockade on pancreas-associated cancer pain.[29,30]

Approach

CT-guided needles are placed on both sides of the L1 vertebral body and radioopaque contrast is injected to ensure precise anatomic location of the needles without intravascular or epidural spread. Once a proper position has been confirmed, the neurolytic solution of either ethyl alcohol or phenol is given through each needle.

Reducing Complications

Complications include transient or permanent spinal cord damage from neurolytic injectate spread to nerve roots, epidural space, or intrathecal space, or vascular

Box 7	
Outcomes and evidence for stellate ganglion block	
Yucel et al,[27] 2009	A prospective study on patients with CRPS type 1 of the upper extremity suggests a significant decrease in visual analog scores and an increase in wrist range of motion 2 wk after stellate ganglion block
Toshniwal et al,[28] 2012	A randomized, controlled trial of 33 patients found significant improvement in neuropathic pain scale scores, edema scores, and range of motion of the upper extremity for both the continuous stellate ganglion block and continuous infraclavicular brachial plexus blocks

Box 8	
Outcomes and evidence for celiac plexus block	
Lieberman & Waldman,[34] 1990	A prospective study using a modified transaortic approach with alcohol for neurolysis of abdominal malignancy pain was used on 124 patients showing 91% of patients reporting marked pain relief
Eisenberg et al,[35] 1995	A meta-analysis of 21 studies suggests that the celiac plexus block can provide long-lasting pain relief for 70%–90% of patients with pancreatic or other intra-abdominal malignancies

damage to the artery of Adamkiewicz.[31,32] CT guidance should be used to confirm exact needle placement in neurolytic procedures (**Box 8**).[33]

PROCEDURE 5: RADIOFREQUENCY ABLATION
Indications

RFA is primarily indicated for patients with axial LBP that has failed to respond to treatment, including facet blocks, which have temporary benefit.[36] Axial LBP is characterized by pain isolated to the back with worsening with standing or prolonged positions.[37]

Approach

This process is performed unilaterally at 2 levels to denervate a single joint. The more painful side is lesioned first and the patient is brought back in 2 to 3 weeks for denervation of the other side, if necessary.[36]

Postprocedural Care

Following the completion of radiofrequency neurotomy, patients are instructed to ice the surgical area and may need analgesic prescription (**Box 9**).[36]

PART II: SPINAL CORD STIMULATION, INTRATHECAL DRUG DELIVERY, AND PERIPHERAL NERVE STIMULATION
Procedure 6: Spinal Cord Stimulation

Indications
Indications for consideration of spinal cord stimulation (SCS) include failed neck or back surgery syndrome (FBSS), neuritis, and chronic regional pain syndrome (CRPS).[40,46] Patients should have regular follow-up visits during the first year to allow proper optimization of stimulation parameters and medications.[46]

Box 9	
Outcomes and evidence for RFA	
Boswell et al,[8] 2007	Systematic review determined the level of evidence for pain relief with RFA to be moderate for both short-term and long-term pain relief
Gofeld et al,[38] 2007	119 patients (68.4%) had good (>50%) or excellent (>80%) pain relief at 10-y follow-up; 174 of 209 had complete data
Park et al,[39] 2014	Compared NRB with RFA and spinal surgery in 371 patients: 74% of patients obtained good to excellent relief with surgery, compared with 71% with RFA and 64% with NRB

Box 10	
Outcomes and evidence for SCS	
North et al,[50] 1995	SCS showed a statistically significant advantage vs reoperation for FBSS
Kumar et al,[47] 2007	48% of the patients having SCS achieved the primary outcome of a ≥50% pain reduction compared with only 9% of the patients having conventional medical management

Approach

All candidates for SCS therapy are required to undergo a trial period usually from 3 to 7 days.[46] A successful trial is defined as greater than or equal to 50% pain relief and/or 50% improvement in function.[47] Alternative waveforms, such as bursting and high-frequency stimulation, should be used if the patient is not getting adequate relief with the trial.[40,48] Before ending a trial in a complex patient, radiographs should be obtained to rule out migration (**Fig. 1**). Earlier treatment with SCS had better outcomes, especially in FBSS and CRPS (**Box 10**).[5,49]

Reducing complications

For reduction of complications, refer to **Table 2**.

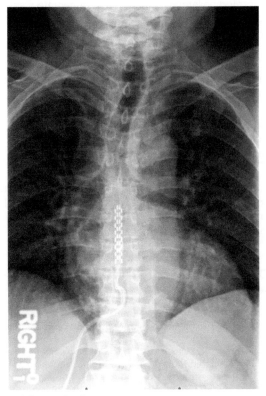

Fig. 1. Example of paddle SCS lead.

Table 2
General care for patients having SCS and IDD

Contraindications	• Anticoagulant, bleeding disorders, bacteremia, impaired mental stability or cognition, psychiatric disorders, immunosuppression, untreated medication or drug abuse/addictions[40]
Patient preparation	• Thorough neuropsychological evaluation to assess the physiologic pain syndrome as well as the patient's emotional aspect of pain[40,41] • For IDD, consider an endocrine evaluation to monitor for disorders like hypogonadotropic hypogonadism, hypocortisolism, and growth hormone deficiency.[42] • Urine analysis, and complete blood count (CBC) preoperatively. We routinely swab the nares of our patients for methicillin-susceptible strains/methicillin-resistant *Staphylococcus aureus* and treat with mupirocin appropriately. Patients should also be taken off immunosuppressants before surgery to reduce infection[40]
Postprocedure care	• Wound inspection within 7 to 14 d after surgery[40] • Occlusive dressing has been shown to increase the rates of infection when applied for more than 24–48 h.[43,44] We remove ours on the first postoperative day • Keep patients flat overnight to limit spinal headaches for IDD. Consider placing patients in a binder to promote healing until follow-up at 10–14 d postsurgery
Reducing complications	Physicians should be attentive for any adverse side effects postprocedure, including: Infections. To reduce infections: ○ Practice meticulous sterile technique such as limiting traffic in and out of the operating room, maintaining adequate ventilation during the surgical procedure, and limiting handling of hardware ○ Weight-based antibiotics (vancomycin or cefazolin) ○ Use bacitracin irrigation during surgery and place vancomycin powder in the wounds ○ Other practices that reduce the rate of infection include making smaller incisions, shaving with clippers rather than razors, and use of alcohol, Povidone-iodine, and chlorhexidine skin preparation[45] ○ For patients with diabetes, coordinate care with treating endocrinologist to alter dosage of medications as necessary Postdural puncture headache: lay flat, hydrate, administer , and/or consider epidural blood patch[5] Hardware malfunction: patients should refrain from vigorous activity as much as possible in the postoperative period to prevent lead migration

PROCEDURE 7: INTRATHECAL PUMPS (INTRATHECAL DRUG DELIVERY)
Indications

Indications for IDD include established pain diagnosis, chronic pain that lasts throughout the day, a pain source that is not easily correctable, patients who have failed to achieve pain relief with traditional pharmacologic and nonpharmacologic modalities, and patients who are intolerant of oral opioids because of severe side effects.[51] IDD is particularly helpful in cancer-related pain.

Approach

There is no standardized definition or method of measuring a successful outcome in a trial.[5,51] Trials may be a 1-time injection via lumbar puncture or can be performed with

Box 11	
Outcomes and evidence for intrathecal pumps	
Duse et al,[56] 2011	Intrathecal morphine improved psychosocial function in patients compared with the standard analgesic therapy
Atli et al,[57] 2010	Long-term intrathecal therapy not only resulted in decreased visual analog scale scores but also reduced the amount of oral opioids needed
Grider et al,[58] 2011	Analgesia was able to be achieved with microdosages (<400 μg/d) of morphine

an epidural catheter over several days. The placebo effect can be better ascertained with a multistep process through an epidural catheter. Further, this route may be able to determine dosing requirements after the IDD is initiated. In patients with cancer pain or a well-documented pain disorder and/or a patient well known to the provider, a single-dose trial may be adequate.

Approach

At present, morphine, baclofen, and ziconotide are US Food and Drug Administration (FDA) approved for IDD. Off-label medications include hydromorphone, fentanyl, sufentanil, bupivacaine, and clonidine. The efficacy of hydromorphone is currently undergoing a phase 3 FDA clinical trial.[52]

Postprocedural Care

It is recommended that IDD starts at the lowest doses and gradually increases to an appropriate level on an outpatient basis, except in the case of cancer pain, for which more aggressive therapy may be required. In addition to recommendations mentioned in **Box 10**, some risk factors that require special attention include respiratory depression and sleep apnea, which are signs of drug overdose.[53]

Reducing Complications

Additional considerations for reducing complications with intrathecal pumps include:

- Urinary retention: catheterization, urinalysis, urology consult; note that ziconotide may cause retention in 8.9% of patients.[54]
- Catheter dislodgement: a low entry site in the lumbar region is recommended to minimize dislodgment because lower entry sites allow minimal movement. The catheter should ascend a minimum of 3 levels.[5,55]
- Respiratory depression: patients at risk for respiratory depression (sleep apnea, smoking, benzodiazepines) should be monitored for adequate ventilation, oxygenation, and consciousness.[5]
- Granuloma formation: using the lowest effective does via intermittent bolus administration is recommended. In addition, as of 2012, ziconotide and fentanyl have no FDA-reported cases of granuloma formation, and thus could be appropriate alternatives (**Box 11**).[5]

SUMMARY

Pain management is a constantly evolving field. The current armamentarium includes spinal injections, nerve blocks, RFA, as well as intrathecal pumps and neuromodulation. A proper history and physical as well as review of imaging findings are essential to selecting the correct procedure.

REFERENCES

1. Schmidt CO, Raspe H, Pfingsten M, et al. Back pain in the German adult population: prevalence, severity, and sociodemographic correlates in a multiregional survey. Spine 2007;32(18):2005–11.
2. Pauza KJ. Education guidelines for interventional spine procedures. Rosemont (IL): American Academy of Physical Medicine and Rehabilitation; 2001.
3. Friedrich JM, Harrast MA. Lumbar epidural steroid injections: indications, contraindications, risks, and benefits. Curr Sports Med Rep 2010;9(1):43–9.
4. Valat JP, Rozenberg S. Local corticosteroid injections for low back pain and sciatica. Joint Bone Spine 2008;75(4):403–7.
5. Deer TR, Prager J, Levy R, et al. Polyanalgesic Consensus Conference 2012: recommendations for the management of pain by intrathecal (intraspinal) drug delivery: report of an interdisciplinary expert panel. Neuromodulation 2012; 15(5):436–64.
6. Manchikanti L, Hirsch JA, Pampati V. Chronic low back pain of facet (zygapophysial) joint origin: is there a difference based on involvement of single or multiple spinal regions? Pain Physician 2003;6(4):399–405.
7. Manchikanti L, Singh V, Pampati V, et al. Is there correlation of facet joint pain in lumbar and cervical spine? An evaluation of prevalence in combined chronic low back and neck pain. Pain Physician 2002;5(4):365–71.
8. Boswell MV, Colson JD, Sehgal N, et al. A systematic review of therapeutic facet joint interventions in chronic spinal pain. Pain Physician 2007;10(1):229–53.
9. Fuchs S, Erbe T, Fischer HL, et al. Intraarticular hyaluronic acid versus glucocorticoid injections for nonradicular pain in the lumbar spine. J Vasc Interv Radiol 2005;16(11):1493–8.
10. Civelek E, Cansever T, Kabatas S, et al. Comparison of effectiveness of facet joint injection and radiofrequency denervation in chronic low back pain. Turk Neurosurg 2012;22(2):200–6.
11. Wilkinson IM, Cohen SP. Epidural steroid injections. Curr Pain Headache Rep 2012;16(1):50–9.
12. Lee JH, An JH, Lee SH. Comparison of the effectiveness of interlaminar and bilateral transforaminal epidural steroid injections in treatment of patients with lumbosacral disc herniation and spinal stenosis. Clin J Pain 2009;25(3): 206–10.
13. Chou R, Atlas SJ, Stanos SP, et al. Nonsurgical interventional therapies for low back pain: a review of the evidence for an American Pain Society clinical practice guideline. Spine 2009;34(10):1078–93.
14. Depalma MJ, Bhargava A, Slipman CW. A critical appraisal of the evidence for selective nerve root injection in the treatment of lumbosacral radiculopathy. Arch Phys Med Rehabil 2005;86(7):1477–83.
15. Roberts ST, Willick SE, Rho ME, et al. Efficacy of lumbosacral transforaminal epidural steroid injections: a systematic review. PM R 2009;1(7):657–68.
16. Benny B, Azari P. The efficacy of lumbosacral transforaminal epidural steroid injections: a comprehensive literature review. J Back Musculoskelet Rehabil 2011;24(2):67–76.
17. Abdi S, Datta S, Trescot AM, et al. Epidural steroids in the management of chronic spinal pain: a systematic review. Pain Physician 2007;10(1):185–212.

18. Carragee EJ, Hurwitz EL, Cheng I, et al. Treatment of neck pain: injections and surgical interventions: results of the Bone and Joint Decade 2000-2010 Task Force on Neck Pain and its Associated Disorders. Spine 2008;33(4 Suppl):S153–69.
19. Hodge J. Facet, nerve root, and epidural block. Semin Ultrasound CT MR 2005; 26(2):98–102.
20. Eckel TS, Bartynski WS. Epidural steroid injections and selective nerve root blocks. Tech Vasc Interv Radiol 2009;12(1):11–21.
21. Ko SB, Vaccaro AR, Chang HJ, et al. An evaluation of the effectiveness of hyaluronidase in the selective nerve root block of radiculopathy: a double blind, controlled clinical trial. Asian Spine J 2015;9(1):83–9.
22. Dam WH. Therapeutic blockade. Acta Chir Scand Suppl 1965;343:89.
23. Walsh JA, Glynn CJ, Cousins MJ, et al. Blood flow, sympathetic activity and pain relief following lumbar sympathetic blockade or surgical sympathectomy. Anaesth Intensive Care 1984;13:18–24.
24. Cameron HU, Park YS, Krestow M, et al. Reflex sympathetic dystrophy following total knee replacement. Contemp Orthop 1994;29(4):279–81.
25. Meier PM, Zurakowski D, Berde CB, et al. Lumbar sympathetic blockade in children with complex regional pain syndromes: a double blind placebo-controlled crossover trial. Anesthesiology 2009;111(2):372–80.
26. Dondelinger RF, Kurdziel JC. Percutaneous phenol block of the upper thoracic sympathetic chain with computed tomography guidance. A new technique. Acta Radiol 1987;28:511–5.
27. Yucel I, Demiraran Y, Ozturan K, et al. Complex regional pain syndrome type 1: efficacy of stellate ganglion block. J Orthop Traumatol 2009;10(4):179–83.
28. Toshniwal G, Sunder R, Thomas R, et al. Management of complex regional pain syndrome type 1 in upper extremity – evaluation of continuous stellate ganglion block and continuous infraclavicular brachial plexus block: a pilot study. Pain Med 2012;13(1):96–106.
29. Wong GY, Schroeder DR, Carns PE, et al. Effect of neurolytic celiac plexus block on pain relief, quality of life, and survival in patients with unresectable pancreatic cancer: a randomized controlled trial. JAMA 2004;291(9):1092–9.
30. Staats PS, Hekmat H, Sauter P, et al. The effects of alcohol celiac plexus block, pain, and mood on longevity in patients with unresectable pancreatic cancer: a double-blinded, randomized, placebo-controlled study. Pain Med 2001;2(1):28–34.
31. Woodham MJ, Hanna MH. Paraplegia after coeliac plexus block. Anaesthesia 1989;44(6):487–9.
32. Davies DD. Incidence of major complications of neurolytic coeliac plexus block. J R Soc Med 1993;86(5):264–6.
33. Ischia S, Ischia A, Polati E, et al. Three posterior percutaneous celiac plexus block techniques. A prospective, randomized study in 61 patients with pancreatic cancer pain. Anesthesiology 1992;76(4):534–40.
34. Lieberman RP, Waldman SD. Celiac plexus neurolysis with modified transaortic approach. Radiology 1990;175(1):274–6.
35. Eisenberg E, Carr DB, Chalmers TC, et al. Neurolytic celiac plexus block for treatment of cancer pain: a meta-analysis. Anesth Analg 1995;80(2):290–5.
36. Calodney A. Radiofrequency denervation of the lumbar zygapophysial joints. Tech Reg Anesth Pain Manag 2004;8(1):35–40.
37. Förster M, Mahn F, Gockel U, et al. Axial low back pain: one painful area–many perceptions and mechanisms. PLoS One 2013;8(7):e68273.
38. Gofeld M, Jitendra J, Faclier G. Radiofrequency denervation of the lumbar zygapophysial joints: 10-year prospective clinical audit. Pain Physician 2007;10(2):291–300.

39. Park CK, Kim SB, Kim MK, et al. Comparison of treatment methods in lumbar spinal stenosis for geriatric patient: nerve block versus radiofrequency neurotomy versus spinal surgery. Korean J Spine 2014;11(3):97–102.

40. Deer TR, Mekhail N, Provenzano D, et al. The appropriate use of neurostimulation of the spinal cord and peripheral nervous system for the treatment of chronic pain and ischemic diseases: the Neuromodulation Appropriateness Consensus Committee. Neuromodulation 2014;17(6):515–50.

41. Campbell CM, Jamison RN, Edwards RR. Psychological screening/phenotyping as predictors for spinal cord stimulation. Curr Pain Headache Rep 2013;17(1):307.

42. Prager J, Deer T, Levy R, et al. Best practices for intrathecal drug delivery for pain. Neuromodulation 2014;17(4):354–72.

43. Hutchinson JJ, Lawrence JC. Wound infection under occlusive dressings. J Hosp Infect 1991;17(2):83–94.

44. Wilkes D. Programmable intrathecal pumps for the management of chronic pain: recommendations for improved efficiency. J Pain Res 2014;7:571–7.

45. Bakay RAE, Smith AP. Deep brain stimulation: complications and attempts at avoiding them. Open Neurosurg J 2011;4:42–52.

46. Atkinson L, Sundaraj SR, Brooker C, et al. Recommendations for patient selection in spinal cord stimulation. J Clin Neurosci 2011;18(10):1295–302.

47. Kumar K, Taylor RS, Jacques L, et al. Spinal cord stimulation versus conventional medical management for neuropathic pain: a multicentre randomised controlled trial in patients with failed back surgery syndrome. Pain 2007;132(1–2):179–88.

48. De Ridder D, Plazier M, Kamerling N, et al. Burst spinal cord stimulation for limb and back pain. World Neurosurg 2013;80(5):642–9.

49. Kumar K, Hunter G, Demeria D. Spinal cord stimulation in treatment of chronic benign pain: challenges in treatment planning and present status, a 22-year experience. Neurosurgery 2006;58(3):481–96.

50. North RB, Kidd DH, Piantadosi S. Spinal cord stimulation versus reoperation for failed back surgery syndrome: a prospective, randomized study design. Acta Neurochir Suppl 1995;64:106–8.

51. Ver Donck A, Vranken JH, Puylaert M, et al. Intrathecal drug administration in chronic pain syndromes. Pain Pract 2014;14(5):461–76.

52. Bolash R, Mekhail N. Intrathecal pain pumps: indications, patient selection, techniques, and outcomes. Neurosurg Clin North Am 2014;25(4):735–42.

53. Coffey RJ, Owens ML, Broste SK, et al. Medical practice perspective: identification and mitigation of risk factors for mortality associated with intrathecal opioids for non-cancer pain. Pain Med 2010;11(7):1001–9.

54. Rauck RL, Wallace MS, Leong MS, et al. A randomized, double-blind, placebo-controlled study of intrathecal ziconotide in adults with severe chronic pain. J Pain Symptom Manage 2006;31(5):393–406.

55. Follett KA, Burchiel K, Deer T, et al. Prevention of intrathecal drug delivery catheter-related complications. Neuromodulation 2003;6(1):32–41.

56. Duse G, Davià G, White PF. Improvement in psychosocial outcomes in chronic pain patients receiving intrathecal morphine infusions. Anesth Analg 2009;109(6):1981–6.

57. Atli A, Theodore BR, Turk DC, et al. Intrathecal opioid therapy for chronic nonmalignant pain: a retrospective cohort study with 3-year follow-up. Pain Med 2010;11(7):1010–6.

58. Grider JS, Harned ME, Etscheidt MA. Patient selection and outcomes using a low-dose intrathecal opioid trialing method for chronic nonmalignant pain. Pain Physician 2011;14(4):343–51.

Common Chronic Pain Conditions

Managing Chronic Headache Disorders

Grace Forde, MD[a],*, Robert A. Duarte, MD[b], Noah Rosen, MD[c,d]

KEYWORDS

- Headaches • Migraines • Treatment • Cluster headaches • Red flags • Primary care
- Botox • Pregnancy

KEY POINTS

- Most women who are of child-bearing age and suffer from headaches have migraines. However, these headaches usually go untreated because of a lack of knowledge on how to make the correct diagnosis.
- There are many treatment options for migraines, both specific and nonspecific. These options include pharmacologic, nonpharmacologic, and interventional. Patients who are experiencing frequent attacks or those who are experiencing disability should be placed on preventative medication.
- Patients who complain of headaches should have a complete evaluation to first rule out any "red flags."
- Most pregnant women experience a reprieve from their migraines. However, if the migraines persist, there are treatment options available.

INITIAL EVALUATION OF HEADACHES

When a clinician evaluates a patient who presents with a complaint of headache, it is imperative to first distinguish between a primary headache (for example, migraine) and a secondary headache (for example, brain tumor). Primary headaches are symptom based and, to date, have no organic or structural abnormality.[1] They are misinterpreted as benign but these headaches cause significant impairment in quality of life. Secondary headaches are etiologically based and can simply be secondary to a febrile

Disclosure Statement: Dr G. Forde is on the speaker's bureau for Allergan.
[a] North American Partners in Pain Management, Department of Pain Medicine, 900 Franklin Avenue, Valley Stream, NY 11580, USA; [b] Department of Neurology, Pain Center, Cushing Neuroscience Institute, North Shore–LIJ Health System, 611 Northern Boulevard, Great Neck, NY 11021, USA; [c] Department of Neurology, North Shore Headache Center, Cushing Neuroscience Institute, Hofstra North Shore LIJ Medical Center, 611 Northern Boulevard, Great Neck, NY 11021, USA; [d] Department of Psychiatry, North Shore Headache Center, Cushing Neuroscience Institute, Hofstra North Shore LIJ Medical Center, 611 Northern Boulevard, Great Neck, NY 11021, USA
* Corresponding author.
E-mail address: neuropain@aol.com

Med Clin N Am 100 (2016) 117–141
http://dx.doi.org/10.1016/j.mcna.2015.09.006   medical.theclinics.com
0025-7125/16/$ – see front matter © 2016 Elsevier Inc. All rights reserved.

illness. Secondary headaches account for less than 10% of headaches in the US population. Despite this low number, one must be diligent in ruling out the secondary causes before diagnosing a primary headache disorder. One approach to help the clinician make the appropriate headache diagnosis is to follow 3 easy steps. Step one[1] requires the clinician to perform a thorough history and a detailed physical examination. A history should include at least onset of headache, prior history and family history of headaches, activity at time of headache, intensity with special attention to severity at onset, location and character of head pain, interference with quality of life, any associated nausea, vomiting, photophobia, phonophobia, osmophobia, eye tearing, nasal congestion, aura symptoms such as scintillating lights, loss of vision, paresthesias, or weakness of an extremity. Response to prior treatment including all current medications and herbal remedies should be documented. An invaluable tool is the headache diary. This diary should be user-friendly and is useful at the initial visit and subsequent visits to monitor progress with the treatment plan. The physical examination will help to confirm the initial diagnostic impression gathered from the history. The key components of a physical examination for headache should begin with documenting blood pressure, heart rate, and respiratory rate. A behavioral assessment should be conducted, observing for sedation/drowsiness, agitation, and pacing. Meningeal signs should be assessed for possible meningitis. Following the mental status examination, motor, sensory, reflexes, and gait testing should be completed. A brief musculoskeletal evaluation should be performed to examine for underlying cervical or temporomandibular joint abnormality.

Step 2 involves identification of "red flags" (**Table 1**).

Martin[2,3] has provided a useful mnemonic, SNOOP4, to assist physicians in remembering the "red flags" for secondary headache disorders. The "red flags" having the most supportive data for identifying secondary headache disorders include (a) headache of sudden onset, (b) headache associated with neurologic signs and symptoms, and (c) headache onset after the age of 50.[4]

In Step 3, the clinician should determine the necessity for ancillary testing. In general, laboratory studies are not useful in making a headache diagnosis.[5] For a baseline, routine complete blood count assessing for infection or anemia should be part of an initial headache workup. Thirty[6] percent of patients with hypothyroidism complain of headache. Therefore, thyroid function test should also be included. Other laboratory testing such as antiphospholipid antibodies should be considered only in individuals with migraine with prolonged aura (>60 minutes), elevated partial thromboplastin time, history of repeated miscarriages, and venous thrombosis. Erythrocyte sedimentation rate (ESR) and C-reactive protein (CRP) should be tested in someone with new or a change in headache over the age of 50. A lumbar puncture (LP) should be done after confirmation of an magnetic resonance imaging (MRI)/computed tomographic (CT) head scan to investigate an infectious process and to measure opening pressure to rule out idiopathic intracranial hypertension (IIH), and hemorrhage.

Neuroimaging recommendations for acute headache as per the American College of Emergency Physicians[7] are as follows: patients presenting to the emergency room with headache and new abnormal neurologic sign; new onset headache; human immunodeficiency virus (HIV) patients with new type of headache; and patients greater than 50 years of age with new type of headache despite a normal neurologic examination. As per the American Academy of Neurology,[8] neuroimaging is not warranted in patients presenting with migraine headaches and a normal neurologic examination. In general, if the clinician does not feel comfortable making the diagnosis of migraine in a patient presenting with an acute headache, a referral to a headache specialist or at least a brain imaging study should be considered.

Table 1
SNOOP4 mnemonic for secondary headache disorders

Mnemonic	Clinical Presentation	Common Secondary Headache Disorder
Systemic	• Unexplained fever, chills, weight loss • New onset headache in patient with malignancy, immunosuppression, or HIV	Primary or metastatic tumors, meningitis, brain abscess, temporal arteritis
Neurologic	• Complaints of motor weakness, sensory loss, diplopia, or ataxia • Abnormal neurologic examination	Malignant, inflammatory, and vascular disorders of the brain
Onset sudden	• Headache reaches peak intensity in <1 min	Vascular events such as SAH (most common), CVA, carotid dissection, cerebral vasoconstriction syndromes, dural venous thrombosis
Onset after age 50 pattern change	• New onset headache after age 50 • Progressive headache (evolution to daily headache) • Precipitated by Valsalva • Postural aggravation • Papilledema	Neoplastic, inflammatory disorders, and temporal arteritis Malignant, inflammatory, and vascular disorders of the brain Chiari malformation, primary and metastatic lessons of brain, hydrocephalus Low pressure headache syndromes, cervicogenic headaches, intracranial hypertension, POTS Malignant and inflammatory disorders of brain, IIH, dural venous thrombosis

Abbreviations: CVA, cerebrovascular accident; POTS, postural orthostatic tachycardia syndrome.
From Martin MT. The diagnostic evaluation of secondary headache disorders. Headache 2011;51(2):347; with permission.

FOUR COMMON SECONDARY HEADACHE DISORDERS

Four common secondary headache disorders are briefly discussed:

1. Subarachnoid hemorrhage
2. Brain tumor headache
3. Idiopathic intracranial hypertension
4. Giant cell arteritiis

Subarachnoid Headache

Patients presenting with their "worst headaches in their life" should be suspected of having subarachnoid hemorrhage (SAH). Typically, these headaches occur after physical exertion but can also be spontaneous in onset. Headaches are often of maximum intensity within 1 minute of onset, or otherwise known as thunderclap headaches (TCH). Headache as the only symptom from SAH accounts for only one-third of patients.[9] Headache relief from an analgesic agent, that is, acetaminophen, ibuprofen, in a patient suspected of having SAH does not rule out the diagnosis of SAH. Other symptoms may include nausea, vomiting, neck pain, focal weakness, and visual disturbances. Patients with SAH can present with a normal neurologic examination. If, however, a patient presents with a third nerve palsy with severe headache, a ruptured aneurysm in the posterior communicating artery must be considered. Sentinel headaches can occur days or weeks preceding the SAH with the highest incidence within 24 hours of bleeding. The cause of the sentinel headache is thought to be due to a small amount of leakage surrounding the aneurysm or simply transient enlargement of the aneurysm before the bleeding. Generally, larger aneurysms (>1 cm) are more likely to bleed than smaller aneurysms. The most common cause of SAH is rupture of saccular aneurysms, but other less common causes include arterial dissections, arteriovenous malformations, vascilitides, and substance abuse.[10]

Once an SAH is in the differential, a CT head scan is of paramount importance to rule out hemorrhage. In up to 5% of patients, head imaging is unremarkable, and a LP is required. In SAH, lumbar puncture shows the presence of red blood cells and xanthochromia if done after 2 hours of onset of symptoms and may last up to 4 weeks. If CT scan of the head and LP results are negative, most authorities would consider a SAH unlikely. Other causes of severe headache include meningitis, cerebral venous sinus thrombosis, intracranial cerebral hemorrhage, and migraine. In cases where mycotic aneurysms are suspected or the symptoms persist, a cerebral angiography should be considered. A CT angiogram has become commonplace in some centers because of its noninvasiveness and its high sensitivity and specificity comparable to cerebral angiography. The headache from SAH can be severe and generally needs intervention. For obvious reasons, nonsteroidal anti-inflammatory drugs (NSAIDs) and aspirin should be avoided. A course of intravenous (IV) steroids can be beneficial in alleviating the head pain. IV morphine may also be considered, but the clinician should closely monitor for respiratory depression and level of alertness.

Brain Tumor Headaches

It has been found that headache, as an isolated symptom, is rare, occurring in only 2% of brain tumor patients. Patients with a prior history of benign headaches, that is, migraine, are more likely to suffer from headaches from a brain tumor compared with patients without a prior history.

The classical presentation of headaches from brain tumors is described as early morning headaches typically being awakened from sleep. It is postulated that a mild CO_2 retention during sleep can lead to vasodilatation and, thereby, causing an increase in intracranial pressure leading to headache.

More commonly, brain tumor headaches cause bilateral, relatively nondescript head pain. If the headache is unilateral, it is invariably on the same side of the tumor. In patients with brain metastasis, headache is the most common symptom. The most common systemic tumors causing metastasis to the brain include breast, lung, skin, kidney, and thyroid.

Differentiating brain tumor headaches from benign headaches can often be a challenge. The history of new onset headache in a patient over the age of 40, a change in headache with a prior history of benign headaches, or a progressive headache over a period of weeks or months with or without an abnormal neurologic examination should raise the possibility of a brain tumor headache.

Idiopathic Intracranial Hypertension: Pseudotumor Cerebri

The most common symptom of IIH is headache, although up to 10% of patients present without head pain.[11,12] The headache itself does not have any distinguishing qualities except that, as in all headaches due to an elevation in intracranial pressure, they can worsen on awakening and with changes in position. Patients are more often overweight women in their reproductive years. In the history-taking, use of oral contraceptives, corticosteroid withdrawal, tetracyclines, and large amounts of vitamin A should be discussed because these have been known to be common predisposing factors. In addition to headache, visual disturbances are common. If IIH is not suspected, vision loss can be a complication of untreated pseudotumor cerebri in up to 25% of patients.[13] Patients will complain of double vision because of bilateral sixth nerve palsies, visual field deficits, and transient episodes of blurred vision known as transient visual obscurations (TVOs). These TVOs are not predictive of permanent visual loss and are not unique to this disorder.[14] Up to 60% of patients with IIH will complain of pulsatile tinnitus due to an elevation in intracranial hypertension.[15] On examination, patients are often obese, and the majority will have papilledema on fundoscopy, although there have been reports of patients with IIH without papilledema. Frequent monitoring of visual field/visual acuity testing and fundoscopy examination by neurology/ophthalmology are essential.

Workup includes a CT or MRI brain scan to rule out other causes of intracranial hypertension, that is, cerebral mass, hydrocephalus, or venous sinus thrombosis. The classic MRI/CT findings are known as slitlike ventricles. However, more commonly, the imaging studies are normal. Following negative imaging studies, a LP should be performed with the patient lying in the lateral recumbent position with the lower extremities extended to detect opening pressure. In order to make the diagnosis, the opening pressure should be greater than 250 mm H_2O. In most cases, the headaches and pulsatile tinnitus from IIH are relieved quickly following the spinal tap procedure because of immediate intracranial pressure reduction. Therefore, an LP can be considered diagnostic and therapeutic. In some cases, repeat LPs can be a primary treatment modality for these patients.

Treatment for IIH

The number one agent to reduce intracranial pressure is Acetazolamide (Diamox) followed by topiramate (Topamax). The proposed mechanism is carbonic anhydrase inhibition resulting in a reduction of cerebrospinal fluid. Weight loss can be an added benefit while using topiramate in this population. Pulsed corticosteroids can be effective but long-term use should be avoided. Surgical approaches include optic nerve sheath decompression and shunting methods.

Giant Cell Ateritis (Temporal Arteritis)

Giant cell arteritis (GCA) is a medium- to large-vessel vasculitis seen primarily in patients over the age of 50, and its incidence rises dramatically with increasing age. The disease is characterized pathologically by granulomatous inflammation of medium- to large-sized arteries presenting with headache experienced by 72% of patients. However, they are only reported by 33% as the initial symptom.[16] The classic headache is described as a sensitive, scalp tenderness in the temporal region. However, the headaches can be located anywhere in the head region. The most serious complaint is blindness, which can lead to permanent, unilateral, or possibly bilateral vision loss as a result of the occlusion of the posterior ciliary arteries with anterior ischemic optic neuropathy.[17] In addition to visual acuity disturbances, they can present with diplopia or ophthalmoplegia in up to one-third of cases. Jaw claudication (pain on chewing) is considered pathognomonic for this condition. GCA, although less common, can affect the central and peripheral nervous system. Polymyalgia rheumatic, characterized by proximal extremity stiffness and achiness, with patients often describing difficulty getting up from a chair, occurs in about 20% of individuals with GCA. Conversely, about one-half of patients with polymyalgia rheumatic will go on to develop GCA.[18]

Workup

Any patient over the age of 50 with new onset headache or a change in their prior headache history should be suspected of having GCA, and measurement of ESR and CRP should be performed immediately. In one study, the ESR was elevated in most patients having a mean value of 85 mm/h.[19] A low ESR (<40 mm/h) was seen in 5% of cases.[20] To properly calculate the ESR measurement for women, the formula is (age + 10)/2 and for men is age/2.[20] An elevated CRP may also be found, and in combination with an elevated ESR, there was a positive predictive value for the diagnosis of GCA. This condition can also be associated with anemia and elevations in liver function tests. Temporal artery biopsy is the gold standard test for GCA. Because there are "skip lesions" present in up to 33% of cases, it is recommended to obtain at least 1-cm length of artery for the biopsy. Further investigations may include color Doppler ultrasonography, angiography, and PET scanning. It is advised that chest imaging or echocardiogram be done, at least every 2 years, to monitor for large vessel complications.

Treatment

Once the diagnosis is suspected, prednisone therapy should be administered. Therapy should not be withheld pending results of a temporal artery biopsy. Treatment consists of prednisone 60 mg per day, up to 80 mg per day if visual loss is occurring, for at least 4 to 6 weeks, with a gradual tapering by 10% of dose per week depending on their clinical improvement and the measurement of ESR/CRP. In addition to CBC, a metabolic profile should be followed closely. Patients should be kept on the lowest dose of prednisone, and, on average, may need to be treated for about 1 year.

MIGRAINE MANAGEMENT

The Landmark Study[21] revealed that of patients presenting to a primary care office with headache and having a normal physical examination, once a secondary headache has been ruled out, 94% of them will fulfill IHS criteria for migraine: 76% for definite migraine and about 18% for probable migraine.

EPIDEMIOLOGY

Millions of Americans suffer from headaches, the most common of which are migraines. In 2013, it was estimated that 28 million Americans (age 12 and older) suffered from migraines. The breakdown is the familiar 3:1 ratio with about 21 million women and 7 million men suffering from this disorder. Migraine is associated with a great amount of disability, and the prevalence peaks in the 25 to 55 age range, which is significant because most of these women have jobs and childcare responsibilities. Migraines are more common than asthma and diabetes combined, yet as of 2013, less than half of the patients were diagnosed (49%). One of the reasons migraines remain undiagnosed is that it is often mistaken for other types of headache disorders, such as sinus and tension headaches.

Migraine features change as girls/women go through their life cycles. They usually start around puberty and subside and even stop after women go through menopause, unless estrogen is added back into the system in the form of hormone replacement therapy or from plant-based estrogen products and soy.

Some women experience migraines for the first time during pregnancy. However, up to 60% to 70% of women with pre-existing migraines report improvement or cessation of migraines during pregnancy, especially from the second trimester on.[22] If no improvement is seen toward the end of the first trimester, then the migraines are likely to continue throughout the entire pregnancy and into the postpartum period.[22]

Migraines following delivery are not uncommon, typically occurring a couple of days postpartum. Women who breast-fed maintained the protective effect of pregnancy until menstruation returned, whereas women who bottle-fed did not achieve that same effect.[22]

Migraines are usually episodic, but can become chronic over time because of a variety of reasons, such as medication and caffeine overuse and increased body mass index.

TREATMENT

The treatment of migraines can be divided into several categories. These categories include abortive, acute, prophylaxis, interventional, and complementary. However, management of migraine triggers and lifestyle changes, particularly encouraging regular meals, regular exercise, sleep hygiene, adequate fluids, avoiding or severely limiting caffeine intake,[23] and control of stress, may help reduce the frequency of attacks without the need for medication.

Patients who experience an aura with their attacks should take medications as soon as the aura starts, to abort the impending migraine. The NSAID and, in some cases, under the direction of their treating physician, a triptan can be used in this manner.

ACUTE TREATMENT

Acute treatment of migraines is designed to relieve the symptom complex of pain and the associated symptoms, such as photophobia, phonophobia, nausea, and vomiting. Ideally, these treatments should provide relief within 2 hours, without recurrence and with minimal adverse events. In 2000, the US Headache Consortium produced an evidence-based guideline for acute treatment and report summary (**Table 2**).[24] The guideline has not been updated.

Triptans are used as first-line agents before analgesics for more severely impacted patients. Nonoral administration of triptans or dihydroergotamine (DHE) is preferred for those who do not respond to oral triptans consistently or have early onset nausea and vomiting.[24]

PROPHYLAXIS

Prevention is not a cure. It is likely that migraines will recur at some point in the patient's life after having been in remission for sometimes several years.

The goal of preventative treatment is to decrease the frequency, severity, and duration of the attacks. These medications can also boost the efficacy of the treatments used acutely to treat the attacks, and there is anecdotal evidence to suggest that they increase the patient's threshold, so they are less susceptible to attacks. Patients who are experiencing 8 or more headache days a month or those who experience disability with their attacks should be on preventative medication. Despite this knowledge, a study done by Lipton and colleagues[25] showed that only about 3% to 13% of patients were receiving preventative medication, whereas more than 25% of migraine patients surveyed would qualify for such treatment.

Preventative treatment can be divided into those used to treat episodic migraines and those used to treat chronic migraines (CM). This distinction is arbitrary because most medications used to treat episodic migraines are also used to treat CM, because there are only 2 medications that are US Food and Drug Administration (FDA) approved for the treatment of CM. These medications are topiramate and onabotulinum toxin A (**Box 1**).

Table 2
Selected acute treatments for migraine reviewed in US Headache Consortium guideline evidence

Drug	Quality of Evidence[a]	Clinical Uses[b]	Types and Relative Risk of Adverse Events[c]
Simple analgesics/combination analgesics/NSAIDs			
Acetaminophen	B	Non-disabling migraine	Nonspecific/infrequent
Aspirin	A	First line: mild to moderate migraine	Gastrointestinal and bleeding/occasional
Acetaminophen, aspirin, caffeine	A	First line: mild to moderate migraine	Cardiovascular, gastrointestinal, and bleeding/occasional
Diclofenac potassium	B	First line: mild to moderate migraine	Gastrointestinal and bleeding/occasional
Flurbiprofen	B	First line: mild to moderate migraine	Gastrointestinal and bleeding/occasional
Ibuprofen	A	First line: mild to moderate migraine	Gastrointestinal and bleeding/occasional
Naproxen	B	First line: mild to moderate migraine	Gastrointestinal and bleeding/occasional
Naproxen sodium	A	First line: mild to moderate migraine	Gastrointestinal and bleeding/occasional
Ketorolac IM	B	Rescue therapy/severe migraine with contraindications to 5HT agonists	Gastrointestinal and bleeding/infrequent
5HT 1B/1D agonists			
Naratriptan	A	Migraine nonresponding to analgesics/moderate to severe migraine	Nausea, paresthesia, chest discomfort/infrequent when used early in attack
Rizatriptan	A	Migraine nonresponding to analgesics/moderate to severe migraine	Nausea, paresthesia, chest discomfort/infrequent when used early in attack
Sumatriptan	A	Migraine nonresponding to analgesics/moderate to severe migraine	Nausea, paresthesia, chest discomfort/infrequent when used early in attack
Zolmitriptan	A	Migraine nonresponding to analgesics/moderate to severe migraine	Nausea, paresthesia, chest discomfort/infrequent when used early in attack
Sumatriptan nasal spray	A	Migraine nonresponding to analgesics/moderate to severe migraine	Nausea, paresthesia, chest discomfort unpleasant taste/occasional
Sumatriptan SC	A	Moderate to severe migraine/oral nonresponders/early-onset nausea	Nausea, paresthesia, chest discomfort/frequent

(continued on next page)

Drug	Quality of Evidence[a]	Clinical Uses[b]	Types and Relative Risk of Adverse Events[c]
DHE: IV/IM/SC	B	Moderate to severe migraine/oral nonresponders/rescue/ headache recurrence/ bridge therapy for CM and MO	Nausea, paresthesia, chest discomfort/frequent
DHE nasal spray	A	Moderate to severe migraine/oral nonresponders/ headache recurrence	Nausea, paresthesia, chest discomfort, nasal congestion/occasional

Table 2
(*continued*)

Abbreviations: MO, medication overuse; SC, subcutaneous.

[a] US Headache Consortium Guideline Evidence Classification. Level A: medications with well-established efficacy; Level B: medications that are probably effective.

[b] Opinion of authors.

[c] After US Consortium Headache Guideline evidence with author opinion.

From Freitag FG, Schloemer F. Medical management of adult headache. Otolaryngol Clin North Am 2014;47:225; with permission.

Medications that are FDA approved to treat episodic migraines, that is, migraines that occur less than 15 days per month, include propranolol, timolol, divalproex sodium, and topiramate (**Table 3**). Other medications that are routinely used, such as the calcium channel blocker verapamil, the tricyclic antidepressants, the SSRIs and SNRIs, are all used off-label (**Table 4**). None of the nonpharmacologic medications (supplements) that are used to treat migraines are FDA approved.

Box 1
Drug prophylaxis of chronic migraine

Highest level evidence (≥2 randomized placebo controlled trials)

Topiramate

Onabotulinum toxin A

Lower quality evidence (1 randomized study)

Sodium valproate

Gabapentin

Tizanidine

Amitriptyline

Lowest quality evidence (open label study)

Atenolol

Memantine

Pregabalin

Zonisamide

The drugs listed have been studied specifically for prophylaxis in CM. However, drugs used for prophylaxis of episodic migraine are often used in CM, even in the absence of data supporting their use in this context.

From Schwedt TJ. Chronic migraine. BMJ 2014;348:g1416; with permission.

Table 3		
Classification of selected migraine preventive therapies (available in the United States)		
Level A: Medications with established efficacy (>2 class I trials)		
Divalproex sodium	Sodium valproate	Topiramate
Metoprolol	Propranolol	Timolol
Level B: Medications are probably effective (1 class I or 2 class II studies)		
Amitriptyline	Venlafaxine	Atenolol
Nadolol	—	—
Level C: Medications are possibly effective (1 class II study)		
Lisinopril	Candesartan	Clonidine
Guanfacine	Carbamazepine	—
Level U: Inadequate or conflicting data to support or refute medication use		
Acetazolamide	Antithrombotics (eg, Coumadin)	Fluvoxamine
Fluoxetine	Gabapentin	Verapamil
Other: Medications that are established as possibly or probably ineffective		
Lamotrigine	Clomipramine	Acebutolol
Clonazepam	Nabumetone	Oxcarbazepine
Telmisartan	Montelukast	—

From Rizzoli P. Preventive pharmacotherapy in migraine. Headache 2014;54(2):366; with permission.

Guidelines have been established by the American Headache Society.

INTERVENTIONAL TREATMENT
Onabotulinum Toxin A

Onabotulinum toxin type A (Botox) is derived from the anaerobic bacteria *Clostridium botulinum*. It has been FDA approved for the treatment of CM since October 2010. CM are defined as greater than 15 headache days a month for more than 3 months and at least 8 of these days have migraine features. These headaches should last at least 4 hours. The injections are done every 12 weeks.

Onabotulinum toxin A plays a role in regulating pain pathways by impairing release of substance P, glutamate, and calcitonin gene related peptide (CGRP). Although the exact mechanism of action of onabotulinum toxin type A in the prophylactic treatment of CM has not been fully elucidated, the current notion is that one component comprises inhibition of neuropeptide and neurotransmitter release from peripheral trigeminal sensory nerve terminals, and this consequently mitigates development of peripheral sensitization and, secondarily, central sensitization (**Fig. 1**).[26]

The most common adverse events were mild to moderate in severity. Only neck pain (8.7%) and muscular weakness (5.5%) were reported in greater than or equal to 5% of patients treated with onabotulinum toxin A. Eyelid and eyebrow ptosis are other side effects that are seen if proper technique is not observed.

PERIPHERAL NERVE STIMULATION FOR THE TREATMENT OF PRIMARY HEADACHES

Despite the advances made in the treatment of headaches over the last few decades, subsets of patients either do not achieve adequate pain relief or cannot tolerate the side effects of typical migraine medications. Electrical stimulation of peripheral nerves via an implantable pulse generator seems to be a good alternative for patients with

Table 4
Selected agents from American Academy guidelines for preventive prescription drugs including NSAIDs, histaminic agents, and nonprescription supplements and vitamins

Drug	Quality of Evidence[a]	Special Clinical Considerations[b]	Types and Relative Risk of Adverse Events[b]
α-agonists			
Clonidine	C	Also used for reducing opioid withdrawal	Fatigue, hypotension/occasional
Guanfacine	C	—	Fatigue, hypotension/occasional
ACE inhibitors			
Lisinopril	C	May be useful for preservation of renal function in patients with diabetes	Dizziness/infrequent
ACE blocking agents			
Candesartan	C	—	Dizziness/infrequent
Antidepressants			
Amitriptyline	B	Coexisting depression	Somnolence, anticholinergic, weight gain/frequent
Venlafaxine	B	Coexisting depression, anxiety, perimenopausal	Sexual dysfunction, mood disorders, especially teenagers/infrequent
Antiepileptic agents			
Carbamazepine	C	Coexisting seizure disorder, trigeminal neuralgia	Aplastic anemia, dizziness, somnolence, extreme caution in women of childbearing potential/frequent
Divalproex sodium/valproate	A	Coexisting mood disorder or seizure disorder	Weight gain, hair loss, tremor, extreme caution in women of childbearing potential/frequent
Topiramate	A	Coexisting seizure disorder	Mood changes, paresthesias, nephrolithiasis, acute glaucoma, weight loss/frequent
β-adrenergic blocking agents			
Atenolol	B	—	Bradycardia, hypotension/occasional
Metoprolol	A	—	Hypotension/infrequent

(continued on next page)

Table 4
(continued)

Drug	Quality of Evidence[a]	Special Clinical Considerations[b]	Types and Relative Risk of Adverse Events[b]
Nadolol	B	—	Hypotension, mood disorders/occasional
Nebivolol	C	—	Hypotension/infrequent
Pindolol	C	Raynaud disease	Hypotension/infrequent
Propranolol	A	Acute anxiety disorder	Hypotension, mood disorder/occasional
Timolol	A	—	Hypotension, mood disorder/occasional
5HT 1B/1D agonists			
Frovatriptan	A	Menstrually associated migraine	Nausea, paresthesia, chest discomfort/infrequent
Naratriptan	B	Menstrually associated migraine	Nausea, paresthesia, chest discomfort/infrequent
Zolmitriptan	B	Menstrually associated migraine	Nausea, paresthesia, chest discomfort/infrequent
Herbal therapies			
Feverfew	B	MIG-99 only formulation shown effective	Gastrointestinal/infrequent
Petasites	A	Petadolux only formulation studied. Processing differences between brands may increase risk of adverse events	Gastrointestinal/infrequent. Other formulations may contain derivatives that are hepatotoxic
Histaminic agents			
Cyproheptadine	C	Children, cluster headache, category B in pregnancy	Sedation, weight gain/occasional
Histamine subcutaneous	B	Cluster headache, must be compounded	Flushing, itching/infrequent
Hormones			
Estrogen (soy isoflavones, dong quai, and black cohosh)/estradiol	C	Menstrually associated migraine	Alteration of menstrual blood loss/occasional

Minerals and vitamins			
Co-Q 10	C	—	Rare
Magnesium	B	Menstrually associated migraine	Gastrointestinal/occasional, based on formulation
Riboflavin	B	—	Urine discoloration/frequent
Nonsteroidal anti-inflammatory drugs			
Flurbiprofen	C	Also menstrually associated migraine	Gastrointestinal and bleeding/occasional
Fenoprofen	B	Also menstrually associated migraine	Gastrointestinal and bleeding/occasional
Ibuprofen	B	Also menstrually associated migraine	Gastrointestinal and bleeding/occasional
Ketoprofen	B	Also menstrually associated migraine	Gastrointestinal and bleeding/occasional
Mefenamic acid	C	Also menstrually associated migraine	Gastrointestinal and bleeding/occasional
Naproxen	B	Also menstrually associated migraine	Lowest risk of cardiovascular disease complications, gastrointestinal and bleeding/occasional
Naproxen sodium	B	Also menstrually associated migraine	Lowest risk of cardiovascular disease complications, gastrointestinal and bleeding/occasional

Abbreviations: ACE, angiotensin-converting enzyme; MIG, migraine.

[a] After the Reports of the Quality Standards Subcommittee of the American Academy of Neurology and the American Headache Society. Level A: medications with well-established efficacy; Level B: medications that are probably effective; Level C: medications that are possibly effective.

[b] Opinion of authors.

From Freitag FG, Schloemer F. Medical management of adult headache. Otolaryngol Clin North Am 2014;47:225–27; with permission.

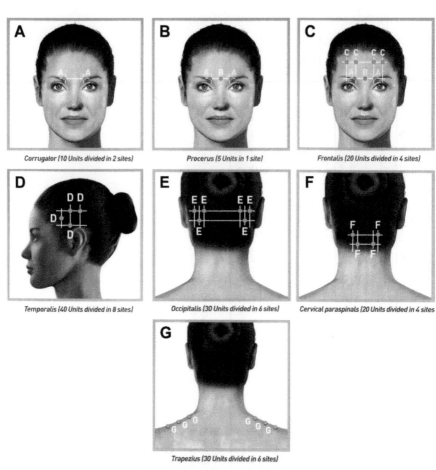

Fig. 1. Botox injection sites for migraines. (*Courtesy of* Allergan USA, Inc, Irvine, CA; with permission. BOTOX® is a registered trademark of Allergan, Inc.)

treatment-refractory headaches.[27] However, this remains an off-label use in the United States. Before the trial, patients should have tried multiple rescue and preventive medications.

The refractory migraine headache (RMH) (**Table 5**) has been defined by the International Classification of Headache Disorders, second edition (ICHD-2).[27] Such headaches should have a significant impact on the patient's function or quality of life.

A trial of rescue medicines should include either a triptan or a DHE intranasal or injectable formulation and either an NSAID or a combination of analgesics. An RMH diagnosis requires that patients fail adequate trials of preventive medicines alone or in combination, from more than 2 of 4 drug classes, including β-blockers, anticonvulsants, tricyclics, and calcium channel blockers. The definition also includes adequate dosage, duration, presence or absence of medication overuse headache (MOH), with or without significant disability, according to the Migraine Disability Assistance Score (MIDAS).

Several clinical trials show considerable evidence supporting the use of peripheral nerve stimulator (PNS) for headaches not responding to conservative therapies.

Table 5
Proposed criteria for definition of refractory migraine and refractory chronic migraine

Criteria	Definition
Primary diagnosis	A. ICHD-II migraine or CM

Refractory	B. Headaches cause significant interference with function or quality of life despite modification of triggers, lifestyle factors, and adequate trials of acute and preventive medicine with established efficacy
	1. Failed adequate trials of preventive medicines, alone or in combination. From at least 2 or 4 drug classes:
	  a. β-blockers
	  b. Anticonvulsants
	  c. Tricyclics
	  d. Calcium channel blockers
	2. Failed adequate trials of abortive medicines from the following classes, unless contraindicated:
	  a. *Both* a triptan *and* DHE intranasal or injectable formulation
	  b. *Either* NSAIDs or combination analgesics

Adequate trial	Period of time during which an appropriate dose of medicine is administered, typically at least 2 mo at optimal or maximum tolerated dose, unless terminated early due to adverse effects
Modifiers	With or without medication overuse, as defined by ICHD-2. With significant disability, as defined by MIDAS 11

Adapted from Lee P, Huh BK. Peripheral nerve stimulation for the treatment of primary headache. Curr Pain Headache Rep 2013;17:319; with permission.

However, the mechanism by which PNS improves headaches or predicts who will benefit from PNS stimulation remains uncertain.[28] The decision to use PNS should be individualized based on patient suffering and disability.

When a trial or permanent PNS implantation is considered, it is important to evaluate cost-effectiveness and psychological evaluation.

A psychological evaluation is essential and should be performed to rule out secondary gain, drug abuse, unresolved legal issues, as well as somatization or untreated depression.

Most chronic headache patients receive nerve blocks such as occipital nerve block or supraorbital nerve block before proceeding with a PNS trial.[29,30] Whether positive response to nerve blocks with short-acting local anesthetics is a predictor of successful PNS trial is debatable.

Contraindications include anatomic defect or infection at the implant site, bleeding tendency, terminal disease, need for a cardiac pacemaker, pregnant or nursing, need for future MRI imaging, and metal allergy.

Infection is a serious complication, and lead migration is the most common complication.

There are many good reviews about neurostimulation in headaches. One such article is "Pearls and pitfalls: Neurostimulation in headaches."[31]

Migraine trigger site deactivation surgery should be considered a last ditch effort in patients with severe disability from chronic refractory migraines.[32]

COMPLEMENTARY THERAPY

There is a growing body of evidence supporting the efficacy of various complementary and alternative medicine approaches in the management of headache disorder. In particular, constituents of *Petasites hybridus* (Butterbur), *Tanacetum Parthenium* (Feverfew), and Ginkgo Biloba have shown antimigraine action in clinical studies.[33]

Petasites is commonly used in migraine prevention in Europe. Although the mechanism of action is not fully understood, it likely acts through calcium channel regulation, and inhibition of peptide leukotriene biosynthesis, thus influencing the inflammatory cascade associated with migraine.[34]

Although the butterbur plant also contains pyrrolizidine alkaloids that are hepatotoxic, carcinogenic, lung toxic, and prothrombotic, these substances are removed in the commercially available preparations, such as Petadolex Petaforce, Petadolor H, Tesalin, and Tussilago.[34] Nonetheless, patients should be advised to use only petasite products that are certified and labeled "PA-free." Butterbur is considered a food in the United States and as such is not subject to FDA approval or standardization of preparation.[34] Butterbur is established as effective for migraine prevention (2 class I studies), and there is level A recommendation for its use from the recent evidence-based guidelines on treatments for episodic migraine prevention in adults.[34]

Feverfew

Traditionally, the herb has been used as an antipyretic, analgesic, and anti-inflammatory, and it was also used for allergies, nausea, and vomiting. Although the mechanism of action is unknown, feverfew (*T parthenium*) has anti-inflammatory activity mediated by inhibition of prostaglandin synthesis. It has effects on vascular smooth muscle, and it is a potent inhibitor of serotonin release from platelets to polymorphonuclear leukocyte granules. Inhibition of histamine release is another mechanism demonstrated.[33]

MANAGEMENT OF MENSTRUAL MIGRAINES

Menstrual migraines are triggered by a drop in estrogen levels during menses. Non-pharmacologic treatment should be incorporated into any treatment plan for menstrual migraine regardless of whether it is menstrually related or pure menstrual migraine. Clinical trials have been done using the triptans, DHE, and naproxen for the acute treatment of menstrual migraine. One consensus is that frovatriptan is the preferred choice in those with frequent next day recurrences after treating an acute attack in the 24 hours prior.[35]

Most patients prefer short-term preventative treatment, that is, the use of preventative medication only during the time of highest migraine risk; this reduces the side effects associated with long-term daily preventative medications. The more common agents that are used include Frovatriptan, Naratriptan, Naproxen, and magnesium. Magnesium 360 mg a day starting on day 15 was superior to placebo in a 2-month trial. In addition, the magnesium group had improvement in premenstrual symptoms.[36]

MANAGEMENT OF MIGRAINES DURING PREGNANCY AND LACTATION

Any medication given during pregnancy should only be considered if the benefit to the mother and fetus outweighs the potential risk (**Table 6**).

Acetaminophen is the analgesic of choice for the short-term relief of mild to moderate pain during pregnancy and lactation. Ibuprofen can be taken during the first and second trimester but should be avoided after 30 weeks of pregnancy because of increased risk of premature closure of the ductus arteriosus and oligohydramnios. NSAIDs can be taken during breast-feeding, and the amount of drug in breast milk is very low. Aspirin can be taken during the first and second trimesters, but use in

Table 6
Drugs used for acute treatment of migraine during pregnancy

FDA category B	
Acetaminophen	—
Diclofenac	3rd trimester: category D
Ibuprofen	3rd trimester: category D
Naproxen	3rd trimester: category D
Meperidine	Category D if prolonged use/high doses at term
Metoclopramide	—
FDA category C	
Aspirin	3rd trimester: category D
Indomethacin	3rd trimester: category D
Mefenamic acid	3rd trimester: category D
Codeine	—
Morphine	—
Tramadol	—
Prochlorperazine	—
Promethazine	—
Almotriptan	—
Eletriptan	—
Frovatriptan	—
Naratriptan	—
Rizatriptan	—
Sumatriptan	—
Zolmitriptan	—
Prednisolone	—
FDA category X	
Ergotamine	—
DHE	—

From MacGregor EA. Migraine in pregnancy and lactation. Neurol Sci 2014;35(Suppl 1):S61–4; with permission.

the third trimester is associated with premature closure of the fetal ductus arteriosus and can increase the risk of prolonged labor, postpartum hemorrhage, and neonatal bleeding. Aspirin is excreted in breast milk, and regular use during breast-feeding can increase the risk of Reye syndrome and impaired platelet function in susceptible infants (**Box 2**).

Antiemetics such as metoclopramide, prochlorperazine, and promethazine can be taken during pregnancy and lactation.

Sumatriptan may be used during pregnancy and breast-feeding if attacks fail to respond to the above treatment. Data from the sumatriptan/naratriptan/treximet pregnancy registry (http://pregnancyregistry.gsk.com/sumatriptan.html) are reassuring and confirm that inadvertent exposure to sumatriptan during pregnancy has not been associated with adverse outcomes, although a small increased risk of specific birth defects cannot be excluded. There are insufficient data regarding other triptans.

Box 2
Drugs for acute treatment of migraine during breast-feeding

Minimal risk

Acetaminophen

Diclofenac

Ibuprofen

Cyclizine

Metoclopramide

Prochlorperazine

Promethazine

Sumatriptan

Benefits likely to outweigh risks

Indometacin

Naproxen

Codeine

Morphine

Meperidine

Tramadol

Eletriptan

Caution

Aspirin

Mefenamic acid

Contraindicated

Ergotamine

DHE

Insufficient data

Almotriptan

Frovatriptan

Naratriptan

Rizatriptan

Zolmitriptan

From MacGregor EA. Migraine in pregnancy and lactation. Neurol Sci 2014;35(Suppl 1):S61–4; with permission.

PROPHYLAXIS

Nonpharmacologic preventives such as acupuncture and biofeedback are useful during pregnancy.[33] Coenzyme Q10 and magnesium supplements have the additional effect of reducing the risk of pre-eclampsia. The drugs of choice during pregnancy and lactations (**Box 3**) are propranolol or metoprolol in the lowest effective doses (**Box 4**). These drugs should be stopped 2 to 3 days before delivery to minimize the risk fetal

---

Box 3
Drugs used for prophylaxis of migraine during pregnancy

FDA category C

Amitriptyline

Citalopram

Escitalopram

Fluoxetine

Sertraline

Venlafaxine

Metoprolol

Nadolol

Propranolol

Timolol

Gabapentin

Botulinum toxin

FDA category D

Atenolol

Topiramate

Candesartan

Lisinopril

FDA category X

Valproic acid

From MacGregor EA. Migraine in pregnancy and lactation. Neurol Sci 2014;35(Suppl 1):S61–4; with permission.

---

bradycardia and decreased uterine contraction. The baby should be monitored for neonatal bradycardia, hypotension, and hypoglycemia.

EMERGENCY TREATMENT

Hydration and minimizing known triggers such as bright light and noise are paramount when patients are in the throes of an acute attack.

Prochlorperazine 10 mg or chlorpromazine 25 to 50 mg by intramuscular (IM) injection together with IV fluids is usually sufficient to abort an attack. IV magnesium sulfate 1 g given over 15 minutes is an alternative and can be given together with IV prochlorperazine.[16] Ketorolac 60 mg IM is usually given in the office with quick, effective relief. Other IV medications, such as Divalproex, Diprovan, and Levetiracetam, can be given in the emergency department or other monitored settings.

TENSION-TYPE HEADACHE

Tension-type headache is the most common form of headache experienced by people with up to 40% of men and women having experienced a tension-type headache in the last year and lifetime prevalence with a range of estimates from 30% to 78%. Despite

> **Box 4**
> **Drugs used for prophylaxis of migraine during breast-feeding**
>
> *Minimal risk*
>
> Amitriptyline
>
> Nortriptyline
>
> Propranolol
>
> Verapamil
>
> Nifedipine
>
> *Benefits likely to outweigh risks*
>
> Metoprolol
>
> Escitalopram
>
> Paroxetine
>
> Sertraline
>
> Venlafaxine
>
> Gabapentin
>
> Topiramate
>
> Valproic acid
>
> *Concern*
>
> Citalopram
>
> Fluoxetine
>
> Atenolol
>
> Nadolol
>
> Timolol
>
> *Contraindicated*
>
> Lithium
>
> *Insufficient data*
>
> Candesartan
>
> Lisinopril
>
> Botulinum toxin
>
> *From* MacGregor EA. Migraine in pregnancy and lactation. Neurol Sci 2014;35(Suppl 1):S61–4; with permission.

being so common and bearing a tremendous socioeconomic impact, little is known about this condition. Previously known as simple headache, tension headache, stress headache, and psychogenic headache, the diagnostic criteria for this condition have changed over the years. Early editions of the International Headache Classification listed it as being "with or without peri cranial tenderness," but now the subcategories simply denote the frequency, that is, infrequent episodic, frequently episodic, and chronic (that is >15 days per month for the last 3 months). Furthermore, the diagnosis requires at least 10 episodes of headache lasting from 30 minutes to 7 days consisting of at least 2 of the following aspects: mild to moderate intensity, dull tightness (non-pulsating), bilateral, and not worsening of movement. Furthermore, the headache should not be associated with nausea, can only be associated with photophobia or phonophobia but not both, and cannot be attributed to another disorder.

Tension-type headache is generally easily treated with simple analgesics, rest, and hydration. It is unusual for patients with this condition to require physician intervention unless they have the rare occurrence of chronic tension-type headache; this may be complicated by medication overuse or other risk factors for chronification. Other associated secondary causes should be considered, including cervicogenic headaches when the headache is more intractable.

CLUSTER HEADACHE

Cluster headaches and the other trigeminal autonomic cephalgias (TAG) are fortunately very rare conditions because they confer some of the worst possible pain an individual may suffer. Cluster headache is the most common of these conditions with a prevalence between 1 in 2000 and 1 in 2500, and a male predominance of 3 to 1 over women. It is colloquially known as suicide headache, and the rate of suicide may be about 8 times that of the general population. Interestingly, the other cephalgias in this group do not necessarily show that male predominance. Each of the (TACs) consists of unilateral severe retrorbital, supraorbital, or periorbital pain along with associated autonomic activation that includes sympathetic and parasympathetic symptoms. These symptoms may include a partial Horner syndrome with miosis, ptosis, conjunctival injection, nasal congestion or drainage, unilateral sweating, as well as a sense of restlessness or agitation.

Cluster headache is generally the most common and occurs in clusters wherein the headache occurs as infrequently as every other day to multiple times per day, lasts from 15 minutes to 3 hours, and is incredibly disabling. Paroxysmal hemicrania has similar characteristics but lasts only minutes to 15 minutes and has an exquisite response to the anti-inflammatory indomethacin, which is part of the definition of the condition. Similarly, hemicrania continua also is indomethacin responsive but is a continuous headache (often of a less severe nature than the other headaches). The final TAC is a Severe Unilateral Neuralgiform Headache with Conjunctival Injection and Tearing (or SUNCT), which is now known to be part of a condition called Severe Unilateral Neuralgiform Headache with Autonomic Features, where the attacks only last seconds but may occur dozens to hundreds of times per day.

The general treatment of cluster headache is abortive treatment with pure oxygen by non-rebreather face mask, subcutaneous or intranasal sumatriptan, or intranasal or oral zolmitriptan, although other agents have been used. Prevention may be indicated with some evidence for verapamil, topiramate, lithium, and valproic acid. The treatment of choice for paroxysmal hemicrania and hemicrania continua is indomethacin, and treatment of SUNCT may include lithium or IV lidocaine but truly remains unknown.

INPATIENT TREATMENT OF MIGRAINE, TENSION HEADACHE, AND CLUSTER AND OTHER AUTONOMIC CEPHALGIAS

Most patients with migraine are able to care for themselves with over-the-counter medications; some seek help from their primary care physician; some are referred to neurologists, with fewer referred to headache specialists. A small number require the level of care that is available in an inpatient setting. This higher-level care is needed infrequently and often occurs in an unplanned and poorly organized manner. Hospitalization rates for migraineurs have been reported to be twice that of rates for a normal population.[37] An inpatient setting can allow for more rapid diagnosis of secondary headache syndromes, provide complex treatment regimens, deliver monitoring for individuals with concomitant medical problems, offer a safe means for detoxification, and (in some cases) allow for a multidisciplinary intervention. A dedicated inpatient treatment program can help manage the most severe, refractory cases. These individuals seem to benefit from advanced and intense levels of care, including inpatient treatment.[38]

Organized inpatient management is rarely available, and a select group of patients seek out magnet hospitals where this service can be delivered. A survey of 174 physicians selected from the membership of the American Association for the Study of Headache (now called the American Headache Society) showed that more than 50% of them used inpatient hospitalization for their patients.[39] However, there are limitations to this level of care, including limited access, risks of medication, psychological burden, and the cost for the patient, the employer, and the insurance company. More often, hospitalization occurs after failed treatment in the emergency room setting, and these individuals are admitted ad hoc with a disorganized treatment plan, an inexperienced staff, and resentment or frustration by the treating team. Clinicians should consider a variety of factors when deciding on a course of therapy; **Box 5** shows current considerations for inpatient criteria.

Some medications used for headache management demand careful observation and may require the patient to be hospitalized. A good history is also necessary because one of the most salient risk factors for the development of chronic daily headache is medication overuse and rebound headache, and this needs to be recognized for effective inpatient care because the individual may require a specific detoxification plan (whether it be from opiates or barbiturates). For example, it is common practice to hospitalize patients who have been overusing large amounts of barbiturate-containing compounds, because withdrawal may not only be psychologically difficult but also can cause autonomic instability, seizure, and death.

Once the decision to hospitalize a patient is made, a treatment plan should be developed. Goals for the hospitalization need to be defined and effectively communicated to the patient. The first step is defining the condition and performing necessary tests to confirm the diagnosis. For example, if the patient has a "thunderclap" onset of a new daily persistent headache, then neuroimaging should be ordered to evaluate a

---

Box 5
Inpatient admission criteria

- Moderate to severe intractable pain with significant associated disability.
- Headache refractory to appropriate aggressive outpatient or emergency room treatment.
- Continuous nausea, vomiting, or diarrhea that interferes with activities.
- Need for supportive medical measures to treat dehydration, electrolyte imbalances, unstable vital signs, or prostration.
- Need for detoxification and treatment of toxicity, dependency and withdrawal from substances that cannot be safely monitored as an outpatient.
- Overutilization of outpatient or emergency room care during crisis.
- Comorbid dangerous medical conditions.
- Potential of dangerous underlying condition causing headache.
- Psychological health considerations interfering in effective treatment.
- Need for rapid improvement and aggressive drug titration in safe environment.

vascular cause of the headache and LP should be performed. Chronic pain conditions, especially headache, may be comorbid with psychiatric or psychological issues. Patients with significant psychiatric comorbidity often have a worse long-term prognosis and lower quality-of-life ratings despite successful reduction of pain level and frequency of headache attacks.[38] It is important to evaluate comorbid psychiatric disorders, and the inpatient environment is a good setting in which to make the diagnoses and initiate treatment.

The core of hospital care for headache patients is medication management. The ability of repetitive IV DHE (**Box 6**) to treat refractory headache conditions has been well documented.[39] After obtaining baseline laboratory studies and electrocardiograms, patients may receive advancing test doses of DHE until a maximum dose of 1 mg every 8 hours is achieved (see **Box 6**).

Other medications have demonstrated efficacy in the treatment of headache pain. Antiemetics such as metoclopramide (10–20 mg IV) can be coadministered to control nausea via an antidopaminergic effect and may have a primary effect on headache pain more than morphine. Other alternatives include the administration of anti-inflammatory agents, both corticosteroids and nonsteroidal anti-inflammatories, such as ketorolac. These potent anti-inflammatories may be coadministered with DHE and antiemetics in order to maximize care. The repeated administration of valproic acid has shown utility, as have IV magnesium and some muscle relaxants. In many cases, multiple medications are used concurrently. Multiple medications may increase the effect on the headache, but it also increases the risk of adverse events and interactions between medications. In a meta-analysis of outcomes of inpatient hospitalization, it was reported that up to 91% of patients reported significant

---

Box 6
Inpatient treatment protocol for intravenous dihydroergotamine

1. Premedicate with metoclopramide 10 mg IV or other antiemetic

2. Administer DHE 0.5 mg IV over 2 to 30 minutes

3. Adjust dosing on the basis of response

4. If nausea and head pain persist, continue treatment for full 9 doses, but:
   a. Giver reduced dose of IV DHE every 8 hours
   b. Change antiemetic
   c. Reduce infusion rate

5. If the initial treatment leads to the patient being free of pain and nausea at the successive doses:
   a. Repeat steps 1 and 2 above
   b. Give total of 8 additional doses

6. If migraine headache pain continues, but the nausea resolves:
   a. Give additional 0.5 mg of IV DHE in 1 hour
   b. Follow with 8 additional doses

      i. Each dose is 1 mg of IV DHE

      ii. Use the same dose of antiemetic

      iii. Give doses every 8 hours
   c. If nausea at higher doses of IV DHE:

      i. Reduce dose of DHE

      ii. Change antiemetic

      iii. Change infusion rate

(>50%) improvement in symptoms at follow-up intervals up to 6 months; at intervals greater than 6 months, up to 71% of patients reported significant improvement.[40]

REFERENCES

1. Levin M. The international classification of headache disorders, 3rd edition (ICHD III)—changes and challenges. Headache 2013;53(8):1383–95.
2. Dodick DW. Pearls: headache. Semin Neurol 2010;3:74–81.
3. Martin MT. The diagnostic evaluation of secondary headache disorders. Headache 2011;51(2):346–52.
4. Loder E, Cardona L. Evaluation for secondary causes for headache: the role of blood and urine testing. Headache 2011;51(2):338–45.
5. Edlow JA, Panagos PD, Godwin SA, et al. Clinical policy: critical issues in the evaluation and management of adult patients presenting to the emergency department with acute headache. Ann Emerg Med 2008;52(4):405–36.
6. Moreau T, Manceau E, Giroud-Baleydier F, et al. Headache in hypothyroidism: prevalence and outcome under thyroid hormone therapy. Cephalgia 1998; 19(10):687–9.
7. Silberstein SD. Practice parameter: evidence-based guidelines for migraine headache (an evidence based-review): report of the Quality Standards Subcommittee of the American Academy of Neurology. Neurology 2000;55(6): 754–62.
8. Brust JCM. Subarachnoid hemorrhage. In: Rowland LP, editor. Merritts textbook of neurology. 8th edition. Philadelphia: Lea and Febiger; 1989. p. 235–43.
9. Kanner R. Subarachnoid hemorrhage. Pain secrets. Philadelphia: Hanley & Belfus, Inc; 1997. p. 57–8.
10. Nelson S, Taylor LP. Headaches in brain tumor patients: primary or secondary? Headache 2014;54(4):776–85.
11. Strominger MB, Weiss GB, Mehler MF. Asymptomatic unilateral papilledema in pseudotumor cerebri. J Clin Neuroopthalmol 1992;12:238–41.
12. Kosmorsky GS. Idiopathic intracranial hypertension: pseudotumor cerebri. Headache 2015;54(2):389–94.
13. Corbett J. Idiopathic intracranial hypertension. J Neuroophthalmol 2012;32:e4–6.
14. Corbett J, Thompson HS. The rational management of idiopathic intrancranial hypertension. Arch Neurol 1989;46:1049–51.
15. Caselli RJ, Hundler GG, Whisnant JP. Neurologic disease in biopsy-proven giant cell (temporal) arteritis. Neurology 1988;38:352, 163–5.
16. Aiello PD, Trauctmann JC, McPhee TJ, et al. Visual prognosis in giant cell arteritis. Opthalmology 1993;100:550–5.
17. Duarte RA. Temporal arteritis. Pain secrets. Philadelphia: Hanley & Belfus Inc; 1997. p. 66–7.
18. Ellis ME, Ralston S. The ESR in the diagnosis and management of the polymyalgia rheumatic/giant cell arteritis syndrome. Ann Rheum Dis 1983;42:168–70.
19. Salvarini C, Hunder GG. Giant cell arteritis with low erythrocyte sedimentation rate: frequency of occurrence in a population-based study. Arthritis Rheum 2001;45:140–5.
20. Miller A, Green M, Robinson D. Simple rule for calculation normal erythrocyte sedimentation rate. BR Med J 1983;286:266.
21. Tepper SJ, Dahlof CGH, Dowson A, et al. Prevalence and diagnosis of migraine in patients consulting their physician with a complaint of headache: data from the Landmark Study. Headache 2004;44:856–64.

22. MacGregor EA. Migraine in pregnancy and lactation. Neurol Sci 2014;35(Suppl): S61–4.
23. Evans RW. Warning: the Excedrin migraine warning label is inadequate to warn consumers of the risk of medication rebound headache. Headache 1999;39(9): 679–80.
24. Freitag FG, Schloemer F. Medical management of adult headache. Otolaryngol Clin North Am 2014;46:221–37.
25. Lipton RB, Bigal ME, Diamond M, et al. Migraine prevalence, disease burden and the need for preventative therapy. Neurology 2007;68:343–9.
26. Whitcup SM, Turkel CC, DeGryse RE, et al. Development of onabotulinumtoxinA for chronic migraine. Ann N Y Acad Sci 2014;1329:67–80.
27. Schulman EA, Lake AE, Goadsby PJ, et al. Defining refractory migraine and re-fractory chronic migraine: proposed criteria from the Refractory Headache Spe-cial Interest Section of the American Headache Society. Headache 2008;48: 778–82.
28. Lee P, Huh BK. Peripheral nerve stimulation for the treatment of primary head-ache. Curr Pain Headache Rep 2013;17:319.
29. Falowski S, Wang D, Sabesan A, et al. Occipital nerve stimulator systems: review of complications and surgical techniques. Neuromodulation 2010;13:121–5.
30. Schwedt TJ, Dodic DW, Trentman TL, et al. Response to occipital nerve block is not useful in predicting efficacy of occipital nerve stimulaton. Cephalalgia 2007; 27:271–4.
31. Jurgens TP, Leone M. Pearls and pitfalls: neurostimulation in headache. Cepha-lalgia 2013;33(8):512–25.
32. Mathew PG. A critical evaluation of migraine trigger site deactivation surgery. Headache 2013;54:142–52.
33. D'Andrea G, Cevoli S, Cologno D. Herbal therapy in migraine. Neurol Sci 2014; 35(Suppl 1):S135–40.
34. Eaton J. Butterbur, herbal help for migraine. Nat Pharm 1998;2:23–4.
35. Silberstein S, Patel S. Menstrual migraine: an update review on hormonal causes, prophylaxis and treatment. Expert Opin Pharmacother 2014;15(14):2063–70.
36. Facchinetti F, Sances G, Borella P, et al. Magnesium prophylaxis of menstrual migraine: effects on intracellular magnesium. Headache 1991;31(5):298–301.
37. Clouse J, Osterhaus J. Healthcare resource use and costs associated with migraine in a managed healthcare setting. Ann Pharmacother 1994;28: 659–64.
38. Freitag FG. Headache clinics and inpatient treatment units for headache. In: Diamond S, Dalessio DJ, Diamond ML, et al, editors. The practicing physician's approach to the treatment of headache. 6th edition. Saunders; 1999. p. 232–42.
39. Lake A, Saper J, Madden S, et al. Comprehensive inpatient treatment for intrac-table migraine: a prospective long-term outcome study. Headache 1993;33: 55–62.
40. Jauslin P, Goadsby PJ, Lance JW. The hospital management of severe migrainous headache. Headache 1991;31:658–60.

Managing Osteoarthritis and Other Chronic Musculoskeletal Pain Disorders

Andrew Dubin, MD

KEYWORDS

- Osteoarthritis • Cartilage • Exercise • Viscosupplementation

KEY POINTS

- Osteoarthritis (OA) is a common problem in society and can lead to significant disability and impairment of a patient's capacity to perform activities of daily living (ADLs).
- Exercise, pharmacology, bracing, and injections play roles in the management of OA.
- Exercise and injections play roles in the management of myofascial pain syndrome.

INTRODUCTION

OA can be viewed as primarily a wear and tear arthritis. Newer information, however, indicates that inflammation may also play a role. Although the initial pathology is primarily the level of the articular cartilage, the disorder encompasses all aspects of the joint. Ultimately, cartilage, synovium, and bone are all involved in the progression of OA and the debility that can be associated with it. Understanding the pathogenesis of OA is essential when considering the various options potentially available to treat the symptoms.[1,2]

ETIOLOGY OF OSTEOARTHRITIS

The function of cartilage is to allow for the smooth movement of many joints in the body. Its maintenance depends on the balance of cartilage matrix turnover. Perturbation in the balance between synthesis and normal degradation leads to deterioration in cartilage. Multiple factors can lead to alterations in this normal balance. Mechanical trauma to the joint, progressive joint instability, and production of inflammatory cytokines can all trigger the development of OA. A remarkable and consistent feature of osteoarthritic joints is the development of osteophytes, which represent new development of both cartilage and bone. Although the exact function of osteophyte formation

The author has no financial disclosures or conflicts of interest to note.
Department of Physical Medicine and Rehabilitation, Albany Medical College, 47 New Scotland Ave, Albany, NY 12208, USA
E-mail address: dubina@mail.amc.edu

Med Clin N Am 100 (2016) 143–150
http://dx.doi.org/10.1016/j.mcna.2015.08.008   medical.theclinics.com
0025-7125/16/$ – see front matter © 2016 Elsevier Inc. All rights reserved.

is unclear, it may serve to stabilize the joint and may also be an attempt to increase the weight-bearing surface of load-bearing joints, such as the hip and knee.[1–4]

TREATMENT OPTIONS
Exercise

Exercise can take on many forms, including both aerobic conditioning and strength training. Patient and physician thoughts regarding exercise and its role are controversial and often based on personal bias. Data from various studies reveal that a combination of light to moderate cardiovascular training in concert with lower extremity strength training can have significant utility in the management of knee OA. Although patients may express concern about activities, such as walking or light running, in the face of knee OA, the benefits of regular aerobic activity have been shown across multiple studies. Failure to engage in regular and routine activity, even as simple as walking, is associated with debility and loss of muscle mass and may accelerate cartilage degradation secondary to altered cartilage matrix characteristics. Lack of physical activity may result in increased joint stiffness, further alteration in gait mechanics, and an increase in the risk to fall and resultant orthopedic trauma. Separate and distinct from the pain of OA is the pain from soft tissue stiffness that results from assuming a sedentary lifestyle in response to the pain. As the activity level decreases, pain increases, much to the chagrin and frustration of both patient and treating physician. Light to moderate aerobic activity may include walking, jogging, and cycling. Although patients may question using walking and or jogging as part of an aerobic conditioning program in the face of knee OA, the compressive and tensile loads that the cartilage is subjected to are well below threshold. Cycling is well tolerated at low to even high intensity levels, and as such may allow for potentially more significant cardiovascular benefit than walking or jogging. Swimming has been suggested as a way to exercise patients with OA. Its major benefit may lie as a bridge form of activity to ultimate land-based exercise. Swimming has been associated with short-term benefit, but long-term benefit has not been conclusively demonstrated.[5]

Resistance or strength training has been shown to decrease pain scores and increase function in multiple studies of knee OA. Typically emphasis is placed on quadriceps strengthening because knee OA is commonly associated with quadriceps weakness and dysfunction. The cookbook recipe of placing patients with knee OA on a regimen of quadriceps strengthening, however, needs to be avoided because patients with malalignment issues may find that quadriceps strengthening increases the compressive forces across the knee joint and increases pain. In this population, hamstring and hip abductor and lower leg muscle strengthening may be of more benefit. As yet, these data are not readily available and may constitute fertile ground for future research.[4,5]

More recent literature has looked at the role of balance and proprioceptive training in patients with lower extremity OA and found a positive correlation. Whether this correlation is secondary to improved strength that results from engaging in balance training activities or is secondary to improvements in balance alone has not been determined and may be difficult to separate.

Weight Reduction

Multiple studies have shown that for weight-bearing joints, obesity has as great an impact on joint OA development as does a history of prior trauma. Weight reduction should constitute a major intervention in the management of lower extremity joint OA. Several studies have shown that maintenance of appropriate body weight may be one of the most significant interventions that can be taken to decrease the risk for development of OA in weight-bearing joints. Even in obese patients, a relationship between reduction in weight and reducing the risk for developing OA in weight-bearing joints has been demonstrated. Aerobic conditioning can also play a role in weight reduction and should be emphasized.[5]

Physical/Occupational Therapy

Physical and occupational therapy has a role in the management of OA. Physical therapy can be used as a way of getting patients with OA involved in a supervised exercise program with progression to a home program as the patient gains strength and confidence in the ability to tolerate exercise. Occupational therapy may be helpful in identifying adaptive equipment that may make performance of ADLs easier and less painful. Equipment, such as reachers, sock-donning aids, button aids, and Velcro closures rather than laced shoes, are examples of adaptive equipment that may aid performance of ADLs. Canes can be used to partially deweigh arthritic lower extremity joints and aid in mobility and balance. Soft neoprene braces may improve proprioceptive feedback, thereby improving walking tolerance. Ankle braces from lace-up to custom polypropylene ankle foot orthoses may improve walking tolerance by stabilizing arthritic ankle joints. Shoe wear modifications can also have utility by supporting or offloading painful joints. Shoe inserts with arch supports can stabilize and disperse the forces over the tarsal bones decreasing the pain of foot joint arthritis.

A typical finding in knee OA is loss of medial joint space manifesting as a bow-legged posture or varus knee position. Use of a lateral foot wedge affixed to the sole of the foot applies a counterforce to take the knee out of its varus posture to a more neutral to slightly valgus posture, which reduces the stress on the stretched lateral collateral knee ligament and partially unloads the painful medial joint space. This combined effect has been shown to result in decreased knee pain.[6] Although improved walking tolerance in the appropriate patient population is more variable and less pronounced compared with a medial unloader brace, a more aggressive form of intervention to unload the medial knee joint, lateral wedging, is a good first option. Medial unloading or varus correction braces may not be well tolerated because significant force is placed through the knee and patients may find the brace straps uncomfortable and restrictive.[6,7]

In cases of more severe knee OA with associated multiplanar instability, a knee ankle foot orthosis with a hinged knee joint and straps to further augment the stabilizing characteristics of the brace may be helpful. These types of braces, however, are not typically tolerated in more active patients owing to the marked mechanical restrictions they impose.

PHARMACOLOGIC OPTIONS
Topical Nonsteroidal Anti-inflammatory Drugs

Topical nonsteroidal anti-inflammatory drugs (NSAIDs) offer the potential advantage of focal targeted application of an anti-inflammatory analgesic agent with at least the theoretic advantage of a decreased side-effect profile. Topical NSAIDs may have utility in managing the pain of OA, both as an analgesic agent and an anti-inflammatory agent. Recent research has revealed that OA, although not a classic inflammatory arthropathy, does have characteristics of secondary synovitis in response to such factors as joint trauma, malalignment, and obesity. Topical NSAIDs have been shown in a meta-analysis to reduce joint pain and improve function, with loss of efficacy with use beyond 4 weeks' duration. Given that the effectiveness of topical NSAIDs seems to wane after 4 weeks, they may have their greatest utility for management of flares of pain.[8]

Acetaminophen can be considered a first-line oral agent for the management of the pain associated with OA. The advantages of acetaminophen are the overall safety profile of the medication. In general acetaminophen is not associated with significant risk of gastrointestinal (GI) or renal toxicity. Caution should be exercised because there is a clear risk for hepatic toxicity with long-term exposure at high doses. Older suggestions were for use of acetaminophen in doses of up to 4 g per day. With newer data showing an increased risk for liver toxicity as doses increase, more recent suggestions to limit the total dose to no more than 1300 to 2600 mg per day are prudent. Monitoring liver function enzymes is appropriate for patients using chronic acetaminophen.

NSAIDs encompass a broad group of medications. Salicylates have a long history in the management of both rheumatoid arthritis and OA. Proprionic acid derivatives, including but not limited to, ibuprofen, flurbiprofen, naproxen, and ketoprofen, have also been used for years. Acetic acid derivatives, such as sulindac, indomethacin, and tolmetin, can also be used. Failure to respond to one class of NSAIDs does not mean that they are ineffective. Changing class from an acetic acid derivative to a proprionic acid derivative or visa versa may at times prove effective. The major drawbacks to NSAIDS, as a class of medications, include the well-documented risks of both GI and renal toxicity. These risks increase with long-term use. The risk for renal toxicity is further increased in patients with underlying diabetes and hypertension. Cyclooxygenase inhibitors may be associated with fewer GI risks compared with classic NSAIDs, but this has only been demonstrated in short-term studies. There are no well-controlled studies to show this holds for long-term use. The risk for renal toxicity does not seem any different. Cyclooxygenase inhibitors carry the same black box warning as NSAIDs. Caution should be the watch word with the long-term use of NSAIDs, including cyclooxygenase inhibitors.[3,8,9]

Given these concerns, controversy exists about the role of NSAIDs in the management of OA. Data from the United Kingdom make note that of 8 million people in the United Kingdom with OA, approximately half of that group takes NSAIDs on a regular basis, contributing to the annual estimated 2000 deaths from NSAID side effects in the United Kingdom. An increased risk for adverse cardiac events led to the withdrawal of several cyclooxygenase inhibitor class NSAIDs and broad class restrictions and precautions in patients with cardiovascular pathology. Given these concerns, the role of NSAIDs in the long-term management of OA needs to be carefully considered and other alternatives need to be fully explored.[9]

Given the concerns over systemic anti-inflammatory medications, the use of ice as a local anti-inflammatory and analgesic makes it an attractive interventional strategy in the management of OA. Cryotherapy has been shown to slow the rate of neural transmission, which may dampen pain signals. The anti-inflammatory effect may also result in pain reduction as well as the direct analgesic effect of cold.

Viscosupplementation (hyaluronic acid [HA]) presents a novel approach in the management of OA in weight-bearing joints. They are Food and Drug Administration approved for use in knee OA. Viscosupplementation has also been trialed in hip OA. Data have been inconsistent regarding the efficacy of viscosupplementation. Work by Migliore and colleagues[10] compared intra-articular hip joint injections with viscosupplementation injection to local anesthetic. Their results indicated significant improvement in pain and function in the viscosupplementation group compared with the local anesthetic group. Although encouraging, the data need to be interpreted with caution. The mechanism by which injection of local anesthetic potentially results in long-term pain modulation is unclear. Theories include dilution of inflammatory cytokines and inhibition of neuropeptide production.[10]

Intra-articular corticosteroid injections have been a mainstay for management of painful OA joints. They are frequently used to manage knee, hip, and shoulder pain associated with OA. Previously published data have shown that corticosteroids and viscosupplementation have equal efficacy up to 4 weeks postinjection. From weeks 5 through 26, however, greater efficacies were noted for HA products. Intra-articular injections of corticosteroids and HA products have similar responses, although the duration of the response seems of longer duration for the HA group. Intra-articular injections of local anesthetic and corticosteroids should be considered a short-term treatment strategy given their relative short duration of effect, and the possibility that long-term exposure to corticosteroids and local anesthetics (cians) may accelerate cartilage damage.[11,12]

Total joint arthroplasty for painful hip or knee OA that is nonresponsive to conservative management remains the definitive intervention. Total joint arthroplasty has been shown in multiple studies to predictably result in improvement of quality of life, pain scores, and function scores. This intervention is not without risks, however. Concerns include deep vein thrombosis, pulmonary embolism, joint infection, hardware failure, early component loosening, and neurovascular injury, including but not limited to sciatic neuropathy in posterolateral approach total hip arthroplasty and possible femoral nerve neuropathy with anterior approach (total hip arthroplasty). Additionally, total knee arthroplasty can be associated with fibular nerve and/or tibial neuropathy at the level of the knee. Incomplete femoral nerve neuropathy has also been documented secondary to edge compression from the tourniquet used during total knee arthroplasty.

ALTERNATIVES

An interesting study has looked at intra-articular botulinum toxin injections for the management of knee pain. Improvements in Western Ontario and McMaster Universities Osteoarthritis Index (WOMAC) and visual analog scale scores were noted, raising the question of the potential role of neurotransmitter antagonists as part of the armamentarium in the future.[11]

Capsaicin creams have been used in pain management. They have demonstrated improvement in pain score for knee OA patients. Their theoretic mechanism of action is through substance P depletion.[11]

Curcumin, also called turmeric, is yellow pigment isolated from the rhizomes of *Curcuma longa*. There is molecular evidence that curcumin has potency for targeting various inflammatory diseases. Various trials are ongoing. Anecdotal evidence and uncontrolled trials seem to point toward potential utility for curcumin of use in the management of pain associated with OA.[13]

Lidocaine patches have been used for management of various painful conditions. They have been used in the management of knee OA. Several open-label trials of lidocaine patches for the treatment of pain associated with knee OA note improvement in WOMAC scores as well as in pain and function scores with short-term use and follow-up. Given the side-effect profile of lidocaine patches, it represents a possible intervention that is helpful with minimal risk. Further studies are needed.

Nonarticular muscular pain generators can arise from bursa, tendons, and muscle and its associated fascial attachments. Bursitis, tendonitis, and myofascial pain syndrome are common causes of pain that bring patients to physicians.

Bursas serve as interfaces between muscle and the underlying bone. In normal function, they allow for smooth movement of muscle over areas of bony prominence. Bursitis is the inflammation of bursa, which impairs the function of the bursa and results in pain secondary to inflammation. Inflammation can occur secondary to acute trauma or low-grade repetitive trauma.

The first line of treatment typically uses anti-inflammatory modalities; ice can be helpful for managing the pain and inflammation of bursitis. Topical NSAIDs can potentially be effective in the management of bursitis for more superficially located bursas, such as the subdeltoid bursa, as opposed to a more deeply situated bursa, like the trochanteric bursa. Medial and lateral epicondylitis may also respond to both ice and topical NSAIDs. A short course of oral anti-inflammatory agents may be helpful but caution should be exercised given the side-effect profile of oral NSAIDs.

Trochanteric bursitis is a common cause of lateral hip pain. The differential diagnosis includes hip OA, referred pain from the lumbar spine, sacroiliac joint referral pain, and a chronic L5-level radiculopathy, to name a few. An injection of corticosteroid with a local anesthetic can be helpful in establishing a diagnosis and in general is well tolerated with a low side-effect profile. Frequent injections should be avoided to decrease the risk of rupture of the gluteus medius tendon.[14]

A common tendonitis is rotator cuff tendonitis. It can result in significant impairment of upper extremity function secondary to pain. As discussed previously, conservative management is the mainstay first-line intervention. Again, corticosteroid injection with local anesthetic can be helpful in more recalcitrant cases to help confirm the diagnosis.

Surgery can be considered in cases of refractory trochanteric bursitis and rotator cuff tendonitis and can be effective.[15]

Physical therapy can be helpful in the management of bursitis and epicondylitis. Range-of-motion exercises and modalities like ultrasound can be helpful. Steroid phonophoresis or iontophoresis can be used as a way to drive topical steroids to the site of inflammation, allowing for more focal application of anti-inflammatory medication, typically corticosteroids, limiting the potential for systemic side effects. In more chronic cases, moist heat with stretching exercises and progression to strengthening can be helpful. Once the inflammation has been quieted, the patient should be progressed through a gradual strengthening program to decrease the likelihood of recurrence. Referral for surgery can be considered in refractory cases of epicondylitis or bursitis but should be approached with caution.

The etiology of myofascial pain syndrome, a chronic soft tissue muscle pain syndrome, is not fully understood. The typical feature, a myofascial trigger point, is theorized to be an area of sensitized nociceptors within muscle. Myofascial pain syndrome can develop after acute trauma or after exposure to long-term repetitive activities. Myofascial pain can develop after traumatic events, such as motor vehicle accidents (MVAs). Rapid cervical flexion/extension eccentric loading-type mechanisms seen in high-energy impact events may cause localized muscle trauma and set the stage for development of myofascial trigger points and the later development of a chronic soft tissue muscle pain syndrome, which can also be seen in sporting activities, such as basketball and football, potentially high-energy impact sports.[16,17]

Given that a majority of individuals involved in MVAs and high-impact sporting events do not develop long-term muscle pain, the question arises as to which factors predispose the approximate 10% of individuals who are involved in MVAs to progress onto chronic muscle pain. Various studies, including electrophysiologic studies seem to indicate that an abnormal increase in acetylcholine contributes to endplate hyperexcitability, which causes localized areas of increased muscle tension, in turn increasing the metabolic demands on the muscle, creating a relative ischemic state, which may result in an increased release of nociceptive neuropeptides, setting the stage for the development of trigger points and subsequent myofascial pain syndrome.[16,17]

Various conditions can be associated with myofascial pain syndrome or may exacerbate the condition. Poor sleep, stress, or superimposed painful conditions, such as radiculopathy, neuropathy, and OA, may exacerbate the problem.

Typically, the first-line intervention is a combination of stretching of the involved muscles with the application of ice or heat whichever is better tolerated. A global conditioning program emphasizing aerobic conditioning and light strength training can be helpful in managing the chronic muscle pain complaints typically noted by patients dealing with myofascial pain. Strengthening of postural muscles may be helpful as well. Relaxation techniques can be used as adjunct therapy in the management of myofascial pain. Acupuncture and massage can be helpful for managing the trigger points because the application of strong pressure over the trigger point may cause hyperstimulation analgesia. The same theory applies to the rationale for trigger point injections with local anesthetic or dry needling. In more refractory patients, the broad class of neuromodulators may be helpful.[16,17]

Medication choices should take into account the potential for myofascial pain to progress to chronic pain. As such, medications with a low risk for renal or GI toxicity should be medications of choice. Medications with abuse potential should be avoided.[16,17]

REFERENCES

1. Sokolove J, Lepus CM. Role of inflammation in the pathogenesis of osteoarthritis: latest findings and interpretations. Ther Adv Musculoskelet Dis 2013;5(2):77–94.
2. Pulsatelli L, Addimanda O, Brusi V, et al. New findings in osteoarthritis: therapeutic implications. Adv Musculoskelet Med 2013;4(1):23–43.
3. Hinton R, Moody R, Davis A, et al. Osteoarthritis: diagnosis and therapeutic considerations. Am Fam Physician 2002;65(5):841–8.
4. Sandell LJ, Aigner T. Articular cartilage and changes in arthritis. An introduction: cell biology of osteoarthritis. Arthritis Res 2001;3:107–13.
5. Esser S, Bailey A. Effects of exercise and physical activity on knee osteoarthritis. Curr Pain Headache Rep 2011;15:423–30.
6. Latham N, Lui C. Strength training in older adults: the benefits for osteoarthritis. Clin Geriatr Med 2010;26(3):445–59.
7. Sattari S, Ashraf AR. Comparison the effect of 3 point valgus stress knee support and lateral wedge insoles in medial compartment knee osteoarthritis. Iran Red Crescent Med J 2011;13(9):624–8.
8. Cooper C. Topical NSAIDs in osteoarthritis. BMJ 2004;329:304–5.
9. Bjordal J. NSAIDs in osteoarthritis: irreplaceable or troublesome guidelines? Br J Sports Med 2006;40:285–6.
10. Migliore A, Massafra U, Bizzi E, et al. Comparative, double blind, controlled study of intra-articular hyaluronic acid (Hyalubrix) injections versus local anesthetic in osteoarthritis of the hip. Arthritis Res Ther 2009;11(6):R183.
11. Iannitti T, Lodi D, Palmieri B. Intra-articular injections for the treatment of osteoarthritis. focus on the clinical use of hyaluronic acid. Drug R D 2011;11(1):13–27.
12. Chu CR, Izzo NJ, Coyle NE, et al. The invitro effects of bupivacaine on articular chondrocytes JBJS Br. 2008;90(6):814–20.
13. Henrotin Y, Priem F, Mobashen A. Curcumin: a new paradigm and theraputic opportunity for the treatment of osteoarthritis: curcumin for osteoarthritis management. Springerplus 2013;2:56.
14. Lustenberger DP, Ng VY, Best TM, et al. Efficacy of treatment of trochanteric bursitis: a systematic review. Clin J Sport Med 2011;21:447–53.

15. Stephens MB, Beutler AI, O'Connor FG. Musculoskeletal injections: a review of the evidence. Am Fam Physician 2008;78(8):971–6.
16. Chowdhury N, Goldstein L. Diagnosis and management of myofascial pain. Practical Pain Management 2012;12(2):48–50.
17. Cagnie B, Castelein B, Pollie F, et al. Evidence for the use of ischemic compression and dry needling in the management of trigger points of the upper trapezius in patients with neck pain. A systematic review. Am J Phys Med Rehabil 2015; 94(7):573–83.

Managing Neuropathic Pain

Robert Carter Wellford Jones III, MD, PhD[a], Erin Lawson, MD[a,b],
Miroslav Backonja, MD[c],*

KEYWORDS

- Neuropathic pain • Neuralgia • Peripheral neuropathy • Radiculopathy
- Anticonvulsants • Interventional treatments • Physical therapy
- Cognitive behavioral therapy

KEY POINTS

- Neuropathic pain (NP) arises from injuries or diseases affecting the somatosensory component of the nervous system at any level of the peripheral nervous system or central nervous system (CNS).
- Regardless of location of injury, NP is diagnosed based on common neurologic signs and symptoms that are revealed by history taking and on physical examination.
- NP is best treated with a combination of multiple therapeutic approaches, which starts with patient education, and the treatments include conservative, complementary, medical, interventional, and surgical treatment modalities.
- Goals of treatment are the same as in pain management in general, and they include improvement in pain control and in coping skills as well as restoration of functional status. Early identification of realistic treatment expectations is the key to building a successful relationship with a patient suffering from NP.
- In most instances when treating chronic NP, the approach to pain management begins with conservative therapies and advances to more interventional ones only when earlier modalities do not meet goals of pain relief and improved function, because risks increase with the invasiveness of the therapies. Most patients with NP benefit most from an individualized, multimodal approach that emphasizes both pain and function.

ASSESSMENT OF NEUROPATHIC PAIN

The identification of NP, as with other medical conditions, relies on obtaining a detailed history and careful physical examination. It ultimately reflects a constellation of signs and symptoms and so, unlike other conditions, there is no specific test that

[a] Center for Pain Medicine, Department of Anesthesiology, Division of Pain Medicine, University of California San Diego, 9444 Medical Center Drive, MC 7651, La Jolla, CA 92093, USA; [b] Lexington Brain and Spine Institute, 811 West Main Street, Suite 201, Lexington, SC 29072, USA; [c] Department of Neurology, University of Wisconsin-Madison, Madison, WI 53706, USA
* Corresponding author.
E-mail address: backonja@neurology.wisc.edu

Med Clin N Am 100 (2016) 151–167
http://dx.doi.org/10.1016/j.mcna.2015.08.009
0025-7125/16/$ – see front matter © 2016 Elsevier Inc. All rights reserved.

medical.theclinics.com

can confirm its presence. In addition, NP can result from a wide variety of causes; therefore, classification of a patient's pain as neuropathic necessitates subsequent investigation of an underlying cause or multiple causes. Fortunately, NP is relatively straightforward to determine and its identification can be quickly mastered by any conscientious medical practitioner.

History

The International Association for the Study of Pain defines NP as "pain caused by a lesion or disease of the somatosensory nervous system."[1] The definition implies that a demonstrable cause should be sought and traced to a sensory component of the nervous system with a corresponding spatial distribution pattern that reflects the affected nerve supply. Examples include dermatomal NP and other sensory symptom distribution caused by disk herniation and impingement on spinal nerve roots, stocking and glove peripheral neuropathy caused by HIV or diabetes, painful extremities in complex regional pain syndrome (CRPS), and wider areas of pain affected multiple sclerosis lesions (**Fig. 1**). Pain associated with all of these lesions share many common features that are crucial elements of the history suggestive of NP. There

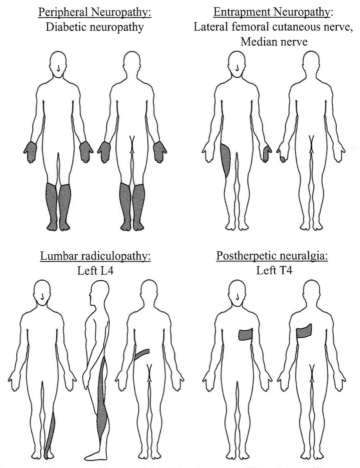

Fig. 1. Representative pain diagrams of 4 distinct neuropathic pain conditions.

are several published screening tools that can capture features of NP and be used to distinguish it from other types of pain (eg, nociceptive). The Leeds Assessment of Neuropathic Symptoms and Signs (LANSS), Neuropathic Pain Questionnaire (NPQ), Douleur Neuropathique 4 Questions, painDETECT, ID Pain, and Standardized Evaluation of Pain (StEP) are examples of such tools developed to identify NP with varying, but relatively strong, sensitivity and specificity.[2] All of these tools are easy to learn and administer and, with the exception of the StEP, freely available.

Several items are important to consider when using one of these NP screening tools. Each tool was validated in different patient populations with distinct types of NP; therefore, each tool may reflect to a greater or lesser degree the patient population of an individual medical practice. The scoring that results from one of these assessment tools should constitute just one line of reasoning in a practitioner's decision-making process to lead to the identification of NP. Some of these assessment tools have been applied to patient populations with pain not typically thought neuropathic in nature, for example, fibromyalgia and knee osteoarthritis, and the scores suggest presence of NP component even in those traditionally non-neuropathic disorders.[3,4] This finding represents either a discriminative inadequacy for the diagnostic accuracy of the tools or an unrecognized neuropathic component to symptoms in these individuals. Additional tools are also available to quantify the severity of NP and help gauge response to treatment. These include the Neuropathic Pain Scale, Neuropathic Pain Symptom Inventory, and Short-Form McGill Pain Questionnaire 2.

Physical Examination

Also implied by the International Association for the Study of Pain definition, although not necessarily obvious, is that a lesion of the nervous system results in neurologic dysfunction that can often be detected on physical examination. The presence of 1 or more physical examination signs helps further substantiate a claim of NP. Signs associated with NP can be categorized as positive or negative in nature and result from derangement of nervous system function as a result of the inciting lesion. Therefore, these signs should be sought in the distribution of the affected painful area. Examples of positive phenomena include allodynia—the sensation of pain to a normally innocuous stimulus (eg, light touch), and hyperalgesia—the sensation of heightened pain to a normally painful stimulus (eg, pinprick). Examples of negative phenomena include the absence of sensation (ie, numbness) and motor weakness. Many of the NP assessment tools, discussed previously, include physical examination components. The LANSS incorporates assessment of hyperalgesia and allodynia on physical examination[5] whereas the NPQ relies on patient report of allodynic phenomena but does not require physical examination testing per se.[6] The StEP involves the most extensive physical examination; however, it also has the highest reported sensitivity and specificity for the identification of low back pain that is neuropathic in nature (>90%[7]).

More extensive testing of nervous system sensory function can be achieved with the use of quantitative sensory testing.[8] This testing involves rigorous and standardized assessment of multiple sensory modalities, including brush, light touch, vibration, heat, cold, and pressure. It is primarily used as a research tool and not required to identify with a high degree of certainty NP in most clinical settings. It can, however, provide important information to researchers on the specific derangements of the nervous system that occur in individual patients and conditions and assess their responsiveness to various treatments.

Diagnostic Testing

The routine use of diagnostic testing is not required for accurate identification of NP in patients.[9] Even when it may not be necessarily clear based on an ambiguous history or physical examination, a presumptive determination of pain as neuropathic in nature can often be presumed and appropriate treatment initiated. Diagnostic testing is invaluable for identifying the underlying cause and must follow any initial determination of NP if the cause is unknown. Testing could include laboratory studies to assess electrolyte disturbances or imaging studies, such as radiograph, CT, or MRI, to identify structural lesions. Electromyography and nerve conduction studies can be helpful as well to determine the presence of abnormal neuromuscular function and clarify the location of the disturbance. The decision to order diagnostic testing and which test to order varies based on the differential diagnosis for each specific patient. It should be stressed that none of these tests verifies the presence or absence of pain but instead serves to uncover a potential cause of their symptoms.

Several additional testing modalities are being developed to aid in the identification of NP and are currently used primarily for research purposes. Histologic and immunochemical examination of skin biopsies obtained from the painful extremity have revealed altered neuronal protein expression and vascularization patterns in patients with CRPS.[10] Functional MRI has been used to characterize brain activation patterns in response to many different types of pain, including NP from postherpetic neuralgia (PHN).[11] The expression pattern of proinflammatory cytokines in plasma is altered in patients with NP.[12] Genetic testing has uncovered heritable traits predisposing to the development of NP.[13] These and other techniques provide invaluable insights toward understanding of NP; however, none is currently able to aid most general medical practitioners in the identification of NP in individual patients.

MANAGEMENT
Pharmacotherapy for Neuropathic Pain

Role of pharmacotherapy as a part of multimodal therapy and treatment planning
Pharmacotherapy is frequently one of the first steps in treatment of pain because of its simplicity and ease of administration. When effective, pharmacotherapy can rapidly provide the basis for implementation of other components of pain management, such as physical therapy modalities and coping skills. Unfortunately, even medications that are approved for the treatment of NP provide only partial pain relief. Medications proved most effective for managing NP most frequently provide only 30% to 50% improvement and in only a subgroup of patients, most often for approximately 40% of patients.[14,15] Because individual medications have limited benefit, medications are often combined in treatment to improve outcome,[16–18] followed by implementation of other modalities. A balanced approach that includes multiple medications and nonpharmacologic treatments should be anticipated from the start as a part of treatment planning.

When initiating treatment, it is critical to clearly communicate to patients the following facts:

- All therapeutic modalities provide partial pain relief rather than a cure.
- Side effects are likely and should be anticipated and managed.
- All medications require titration (discussed later).
- Combinations of medications are most likely with 1 medication initiated at a time.
- Some therapeutic interventions, such as physical therapy and learning psychological coping skills, are best initiated early.

- Outcomes are best when working with the entire pain team.
- The goals of pain treatment include decreasing and controlling pain and other associated symptoms (such as anxiety, depression, and insomnia), gaining coping skills, and improving function.[19]

General principles of pharmacotherapy for NP include

- Initiating therapy at lowest approved and available doses
- Slow upward dose titration to the analgesic effect or recommended dose with the minimum side effects
- Careful and routine monitoring of analgesic effects and side effects
- Discontinuation of medications determined ineffective in relieving NP or causing intolerable side effects
- Avoiding withdrawal effects or exacerbation of any symptoms while discontinuing medications by slow taper off

Each class of pharmacologic agents has its specific properties, with advantages and disadvantages for routine clinical practice, and they are discussed (**Fig. 2, Table 1**).

Topical agents
Topical agents as a class have the advantage of providing localized pain relief with minimal if any systemic side effects, which appeals to many patients. As such, this modality of treatment should be considered early if not first.

Local anesthetics Topical local anesthetics have long been used, even prior to support by randomized trials. Eventually, randomized trials led to approval of the lidocaine-based Lidoderm patch (700 mg of lidocaine in the matrix) for PHN.[20] Lidocaine patch is applied to the area of pain for 12 hours and then removed for 12 hours. Up to 3

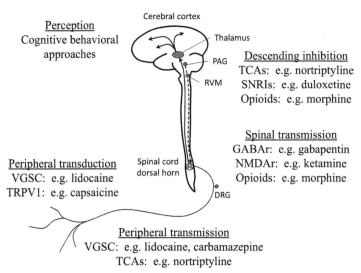

Fig. 2. Site of action of commonly used neuropathic pain interventions. Dashed lines indicate descending pathways and solid lines indicate ascending pathways. DRG, dorsal root ganglion; PAG, periaqueductal gray; RVM, rostroventral medulla; VGSC, voltage-gated sodium channel; GABAr, gamma aminobutyric acid receptor; NMDAr, N-methyl D-aspartate receptor; SNRI, serotonin norepinephrine reuptake inhibitor; TCA, tricyclic antidepressant; TRPV, transient receptor potential vanilloid channel.

Table 1
Pharmacologic agents with demonstrated analgesic efficacy for neuropathic pain

Drug	Dose	Indication for Neuropathic Pain	Common Side Effects
Tricyclic antidepressants	50–100 mg/d	Peripheral and central NP	Sedation, dizziness, orthostatic hypotension, urinary retention, constipation
Duloxetine (Cymbalta[a])	60–120 mg/d	NP associated with diabetes; also for musculoskeletal pain	Nausea, vomiting, dizziness, agitation
Pregabalin (Lyrica[a])	75–600 mg/d divided	NP associated with diabetic peripheral neuropathy; PHN; pain associated with spinal cord injury	Sedation, balance instability, weight gain
Gabapentin (Neurontin[a])	300–3600 mg daily divided	PHN	Sedation, balance instability, weight gain
Gabapentin extended-release (Gralise[a])	300–1800 mg once daily	PHN	Sedation, balance instability, weight gain
Carbamazepine (Tegretol[a])	100–800 mg daily in divided doses	NP from TN	Dizziness; risk of agranulocytosis and aplastic anemia
Lidocaine patch (Lidoderm[a])	1–3 Patches per day, 12 h on then 12 h off	PHN	Minimal transient skin irritation
Systemic lidocaine	500 mg in 250 mL of Normal saline over 30 min; infusion stopped if and when side effects occur	Peripheral and central NP	Transient sedation, dizziness, nausea
Capsaicin cream	0.025%–1%; 3–4 Times per day	Peripheral NP	Transient worsening of pain with application and skin redness
Capsaicin patch (Qutenza[a])	1 Patch for 30–60 min every 3 mo	HIV-associated peripheral neuropathy; PHN	Transient worsening of pain with application and skin redness
Cannabis	Smoked or oral spray	Peripheral and central NP	Sedation, balance instability, weight gain, psychosis

[a] FDA-approved therapies for indicated NP disorders.

patches may be used at once. Mild skin irritation, which resolves quickly with removal, is the most common side effect. Although approved for PHN, lidocaine patches are used in other settings, such as diabetic painful neuropathy (DPN), where even in presence of sensory loss patients report pain relief.[21]

Capsaicin Topical application of capsaicin cream has been used for decades to relieve NP of DPN and PHN, but difficulty of multiple daily applications deters wider use. More recently, a series of studies led to approval of a topical capsaicin patch in the United States for indication of PHN and in Europe for peripheral NP excluding DPN.[22,23] The patch is applied to the area of pain and associated allodynia for 30 to 60 minutes. Studies demonstrated prolonged, up to 3 months', pain relief. Discomfort from application of the capsaicin patch is well tolerated and associated dermal reaction resolves shortly after removal of the patch.[24] This form of therapy could be considered early, because the prolonged pain relief allows patients to tolerate other forms of pain management, such as physical modalities. Furthermore, the less severe residual pain after capsaicin treatment may be more responsive to other medications.

Topical nonsteroidal anti-inflammatory drugs and other compounded preparations Patients with NP tend to benefit little from oral nonsteroidal anti-inflammatory drugs. Not surprisingly there is no clinical trials evidence for efficacy of nonsteroidal anti-inflammatory drugs orally or topically in relieving NP.[25] Many physicians and pharmacies, however, devise compounding preparations, either as single agents or as various combinations of drugs, that are known to have preclinical and clinical effect on nociception and with that justification make those topical preparations. Efficacy of this common method of therapy has been studied on a limited basis.

Intradermal injections

Botulinum toxin A few recent studies, mainly conducted outside of the United States, showed positive results with botulinum toxin when used for treatment of NP disorders, such as PHN, DPN, focal traumatic neuralgias, and trigeminal neuralgia (TN).[26,27] Best results for efficacy are for PHN and TN, but all of these were small studies and replication in larger trials is necessary to better establish effect of this therapy. No significant side effects were reported. Routine use of botulinum toxin requires further standardization and answering basic questions, such as sites for injection and dose at each site.

Medications for systemic administration

Oral medications provide a systemic effect. Because they were available and most conducive to clinical trials methodology and drug development, oral medications have been most heavily investigated for NP. Despite decades of involvement of many investigators and companies, only a few medications have been developed and are currently approved. Ease of administration by oral route makes this type of therapy appealing; however, frequently bothersome side effects limit utility.

Neuromodulating medications The group of neuromodulating medications relieves pain and associated symptoms by modulating the hyperexcitable state of injured neurons. Neuromodulating medications act on different receptors and channel systems at various levels of the neuroaxis, from the peripheral nervous system to CNS.[28] Many of these drugs were originally designed for other indications, such as treatment of depression or seizures, but they found largest utility in treatment of NP. Gabapentin and pregabalin are such examples.

Similar to other areas of medicine, in the portfolio of positive studies for these NP drugs, there are a few published and unpublished studies with negative results.[29] The challenges of development of new therapies for NP is something that should be expected for medical field dealing with a complex medical diagnostic group.

Several recent studies comparing specific agents from the class of neuromodulating drugs found no significant differences.[25] These findings imply that the choice of which medication to choose depends on complete assessment of the patient and maximizing treatment not only of pain but also of associated comorbidities and minimizing side effects.

Anticonvulsants One of the oldest treatment examples for NP was carbamazepine for TN.[30] Despite early demonstration of its positive effect, its use has been limited by narrow therapeutic range and many side effects. Side effects are a common limitation among all of the systemically administered drugs.

Gabapentin and pregabalin exhort their therapeutic effect by acting on the alpha-2-delta subunit of Ca^{++} channels on central sensory neurons.[31] Their efficacy has been established in many clinical trials across many NP diagnoses, notably in PHN and PDN,[32,33] for which they carry Food and Drug Administration (FDA) approval in the United States. Their efficacy in relieving NP in other diagnoses of peripheral and central NP led to approval in Europe for a broader NP indication. In the United States, pregabalin is also approved for pain from spinal cord injury.[34] Main side effects include those related to the CNS, such as dizziness, incoordination, and mental clouding, although other systemic side effects, such as weight gain and peripheral edema, are reasons many patients do not tolerate these drugs.[35]

Other anticonvulsant drugs were studied for relief of NP, such as lamotrigine, topiramate, and oxcarbazepine, but they had more negative than positive outcomes, so most of the consensus recommendations and guidelines publications recommend against using these in medical practice.[25,32]

Antidepressants Tricyclic antidepressants were the earliest class of drugs proved effective for NP.[36] Familiarity with this class of drugs for treatment of depression and insomnia, which are common comorbidities with NP, makes it one of the drug classes identified as first-line therapy for NP.[25] Adverse effects, however, such as sedation, dizziness, and orthostatic hypotension, limit use.

Other medications, including those with positive limited clinical trials and clinical experience: intravenous lidocaine and cannabis There exist systemic treatments for NP that are not dosed orally yet have shown efficacy in clinical trials. Examples include IV lidocaine[37] and marijuana, either as inhaled or as intraoral spray.

IV lidocaine has shown efficacy relieving peripheral and central NP, mostly in smaller-investigator single-center studies, so robustness of these data is lacking. Difficulty of IV administration limits applicability. The side effects (dizziness, paresthesia, and sedation) from this therapy are transient and resolve quickly because these are single infusions. The most commonly used dose is 500 mg administered over 30 minutes.

Marijuana was studied for various indications, including pain from HIV-associated neuropathy[38] and for multiple sclerosis[39] (for which it received approval in the United Kingdom and Canada). The main concern is that for either method of delivery the bioavailability of active substances is poor, so better methods are necessary. Side effects are mainly CNS related, and many patients develop tolerance to those effects. Although medicinal marijuana is approved in approximately half of the states in the United States, it is still an illegal substance at the federal level, which is being addressed in Congress.

Opioids Opioids have consistent positive results in clinical trials as effective for relief of NP.[25] Multiple adverse effects, however, across many organ systems, and the epidemic of opioid overdose deaths due to misuse and abuse make this class of drugs second- or third-line therapy for NP in most recommendations in the United States and Europe.[25] In addition there is a concern about the long-term efficacy for NP.[40] As a result of the wide distribution of μ-opioid receptors across many organ systems, the side-effect profile of opioids is large. The most significant side effects include CNS (leading to addiction in susceptible patients, sleep disturbance, and depression), gastrointestinal (resulting in constipation), immune (hypofunction), endocrine, and reproductive (most prominent, hypogonadism). These potential side effects raise concerns about wider prescribing.

The basic principles when prescribing opioids for treatment of NP are to establish treatment goals and convert administration to a long-acting preparation as soon as a stable dose is established. Stabilizing serum levels of drug may help mitigate some side effects. In addition, avoiding short-acting preparations avoids peaks and valleys of drug levels, which could be associated with intermittent mini-withdrawals and associated pain and anxiety. Most importantly, extended-release preparations allow patients to concentrate on nondrug methods of pain management rather than focusing on opioid dosing. A more detailed discussion about opioids is provided in an article elsewhere this issue.

Nonpharmacologic Treatment of Neuropathic Pain

Cognitive-behavioral therapy

No single pharmacologic or invasive intervention eliminates symptoms of NP completely; management approaches commonly involve the application of varied treatment strategies in an effort to alleviate symptoms. Goals of therapy include not only reduced pain but also improved physical function, diminished psychological distress, and heightened overall quality of life. It is imperative for physicians to explain these goals to patients, establish appropriate expectations for treatment, and engage patients as active participants in treatment. It is further critical that patients understand the benefits of multidisciplinary treatment, facilitating acceptance of and active participation in this varied approach. Patients treated in multidisciplinary pain centers have been shown to have decreased use of opioids, reduced pain intensity, and improved health-related quality of life compared with patients managed by general practitioners even when adhering to a pain management plan delineated by a pain specialist.[41] Psychology, neurology, physical therapy, occupational therapy, and social support all play an important role in the ultimate outcome of patients with chronic pain.

Addressing the psychological component of chronic NP is central to success. Providers can help patients by focusing on well behavior, functionality, and normal participation in activities. Pain catastrophizing, that is, exaggerating the degree and effect of pain experienced, is a recognized predictor of poor response to pharmacotherapy and greater likelihood of discontinuation of treatment; catastrophizing also predicts longer duration of pain, greater disability, and poorer quality of life.[42] Cognitive behavioral therapy directly addresses this maladaptive behavior, helping patients change thoughts and emotions through training in coping skills and/or conscious confrontation of deleterious thoughts and behaviors.[43] Cognitive behavioral therapy has been shown to provide benefit in patients with HIV-related peripheral neuropathy, improving pain and reducing pain-related interference with functioning in these patients.[44] Furthermore, multidisciplinary cognitive behavioral programs have been shown to provide a durable improvement in coping, pain intensity, pain related behavior, anxiety, and participation for patients suffering with chronic neuropathic spinal cord injury pain.[45]

Support groups
Support groups serve as an outlet for patients and facilitate patient engagement in the treatment strategy. Interacting with other patients suffering in similar ways allows patients to share coping techniques and should provide a supportive environment for positive reinforcement to encourage improved functioning. Psychoeducational wellness programs that increase awareness of social, intellectual, emotional, and spiritual factors are effective in improving the overall quality of life and well-being of individuals with pain from multiple sclerosis.[46]

Physical therapy modalities and other methods of active engagement
NP often leads to decreased physical activity and functionality. Diabetic neuropathy, for example, can limit activity due to numbness of the feet. Other NP conditions may lead to loss of function due to guarding and avoidance behaviors. Effective treatment must target both improvement in symptoms and functional restoration and mobilization. A multidisciplinary approach to diabetic neuropathy is important in treating ulcers, contractures, and loss of sensation. Exercise training can improve perceived functional limitations, blood glucose regulation, and muscle strength in patients with diabetic neuropathy.[47] Transcutaneous electrical nerve stimulation (TENS), a treatment modality commonly used by physical therapists, may be applied to improve chronic NP, including that of painful diabetic neuropathy.[48] Physical therapy for functional restoration is also generally accepted as the most important treatment of CRPS.

Other methods of physical engagement include tai chi and yoga. Tai chi has proved beneficial for many chronic pain conditions. A major benefit to tai chi is that it empowers patients, requiring that they take an active role in their outcome. Tai chi improves hemoglobin A_{1C} and plantar sensation in patients with diabetic peripheral neuropathy.[49] In addition, yoga has been shown to improve glycemic control and nerve function in patients with diabetic neuropathy.[50]

Interventional nerve blocks for neuropathic pain
The entire extent of the human body receives sensory innervation and, therefore, NP involving a specific dermatomal distribution may be amenable to targeted blockade of the implicated nerve supply. In general, these nerve block techniques should be reserved for patients who fail more conservative therapies due to increased risks of infection, bleeding, potential nerve damage, and other risks associated with interventional techniques. In general, these risks are low, especially in the case of peripheral blocks, and should be performed by physicians with sufficient training and experience.

Peripheral nerve blocks for peripheral neuralgias and trigeminal neuralgia
Peripheral nerve blocks with local anesthetics and steroids are a useful tool for the treatment of many peripheral neuralgias. NP of the face and head, including occipital neuralgia and supraorbital or supratrochlear neuralgia, is easily targeted using anatomic landmarks and simple nerve blocks with low risks of adverse events. Chronic neuralgias of the trunk or limbs, such as inguinal neuralgia and meralgia paresthetica, are similarly easily targeted.

Intercostal neuralgia and chronic NP after trauma or mastectomy may respond to intercostal nerve blocks. Patients with pain due to PHN may also benefit from intercostal nerve blocks. Although it is possible to perform intercostal nerve blocks using anatomic landmarks, risks are lowered by the use of image guidance, either with ultrasound or fluoroscopy.

Pain due to TN or PHN may be mitigated with gasserian ganglion blockade. This nerve block may be performed via needle insertion through the cheek to inject local anesthetic onto the gasserian ganglion in the foramen ovale. This approach has the associated risk of total spinal anesthesia via local anesthetic, facial swelling or bruising from vessel trauma, or meningitis. Another approach to treating TN is sphenopalatine galnglion block through intranasal local anesthetic. In this approach, local anesthetic accesses the ganglion by diffusing through the nasal mucosa. Risks of the latter approach are minimal, because this is a topical application through a needleless technique.

Sympathetic nerve blocks for complex regional pain syndrome

Sympathetic blockade is one component applied within a multimodal approach that may benefit NP in patients with CRPS. Sympathetic blockade for the treatment of CRPS aims to improve pain and range of motion to facilitate full participation in physical therapy. The most common sympathetic blocks performed for patients with CRPS are stellate ganglion blocks and lumbar sympathetic blocks for upper extremity and lower extremity CRPS, respectively. Thoracic sympathetic block has also been shown to improve pain and depression scores in patients with chronic NP due to CRPS type I of the upper extremities.[51] Although frequently effective, not all patients with CRPS types I and II respond favorably to sympathetic blocks. Some patients with CRPS type I in particular may experience transient increases in pain. Some clinical features, such as allodynia and hypoesthesia, may help predict which patients will not benefit from sympathetic blockade.[52] It is reasonable to apply this interventional approach in an attempt to improve functionality, but it should be repeated only if effective.

Epidural steroid injections for radiculopathy

Epidural steroid injections are a well-established interventional treatment of patients with neuropathic radicular pain. Intralaminar, caudal, and transforaminal epidural steroid injections of the cervical, thoracic, or lumbar spine may provide relief of radicular NP.[53] There is moderate evidence for cervical and lumbar tranasforaminal epidural steroid injections and caudal epidural steroid injections for long-term improvement in nerve root pain.[54] Extreme caution should be taken when performing cervical transforaminal epidural steroid injections given the high risk of devastating neurologic complications and recent warnings issued by the FDA regarding this technique. The authors advocate for using nonparticulate steroids when performing transforaminal injections at any spinal level due to evidence suggesting the risk of infarct is lower with these preparations than particulate ones[55] and careful selection of both patients and performing providers when considering cervical transforaminal interventions specifically.

Potential complications Interventional techniques are only one tool in a multifaceted multidisciplinary approach and rarely are solely effective at eradicating NP. The selection of an interventional approach to the treatment of NP should be weighed against potential risks and in general reserved for patients who have failed to benefit from more conservative treatments. Risks of nerve blocks range from simply lack of benefit or temporary exacerbation of pain to frank nerve, vascular, or organ injury either through needle trauma or bleeding. Another risk of both peripheral and sympathetic nerve blocks is local anesthetic toxicity. Thorough training and proper use of image guidance can decrease but not eliminate risks—intercostal nerve blocks risk pneumothorax, lumbar sympathetic nerve blocks can cause hypotension, and stellate ganglion blocks incur added risks of potential seizure, stroke, or temporary respiratory paralysis due to the proximal location of the spinal artery as well as cervical intrathecal space.

In addition to expected side effects of steroids, such as elevated blood sugar, osteoporosis, osteonecrosis, and adrenal suppression, epidural steroid injections also carry rare potential risk of paralysis, stroke, and death. The FDA in 2014 began requiring a warning label on injectable corticosteroids describing risks of rare but serious adverse events, including loss of vision, stroke, paralysis, and death.

Neurolysis

One major drawback to nerve blockade with local anesthetics is that it is often a temporary solution. Typically, nerve blocks provide weeks to several months of pain relief at best. In most patients, a more long-term solution is desirable. Neurolysis with conventional radiofrequency (RF) or chemical agents can offer a more durable benefit. Ultimately, the risks associated with neurolysis, including potential for worsening of NP, limit its applicability in the chronic noncancer pain population. In this population, application of pulsed RF (PRF) treatment offers an effective, viable option.

Pulsed Radiofrequency Treatment of Neuropathic Noncancer Pain

Treatment with PRF uses intermittent high-frequency current to apply lower temperatures (<42°C) to nerves. PRF is a safer option than conventional continuous high-temperature RF ablation or chemical neurolysis in that by maintaining temperatures below 42°C, nerves are not actually coagulated and the potential for neuronal damage is minimized.[56] PRF is often selected in the treatment of noncancer pain due to this safety profile. It is also an appealing option for peripheral nerves that risk painful neuritis as a possible complication from standard continuous RF ablation or chemical neurolysis. In addition, peripheral nerves with motor components can be safely treated with PRF without affecting motor function whereas conventional RF ablation certainly results in paresis. One drawback to PRF is that the durability of effect is somewhat limited. Typically, PRF provides pain relief lasting up to 4 months compared with approximately 12 months for conventional RF ablation. Another drawback to PRF is that it is considered investigational and not payable by many insurance carriers, including Medicare and Medicaid. Pulsed RF is beneficial in peripheral nerves, including treatment of chronic occipital neuralgia.[57] PRF applied to the dorsal root ganglion improves pain due to radiculopathy.[58]

Radiofrequency ablation and neurolytics for cancer pain of sympathetic ganglia

Ablation with conventional RF or chemical neurolysis may be applied to the sympathetic ganglia to treat intractable NP or other cancer-related pain. Alcohol, glycerol, or phenol applied to sympathetic ganglia can ameliorate regional pain. For patients treated with palliative intent, relief from debilitating pain with neurolytic sympathetic blockade can significantly improve quality of life.[59] This is a valid approach in several clinical settings, with neurolysis of the celiac or splanchnic plexus, lumbar sympathetic plexus, and superior hypogastric plexus targeting abdominal pain, lower extremity pain, and pelvic pain, respectively. RF ablation or chemical neurolysis of the gasserian ganglion may also be applied to treat intractable debilitating TN.

Potential complications Conventional continuous high temperature RF ablation applies therapeutic temperatures of 80°C in an effort to coagulate nerves. This temperature, if misapplied to tissues or nerves not intended as targets, can cause paralysis of motor nerves or painful neuralgias due to neuroma formation. Chemical neurolysis of sympathetic ganglia is typically reserved for refractory cancer pain due to the inherent risks of the procedure. Because chemical neurolytics are liquids, they may spread in the body to other local tissues, nerves, or blood vessels. Possible side effects ultimately include paralysis or painful neuritis.

Spinal cord and pripheral nerve stimulation
Dorsal column spinal cord stimulation (SCS) is approved for the treatment of chronic refractory pain of the body or limbs, intractable low back pain and leg pain, and pain associated with failed back surgery syndrome. SCS improves health-related quality of life and provides better pain relief than conventional medical management for selected patients with NP due to failed back surgery syndrome.[60]

SCS should be considered for patients with neuropathic radicular pain from failed back surgery syndrome as well as patients with CRPS who have failed more conservative treatments.[61] SCS may also be considered for patients with traumatic and brachial plexus neuropathy.[61] Stimulation of the dorsal root ganglion can also reduce chronic pain.[62]

Potential complications Potential complications of SCS include ineffective pain control, discomfort at the generator site, overstimulation, migration of leads causing both inadequate stimulation over painful sites and unintended stimulation over nonpainful areas, infection, dural puncture, cerebrospinal fluid leak, or device malfunction requiring surgical removal or repositioning. Historically, presence of an implanted SCS precluded MRI scanning of the patient. There are now some exceptions, however, that allow MRI scanning.

Intrathecal drug delivery
Intrathecal delivery of analgesic medication is a technique typically reserved for patients with chronic malignant and nonmalignant pain that is refractory to more conservative measures. Recent guidelines on intrathecal drug delivery identify several different types of medications that are recommended for the treatment of NP both through clinical experience and experimental evidence, when available.[63] Ziconotide, a voltage-gated calcium channel antagonist isolated from the cone snail, is one of the few intrathecal medications with an FDA indication for the treatment of pain and has demonstrated efficacy for NP.[64–66]

Acupuncture and other methods of integrative medicine
Complementary and integrative medicine (CIM) includes nonconventional treatments, such as acupuncture, meditation, massage, cupping, movement therapies, and relaxation techniques, that may be used in conjunction with or in place of other medical treatments. CAM therapy has been shown effective in reducing chronic PHN pain.[67]

Acupuncture can improve diabetic peripheral neuropathy.[68] Electroacupuncture has been shown to modulate NP by stimulating spinal opioid receptors, activating spinal norepinephrine α_2-adrenoceptors and serotonin 5-HT$_{1A}$ receptors and inhibiting nerve injury–induced GluN1 expression in the spinal cord.[69] Furthermore, electroacupuncture decreases spinal levels of the excitatory amino acids glutamate, aspartate, and glutamine and increases spinal levels of inhibitory amino acids glycine, γ-aminobutyric acid, and taurine.[69,70]

Whole-body vibration therapy has been shown to improve diabetic NP.[71] Reflexology has been shown to improve paresthesias.[72]

Potential complications In general, CIM treatments, including acupuncture, are low-risk measures that can provide substantial relief in certain patients. Often, they are supplementary and may not provide complete relief of pain. Rarely, acupuncture may cause perforation of blood vessels, pneumothorax, or organ puncture depending on location and depth of needle placement. Spinal hematoma is a rare complication reported in the literature after muscle needling.[73]

SUMMARY

NP is complex and dynamic in presentation and its underlying mechanisms are still being investigated. Despite this complexity and lack of full understanding, modern principles of multidisciplinary and multimodal approach still can and do provide reasonable degree of pain relief to a majority of patients suffering from NP.

REFERENCES

1. Treede RD, Jensen TS, Campbell JN, et al. Neuropathic pain: redefinition and a grading system for clinical and research purposes. Neurology 2008;70(18): 1630–5.
2. Jones RC, Backonja MM. Review of neuropathic pain screening and assessment tools. Curr Pain Headache Rep 2013;17(9):363.
3. Gauffin J, Hankama T, Kautiainen H, et al. Neuropathic pain and use of PainDETECT in patients with fibromyalgia: a cohort study. BMC Neurol 2013;13:21.
4. Ohtori S, Orita S, Yamashita M, et al. Existence of a neuropathic pain component in patients with osteoarthritis of the knee. Yonsei Med J 2012;53(4):801–5.
5. Bennett M. The LANSS pain scale: the leeds assessment of neuropathic symptoms and signs. Pain 2001;92(1–2):147–57.
6. Krause SJ, Backonja M-M. Development of a neuropathic pain questionnaire. Clin J Pain 2003;19(5):306–14.
7. Scholz J, Mannion RJ, Hord DE, et al. A novel tool for the assessment of pain: validation in low back pain. PLoS Med 2009;6(4):e1000047.
8. Backonja MM, Attal N, Baron R, et al. Value of quantitative sensory testing in neurological and pain disorders: NeuPSIG consensus. Pain 2013;154(9):1807–19.
9. Haanpää M, Attal N, Backonja M, et al. NeuPSIG guidelines on neuropathic pain assessment. Pain 2011;152(1):14–27.
10. Albrecht PJ, Hou Q, Argoff CE, et al. Excessive peptidergic sensory innervation of cutaneous arteriole-venule shunts (AVS) in the palmar glabrous skin of fibromyalgia patients: implications for widespread deep tissue pain and fatigue. Pain Med 2013;14(6):895–915.
11. Liu J, Hao Y, Du M, et al. Quantitative cerebral blood flow mapping and functional connectivity of postherpetic neuralgia pain: a perfusion fMRI study. Pain 2013; 154(1):110–8.
12. Backonja MM, Coe CL, Muller DA, et al. Altered cytokine levels in the blood and cerebrospinal fluid of chronic pain patients. J Neuroimmunol 2008;195(1–2): 157–63.
13. Meng W, Deshmukh HA, van Zuydam NR, et al. A genome-wide association study suggests an association of Chr8p21.3 (GFRA2) with diabetic neuropathic pain. Eur J Pain 2015;19(3):392–9.
14. Finnerup NB, Sindrup SH, Jensen TS. The evidence for pharmacological treatment of neuropathic pain. Pain 2010;150(3):573–81.
15. Dworkin RH, Jensen MP, Gould E, et al. Treatment satisfaction in osteoarthritis and chronic low back pain: the role of pain, physical and emotional functioning, sleep, and adverse events. J Pain 2011;12(4):416–24.
16. Backonja M-M, Irving G, Argoff C. Rational multidrug therapy in the treatment of neuropathic pain. Curr Pain Headache Rep 2006;10(1):34–8.
17. Mao J, Gold MS, Backonja MM. Combination drug therapy for chronic pain: a call for more clinical studies. J Pain 2011;12(2):157–66.
18. Gilron I, Jensen TS, Dickenson AH. Combination pharmacotherapy for management of chronic pain: from bench to bedside. Lancet Neurol 2013;12(11):1084–95.

19. Argoff CE, Cole BE, Fishbain DA, et al. Diabetic peripheral neuropathic pain: clinical and quality-of-life issues. Mayo Clin Proc 2006;81(4 Suppl):S3–11.

20. Galer BS, Rowbotham MC, Perander J, et al. Topical lidocaine patch relieves postherpetic neuralgia more effectively than a vehicle topical patch: results of an enriched enrollment study. Pain 1999;80(3):533–8.

21. Baron R, Mahn F. Types of topical treatment for peripheral neuropathic pain : mechanism of action and indications. Schmerz 2010;24(4):317–25.

22. Backonja M, Wallace MS, Blonsky ER, et al. NGX-4010, a high-concentration capsaicin patch, for the treatment of postherpetic neuralgia: a randomised, double-blind study. Lancet Neurol 2008;7(12):1106–12.

23. Simpson DM, Gazda S, Brown S, et al. Long-term safety of NGX-4010, a high-concentration capsaicin patch, in patients with peripheral neuropathic pain. J Pain Symptom Manage 2010;39(6):1053–64.

24. Irving GA, Backonja MM, Dunteman E, et al. A multicenter, randomized, double-blind, controlled study of NGX-4010, a high-concentration capsaicin patch, for the treatment of postherpetic neuralgia. Pain Med 2011;12(1):99–109.

25. Finnerup NB, Attal N, Haroutounian S, et al. Pharmacotherapy for neuropathic pain in adults: a systematic review and meta-analysis. Lancet Neurol 2015; 14(2):162–73.

26. Brown EA, Schutz SG, Simpson DM. Botulinum toxin for neuropathic pain and spasticity: an overview. Pain Manag 2014;4(2):129–51.

27. Hu Y, Guan X, Fan L, et al. Therapeutic efficacy and safety of botulinum toxin type A in trigeminal neuralgia: a systematic review. J Headache Pain 2013;14:72.

28. Jensen TS, Finnerup NB. Neuropathic pain treatment: a further step forward. Lancet 2009;374(9697):1218–9.

29. Smith SM, Wang AT, Pereira A, et al. Discrepancies between registered and published primary outcome specifications in analgesic trials: ACTTION systematic review and recommendations. Pain 2013;154(12):2769–74.

30. Burke WJ, Grant JM, Selby G. The treatment of trigeminal neuralgia: a clinical trial of carbamazepine. Med J Aust 1965;1(14):494–8.

31. Lana B, Schlick B, Martin S, et al. Differential upregulation in DRG neurons of an alpha2delta-1 splice variant with a lower affinity for gabapentin after peripheral sensory nerve injury. Pain 2014;155(3):522–33.

32. Bril V, England J, Franklin GM, et al. Evidence-based guideline: treatment of painful diabetic neuropathy: report of the American Academy of Neurology, the American Association of Neuromuscular and Electrodiagnostic Medicine, and the American Academy of Physical Medicine and Rehabilitation. Neurology 2011; 76(20):1758–65.

33. Johnson RW, Rice AS. Clinical practice. Postherpetic neuralgia. N Engl J Med 2014;371(16):1526–33.

34. Parsons B, Sanin L, Yang R, et al. Efficacy and safety of pregabalin in patients with spinal cord injury: a pooled analysis. Curr Med Res Opin 2013;29(12):1675–83.

35. Toth C. Substitution of gabapentin therapy with pregabalin therapy in neuropathic pain due to peripheral neuropathy. Pain Med 2010;11(3):456–65.

36. Max MB. Treatment of post-herpetic neuralgia: antidepressants. Ann Neurol 1994;35(Suppl):S50–3.

37. Tremont-Lukats IW, Hutson PR, Backonja MM. A randomized, double-masked, placebo-controlled pilot trial of extended IV lidocaine infusion for relief of ongoing neuropathic pain. Clin J Pain 2006;22(3):266–71.

38. Abrams DI, Jay CA, Shade SB, et al. Cannabis in painful HIV-associated sensory neuropathy: a randomized placebo-controlled trial. Neurology 2007;68(7):515–21.

39. Zajicek JP, Hobart JC, Slade A, et al. Multiple sclerosis and extract of cannabis: results of the MUSEC trial. J Neurol Neurosurg Psychiatr 2012;83(11):1125–32.
40. Ballantyne JC, Mao J. Opioid therapy for chronic pain. N Engl J Med 2003; 349(20):1943–53.
41. Becker N, Sjøgren P, Bech P, et al. Treatment outcome of chronic non-malignant pain patients managed in a danish multidisciplinary pain centre compared to general practice: a randomised controlled trial. Pain 2000;84(2–3):203–11.
42. Toth C, Brady S, Hatfield M. The importance of catastrophizing for successful pharmacological treatment of peripheral neuropathic pain. J Pain Res 2014;7:327.
43. Turk DC, Audette J, Levy RM, et al. Assessment and treatment of psychosocial comorbidities in patients with neuropathic pain. Mayo Clin Proc 2010;85(3 Suppl):S42–50.
44. Evans S, Fishman B, Spielman L, et al. Randomized trial of cognitive behavior therapy versus supportive psychotherapy for HIV-related peripheral neuropathic pain. Psychosomatics 2003;44(1):44–50.
45. Heutink M, Post MW, Luthart P, et al. Long-term outcomes of a multidisciplinary cognitive behavioural programme for coping with chronic neuropathic spinal cord injury pain. J Rehabil Med 2014;46(6):540–5.
46. McGuire KB, Stojanovic-Radic J, Strober L, et al. Development and effectiveness of a psychoeducational wellness program for people with multiple sclerosis: description and outcomes. Int J MS Care 2015;17(1):1–8.
47. Otterman NM, van Schie CHM, van der Schaaf M, et al. An exercise programme for patients with diabetic complications: a study on feasibility and preliminary effectiveness. Diabet Med 2011;28(2):212–7.
48. Kumar D, Marshall HJ. Diabetic peripheral neuropathy: amelioration of pain with transcutaneous electrostimulation. Diabetes Care 1997;20(11):1702–5.
49. Richerson S, Rosendale K. Does Tai Chi improve plantar sensory ability? A pilot study. Diabetes Technol Ther 2007;9(3):276–86.
50. Malhotra V, Singh S, Singh KP, et al. Study of yoga asanas in assessment of pulmonary function in NIDDM patients. Indian J Physiol Pharmacol 2002;46(3):313–20.
51. de Oliveira Rocha R, Teixeira MJ, Yeng LT, et al. Thoracic sympathetic block for the treatment of complex regional pain syndrome type I: a double-blind randomized controlled study. Pain 2014;155(11):2274–81.
52. van Eijs F, Geurts J, van Kleef M, et al. Predictors of pain relieving response to sympathetic blockade in complex regional pain syndrome type 1. Anesthesiology 2012;116(1):113–21.
53. Ackerman WE, Ahmad M. The efficacy of lumbar epidural steroid injections in patients with lumbar disc herniations. Anesth Analg 2007;104(5):1217–22.
54. Abdi S, Datta S, Trescot AM, et al. Epidural steroids in the management of chronic spinal pain: a systematic review. Pain Physician 2007;10(1):185–212.
55. Dawley JD, Moeller-Bertram T, Wallace MS, et al. Intra-arterial injection in the rat brain. Spine 2009;34(16):1638–43.
56. Byrd D, Mackey S. Pulsed radiofrequency for chronic pain. Curr Pain Headache Rep 2008;12(1):37–41.
57. Huang JHY, Galvagno SM, Hameed M, et al. Occipital nerve pulsed radiofrequency treatment: a multi-center study evaluating predictors of outcome. Pain Med 2012;13(4):489–97.
58. van Boxem K, de Meij N, Kessels A, et al. Pulsed radiofrequency for chronic intractable lumbosacral radicular pain: a six-month cohort study. Pain Med 2015;16(6):1155–62.

59. de Oliveira R, Reis dos MP, Prado WA. The effects of early or late neurolytic sympathetic plexus block on the management of abdominal or pelvic cancer pain. Pain 2004;110(1–2):400–8.

60. Kumar K, Taylor RS, Jacques L, et al. Spinal cord stimulation versus conventional medical management for neuropathic pain: a multicentre randomised controlled trial in patients with failed back surgery syndrome. Pain 2007;132(1–2):179–88.

61. Mailis A, Taenzer P. Evidence-based guideline for neuropathic pain interventional treatments: spinal cord stimulation, intravenous infusions, epidural injections and nerve blocks. Pain Res Manag 2012;17(3):150–8.

62. Deer TR, Grigsby E, Weiner RL, et al. A prospective study of dorsal root ganglion stimulation for the relief of chronic pain. Neuromodulation 2013;16(1):67–71.

63. Deer TR, Prager J, Levy R, et al. Polyanalgesic consensus conference 2012: recommendations for the management of pain by intrathecal (intraspinal) drug delivery: report of an interdisciplinary expert panel. Neuromodulation 2012;15(5):436–66.

64. Rauck RL, Wallace MS, Leong MS, et al. A randomized, double-blind, placebo-controlled study of intrathecal ziconotide in adults with severe chronic pain. J Pain Symptom Manage 2006;31(5):393–406.

65. Staats PS, Yearwood T, Charapata SG, et al. Intrathecal ziconotide in the treatment of refractory pain in patients with cancer or AIDS. JAMA 2004;291(1):63–70.

66. Wallace MS, Charapata SG, Fisher R, et al. Intrathecal ziconotide in the treatment of chronic nonmalignant pain: a randomized, double-blind, placebo-controlled clinical trial. Neuromodulation 2006;9(2):75–86.

67. Hui F, Boyle E, Vayda E, et al. A randomized controlled trial of a multifaceted integrated complementary-alternative therapy for chronic herpes zoster-related pain. Altern Med Rev 2012;17(1):57–68.

68. Zhang C, Ma Y-X, Yan Y. Clinical effects of acupuncture for diabetic peripheral neuropathy. J Tradit Chin Med 2010;30(1):13–4.

69. Zhang R, Lao L, Ren K, et al. Mechanisms of acupuncture-electroacupuncture on persistent pain. Anesthesiology 2014;120(2):482–503.

70. Yan LP, Wu XT, Yin ZY, et al. Effect of electroacupuncture on the levels of amino acid neurotransmitters in the spinal cord in rats with chronic constrictive injury. Zhen Ci Yan Jiu 2011;36:353–6.

71. Hong J, Barnes M, Kessler N. Case study: use of vibration therapy in the treatment of diabetic peripheral small fiber neuropathy. J Body Mov Ther 2013;17(2):235–8.

72. Yadav V, Narayanaswami P. Complementary and alternative medical therapies in multiple sclerosis–the American Academy of Neurology guidelines: a commentary. Clin Ther 2014;36(12):1972–8.

73. Ji GY, Oh CH, Choi W-S, et al. Three cases of hemiplegia after cervical paraspinal muscle needling. Spine J 2015;15(3):e9–13.

Acute and Chronic Low Back Pain

 CrossMark

Nathan Patrick, MD, Eric Emanski, MD, Mark A. Knaub, MD*

KEYWORDS

- Acute low back pain • Chronic low back pain • Patient education
- Treatment protocols

KEY POINTS

- Numerous factors put patients at risk for the development of chronic back pain, including age, educational status, psychosocial factors, occupational factors, and obesity.
- Evaluation of patients with back pain includes completing an appropriate history (including red-flag symptoms), performing a comprehensive physical examination, and, in some scenarios, obtaining imaging in the form of plain radiographs and magnetic resonance imaging.
- Treatment of an acute episode of back pain includes relative rest, activity modification, nonsteroidal anti-inflammatories, and physical therapy.
- Patient education is also imperative, as these patients are at risk for further episodes of back pain in the future.
- Chronic back pain (>6 months' duration) develops in a small percentage of patients. Clinicians' ability to diagnose the exact pathologic source of these symptoms is severely limited, making a cure unlikely. Treatment of these patients should be supportive, the goal being to improve pain and function rather than to "cure" the patient's condition.

MAGNITUDE OF THE PROBLEM

Low back pain is an extremely common problem that affects at least 80% of all individuals at some point in their lifetime, and is the fifth most common reason for all physician visits in the United States.[1–3] Approximately 1 in 4 adults in the United States reported having low back pain that lasted at least 24 hours within the previous 3 months, and 7.6% reported at least 1 episode of severe acute low back pain within a 1-year period.[4,5] In addition, low back pain is a leading cause of activity limitation and work absence (second only to upper respiratory conditions) throughout much of the world, resulting in a vast economic burden on individuals, families, communities, industry, and governments.[6–9] In 1998, total incremental direct health care costs attributable to low back pain in the United States were estimated at $26.3 billion.[10]

This article originally appeared in Medical Clinics, Volume 98, Issue 4, July 2014.
Department of Orthopaedic Surgery, Penn State–Milton S. Hershey Medical Center, 30 Hope Drive, Building A, Hershey, PA 17033, USA
* Corresponding author.
E-mail address: mknaub@hmc.psu.edu

Med Clin N Am 100 (2016) 169–181
http://dx.doi.org/10.1016/j.mcna.2015.08.015   **medical.theclinics.com**

Furthermore, indirect costs related to days lost from work are substantial, with nearly 2% of the work force of the United States compensated for back injuries each year.[11]

RISK AND PROGNOSTIC FACTORS

Factors that play a role in the development of back pain include age, educational status, psychosocial factors, job satisfaction, occupational factors, and obesity. Age is one of the most common factors in the development of low back pain, with most studies finding the highest incidence in the third decade of life and overall prevalence increasing until age 60 to 65 years. However, there is recent evidence that prevalence continues to increase with age with more severe forms of back pain.[1,12] Other studies show that back pain in the adolescent population has become increasingly common.[13]

An increased prevalence of low back pain is associated with patients of low educational status.[1] Lower educational levels are a strong predictor of more prolonged episode duration and poorer outcomes.[14] Psychosocial factors such as stress, anxiety, depression, and certain types of pain behavior are associated with greater rates of low back pain. The presence of these conditions also increases the risk that a patient's episode of back pain will last long enough to be considered chronic.[1,15] Likewise, patients who are dissatisfied with their work situation are at risk of having an acute episode of back pain transition to a chronic situation.[16] Occupational factors, specifically the physical demands of work, are also associated with an increased prevalence of low back pain. Matsui and colleagues[17] found the point prevalence of low back pain to be 39% in manual workers, whereas it was found in only 18.3% of those with sedentary occupations. A more recent systematic review found manual handling, bending, twisting, and whole-body vibration to be risk factors for low back pain.[18] Lastly, obesity, or a body mass index of more than 30 kg/m^2, has been connected with an increased incidence of low back pain.[1,19]

PRESENTATION

For most patients, an episode of acute low back pain is a self-limited condition that does not require any active medical treatment.[5] Among those who do seek medical care, their symptoms and disability improve rapidly and most are able to return to work and normal activities within the first month.[20] Up to 1 in 3 of these patients, however, report persistent back pain of at least moderate intensity 1 year after an acute episode, and 1 in 5 reports substantial limitations in activity.[21]

Initial evaluation of patients with back pain should begin with a focused history. Key aspects of this should include: duration of symptoms; description of the pain (location, severity, timing, radiation, and so forth); presence of neurologic symptoms (weakness or alterations in sensation or pain) or changes in bowel and bladder function; evidence of any recent or current infection (fever, chills, sweats, and so forth); previous treatments; and pertinent medical history (cancer, infection, osteoporosis, fractures, endocrine disorders). Key facets of the history are listed in **Box 1**. Some historical facts, referred to by many as red-flag symptoms, may be a harbinger of a dangerous clinical situation (**Box 2**). When present, these symptoms should raise the level of suspicion of the provider that this patient is presenting with more than a simple, benign episode of acute low back pain. In patients presenting with 1 or more of these red flags, there is a 10% chance that they have a serious underlying source of their symptoms of low back pain. These patients should have plain radiographs taken of their lumbar spine to rule out serious structural abnormality. In a patient in whom an infectious cause is considered, plain radiographs may be normal early in the disease process. A white blood cell

---

Box 1
Historical factors that must be considered in the evaluation of a patient with low back pain

Duration

Acute low back pain: less than 4 weeks

Subacute low back pain: 4 weeks to 3 months

Chronic low back pain: more than 3 months

Pain Description

Location (cervical, thoracic, lumbar, sacral)

Severity (pain scale, type of pain, activities affected)

Timing (morning, evening, constant, intermittent)

Aggravating and relieving factors (ambulation/rest, sitting/standing/laying, inclines/declines, back flexion/extension)

Radiation (dermatomal or nondermatomal)

Deficits

Motor weakness

Sensory changes (numbness, tingling, paresthesias, dermatomal or nondermatomal)

Urinary or bowel incontinence, urgency, or frequency

Risk Factors

Age

Educational status

Psychosocial factors

Occupation

Body mass index

Medical History

Cancer

Recent or current infection

Osteoporosis and history of other fractures

Endocrine disorders

Previous spinal surgeries

---

count, erythrocyte sedimentation rate, and C-reactive protein should be obtained. Elevation of these inflammatory parameters should prompt evaluation with magnetic resonance imaging (MRI), with and without contrast, of the lumbar spine.

Patient-completed pain diagrams are useful adjuncts in evaluating patients with acute or chronic low back pain, and are especially useful for those with radicular complaints. Patient outcomes measures such as the Oswestry Disability Index can give insight into how patients' symptoms are affecting their life, and can be useful to track treatment progress.

PHYSICAL EXAMINATION

Physical examination of the patient with low back pain is a necessity during the office visit. The examination should focus on determining the presence and severity of

---

Box 2
Red-flag symptoms

The presence of any of these historical factors in a patient presenting with low back pain may indicate a serious underlying disorder and should prompt a more rapid and thorough evaluation of the patient.

Age >50 years

Systemic symptoms: fever, chills, night sweats, fatigue, decreased appetite, unintentional weight loss

History of malignancy

Nonmechanical pain (pain that gets worse with rest): night pain

Recent or current bacterial infection, especially skin infection or urinary tract infection

Immunosuppression

History of intravenous drug use

Failure of response to initial treatment/therapy

Prolonged corticosteroid use or diagnosis of osteoporosis

Trauma

---

neurologic involvement. At the conclusion of the visit, the clinician should also attempt to place the patient's back pain into 1 of 3 categories: nonspecific low back pain, back pain associated with radiculopathy or spinal stenosis, or back pain associated with a specific spinal cause.[22,23] **Table 1** lists common spinal causes of back pain with associated historical and physical examination findings, in addition to imaging recommendations. Although the physical examination is an essential part of the visit, it rarely provides the clinician with a specific diagnosis for the cause of the patient's symptoms. An examination begins with observation of the patient, typically starting when the clinician enters the examination room and involves noting how the patient acts during the history taking. Visual inspection of the patient's thoracic and lumbar spine, and the posterior pelvis, is accomplished by having the patient in a gown. Assessment for any skin abnormalities or asymmetry around the lumbar spine should be performed. Palpation of the bony elements of the spine and the posterior pelvis in addition to the paraspinal muscles can help localize the patient's complaints. Obvious deformities such as significant scoliosis or a high-grade spondylolisthesis may be discovered with observation and/or palpation in a nonobese patient. Assessment of spinal motion can be difficult in a patient with acute low back pain, but should be attempted. Limitations in specific directions should be noted, as should any worsening of symptoms with specific motions. Unfortunately, the assessment of motion has not proved to be reliable between observers and does not provide the clinician with a specific diagnosis.

A complete neurologic examination is performed, and should include both upper and lower extremity function. Subtle examination findings in the upper extremities, such as hyperreflexia or a positive Hofmann sign, could indicate a more proximal cause (cervical spinal cord compression/dysfunction) of a patient's lower extremity neurologic complaints or bowel/bladder dysfunction. Manual muscle strength testing should be performed of the major muscle groups of the lower extremity to include the myotomes of the lumbar nerve roots (**Table 2**). Muscle strength should be recorded using a scale of 0 to 5 (**Table 3**). Sensory examination should be performed with reference to the lumbar dermatomes (see **Table 2**). Side-to-side comparison of sensation to light touch and pinprick should be performed in all patients. Assessment of proprioception and vibration sense can be included in select patients in whom central processes or lesions are suspected. Patellar and Achilles deep tendon reflexes are helpful in differentiating central nervous system abnormalities (indicated by hyperactive reflexes) from lumbar nerve root or peripheral nerve problems (hypoactive reflexes expected). The presence of a Babinski sign (upward-moving great toe when the plantar-lateral surface of the foot is scraped) should alert the examiner to the probability of a more central issue. Functional muscle strength should be assessed by asking the patient to stand from a seated position without the assistance of the upper extremities (assessing functional strength of quadriceps). Asking the patient to squat from a standing position can also assess the functional strength of the quadriceps. Having the patient stand on the heels and toes can assess the strength of the ankle dorsiflexor and plantarflexor musculature. A single-leg toe raise can be used to diagnose subtle weakness of the gastrocnemius-soleus complex.

Straight-leg raise (SLR) and cross-SLR tests are not useful in patients with complaints of only low back pain. Nearly all patients with low back pain will have an increase in their symptoms with these maneuvers. These tests are helpful in patients with radiating leg pain in an attempt to differentiate true radiculopathy from other causes of leg pain. For an SLR test to be considered positive, the patient must have a reproduction of the radiating leg pain distal to the knee on the side that is being tested. A positive cross-SLR test occurs when the patient's radicular pain below the knee is reproduced while the contralateral leg is extended at the hip and knee. Positive results for the SLR test have high sensitivity (91%; 95% confidence interval [CI] 82%–94%) but is not specific (26%; 95% CI 16%–38%) for identifying a disc herniation. The cross-SLR test is more specific (88%; 95% CI 86%–90%) but not sensitive (29%; CI 24%–34%).[24] Both SLR and cross-SLR tests are designed to evaluate for compression of the lower (L4-S1) lumbar nerve roots. The femoral stretch test is a similar provocative maneuver that aims to create tension in the upper lumbar roots (L2 and L3) in an attempt to reproduce L2 or L3 radicular symptoms in the anterior thigh.

The physical examination must also evaluate for other potential sources of the patient's pain. Nonmusculoskeletal causes of back pain should be considered, as should nonspinal, musculoskeletal causes. A partial list of nonmusculoskeletal abnormalities that may cause back pain is shown in **Box 3**. The sacroiliac (SI) joints and the hips should be examined to assess whether these structures are contributing to a patient's symptoms. Simple internal and external rotation of the hip in either the supine or seated position places the hip joint through a range of motion that will likely reproduce the patient's pain if it is originating in the hip joint. The SI joint can be loaded or stressed with the Patrick test or the FABER test, whereby the patient's hip is placed into flexion, abduction, and external rotation. This test is typically performed with the patient in the supine position and the lower extremity placed into a "figure-4" position. The Patrick test is positive if it reproduces the patient's back pain on the side that is being examined. A positive test, though not diagnostic of an SI joint problem, should at least alert the examiner to the possibility that the SI joint may be contributing to the patient's symptoms.

Psychosocial issues play an important role in both acute and chronic low back pain. Patients with abnormal psychometric profiles are at greater risk for development of chronic back pain. In addition, they are more likely to be functionally affected (or disabled) by their symptoms of back pain. Screening for depression can be performed in an attempt to identify patients who are at risk. Psychological overlay is often found in these patients, which can cloud their physical examination. Assessing for Waddell signs can be useful in determining if there is a nonorganic cause of the patient's symptoms.[25,26] The presence of 1 or more of these findings on examination increases the

Table 1
Common spinal causes of back pain with associated historical factors, physical examination findings, recommended imaging modalities, and any additional diagnostic testing

Etiology	Key Features	Imaging	Additional Studies
Muscle strain	General ache or muscle spasms in the lower back, may radiate to buttock or posterior thighs; worse with increasing activity or bending	None	None
Disc herniation	Pain originating in the lower back with dermatomal radiation to the lower extremity; relieved by standing and worsened with sitting; may be accompanied by motor/sensory changes	Symptoms present <1 mo: none; Symptoms present >1 mo or severe/progressive: MRI	None
Lumbar spondylosis	Generalized back pain worse immediately after waking up; improvement throughout the day; pain fluctuates with activity and may worsen with extension of the spine	Symptoms present <1 mo: plain radiographs	None
Spinal stenosis with neurogenic claudication	Back pain with radiculopathy that is often worsened with extension/standing and improved with flexion/sitting; may be accompanied by motor/sensory changes	Symptoms present <1 mo: none; Symptoms present >1 mo or severe/progressive: MRI	None
Spondylolisthesis	Back pain that may radiate down one or both legs and is exacerbated by flexion and extension; may be accompanied by motor/sensory changes	Symptoms present <1 mo: none; Symptoms >1 mo or severe/progressive: plain radiographs	None
Spondylolysis: stress reaction or stress fracture of pars interarticularis	One of the most common causes of back pain in children and adolescents	Symptoms present <1 mo: none; Symptoms >1 mo or severe/progressive: plain radiographs	None

(continued on next page)

Table 1
(continued)

Etiology	Key Features	Imaging	Additional Studies
Ankylosing spondylitis	More common in young males; morning stiffness; low back pain that often radiates to the buttock and improves with exercise	Anterior-posterior pelvis radiographs	ESR, CRP, HLA-B27
Infection: epidural abscess ± osteomyelitis	Severe pain with an insidious onset that is unrelenting in nature; night pain; presence of constitutional symptoms; history of recent infection; may have radiculopathy or be accompanied by motor/sensory changes	Plain radiographs and MRI	CBC, ESR, CRP
Malignancy	History of cancer with new onset of low back pain; unexplained weight loss; age >50 y; may have radiculopathy or be accompanied by motor/sensory changes	Plain radiographs and MRI	CBC, ESR, CRP, PTH, TSH, SPEP, UA, UPEP
Cauda equina syndrome	Urinary retention or fecal incontinence; decreased rectal tone; saddle anesthesia; may be accompanied by weakness	MRI	None
Conus medullaris syndrome	Same as cauda equina, but often accompanied by upper motor neuron signs (hyperreflexia, clonus, etc)	MRI	None
Vertebral compression fracture	History of osteoporosis or corticosteroid use; older age	Plain radiographs	1,25-Dihydroxyvitamin D_3
Trauma	Variable examination pending the severity of the injury; may be accompanied by motor/sensory changes	Lumbosacral radiographs, CT, ± MRI	None

Abbreviations: CBC, complete blood count; CRP, C-reactive protein; CT, computed tomography; ESR, erythrocyte sedimentation rate; HLA-B27, human leukocyte antigen B27; MRI, magnetic resonance imaging; PTH, parathyroid hormone; SPEP, serum protein electrophoresis; TSH, thyroid-stimulating hormone; UA, urinalysis; UPEP, urine protein electrophoresis.

Table 2			
Lower extremity myotomes, dermatomes, and reflexes by lumbar nerve root			
Lumbar Nerve Root	Muscle Group	Sensory Distribution	Deep Tendon Reflex
L2	Hip flexor	Anterior medial thigh	None
L3	Quadriceps	Anterior thigh to knee	Patellar
L4	Anterior tibialis	Medial calf/ankle	Patellar
L5	Extensor hallicus longus	Lateral ankle/dorsum of foot	None
S1	Gastrocnemius/soleus/peroneals	Plantar-lateral foot	Achilles

possibility that the patient has a nonstructural source of the symptoms (**Box 4**). As a word of caution, the presence of Waddell signs does not exclude an organic cause of low back pain; rather, it points to the need for further psychological evaluation of the patient.

IMAGING

Evidenced-based treatment guidelines have long established that most patients presenting with an episode of acute low back pain do not need any imaging. Most of these patients will have improvement in their clinical symptoms within a few days to a week, even in the absence of any active treatment. In addition, imaging (including MRI) is not likely to reveal an exact pathologic diagnosis in the most patients. Overutilization of imaging in the evaluation of acute low back pain leads to increased health care expenditures in a patient population that will likely improve on its own. In addition, imaging in these patients frequently leads to the diagnosis of degenerative disc disease, which allows the patient to adopt the sick role. The thought that one has a "disease" leads the patient to change his or her behavior, and many begin to exhibit fear-avoidance behavior. This term refers to patients' fear that they are going to do something that will injury or worsen their "diseased" back; therefore they decrease their physical activity, which culminates in being detrimental to their recovery. The preferred approach is to reassure patients that they will likely get better without any active medical intervention and that imaging, including MRI, will not reveal an exact pathologic diagnosis in most patients.

Imaging is indicated in patients who present with red-flag symptoms or in those whose symptoms persist despite 4 to 6 weeks of conservative treatment. Standing plain radiographs of the lumbar spine are the initial imaging modality of choice. Though not likely to reveal the exact pathologic cause of a patient's symptoms, these

Table 3	
Grading system for muscle power on manual muscle strength testing	
Grade	Description
0	No contraction
1	Muscle flicker/twitch
2	Able to fire muscle with gravity removed
3	Able to fire muscle against force of gravity
4	Able to fire muscle against some resistance
5	Normal strength against resistance

Box 3
Nonmusculoskeletal causes of back pain

Nonmusculoskeletal causes of pain must be considered in patients being evaluated for back pain.

Genitourinary

  Nephrolithiasis

  Pyelonephritis

  Prostatitis

  Endometriosis

  Ovarian cysts

Gastrointestinal

  Esophagitis

  Gastritis and peptic ulcer disease

  Cholelithiasis and cholecystitis

  Pancreatitis

  Diverticulitis

  Other intra-abdominal infections

Cardiovascular

  Abdominal or thoracic aortic aneurysm

  Cardiac ischemia or myocardial infarction

Neurologic

  Intramedullary spinal cord tumors

---

images will rule out troubling disorder such as fracture, tumor, or infection. With these diagnoses largely excluded with plain radiographs, most patients with low back pain do not require further imaging. MRI should be used in patients with neurologic complaints or in those for whom the clinician has a high level of suspicion for an occult

---

Box 4
Signs of nonorganic abnormality

Waddell's signs, when present, can indicate a psychological component of chronic low back pain.

Tenderness tests: superficial and/or diffuse tenderness and/or nonanatomic tenderness

Simulation tests: based on movements, which produce pain, without actually causing that movement, such as axial loading on the top of the head causing low back pain and pain on simulated lumbar spine rotation

Distraction tests: positive tests are rechecked when the patient's attention is distracted, such as a straight leg raise test with the patient in a seated position

Regional disturbances: regional strength or sensory changes that do not follow accepted neuroanatomy

Overreaction: subjective signs regarding the patient's demeanor and overreaction to testing

From Waddell G, McCulloch J, Kummel E, et al. Nonorganic physical signs in low-back pain. Spine 1980;5:117–25.

fracture, tumor, or early infection. MRI is a highly sensitive imaging modality, but lacks specificity when a patient's complaint is axial pain. Degenerative changes are found in many asymptomatic subjects, and these changes increase in frequency with increasing age. Therefore, it is impossible to attribute a patient's back pain to a degenerative disc or an arthritic facet joint, given that they are present in most asymptomatic subjects.

Other imaging modalities that are used in patients with back pain include computed tomography, myelography, and bone scans. The indications for these tests are limited and fall outside the scope of this article. Provocative lumbar discography is a highly debated topic within the community of spine care providers. The senior author believes that discography has poor positive predictive value for successful surgical outcomes when it is used to determine whether a patient is a candidate for surgical intervention for axial low back pain. As a result, discography is not used during the evaluation of patients with chronic low back pain. Other spine surgeons routinely use discography to determine if a patient is a candidate for spinal fusion for "discogenic" low back pain, and many patients agree to have this diagnostic test performed and subsequently undergo spinal fusion in an attempt to improve their axial low back pain. Successful outcomes occur in only 40% to 60% of patients undergoing this type of procedure. Because of these poor results, the senior author does not perform spinal fusion procedures on patients with isolated low back pain and only degenerative changes on imaging.

TREATMENT

An exhaustive discussion of the treatment options available for acute and chronic low back pain is beyond the scope of this article. Most acute episodes of low back pain will resolve within 6 to 8 weeks even in the absence of active treatment. Relative rest, activity modification, nonsteroidal anti-inflammatory drugs (NSAIDs), chiropractic manipulation, and physical therapy are all treatment options in the acute and subacute phase of this clinical syndrome. These treatment modalities probably do not result in a significant change in the natural history of the condition, but do provide the patient with some active treatment modalities while the episode runs its natural course. Initial management of an episode of low back pain should include relative rest, cessation of pain-provoking activities, and a limited course of medications. NSAIDs, acetaminophen, tramadol, muscle relaxants, antidepressants, and opioids are frequently used in the treatment of both acute and chronic back pain. In patients with chronic axial pain, the use of simple analgesics, such as acetaminophen or tramadol, in combination with an antidepressant, appears to have the greatest efficacy.[27] Long-term opioid use for the treatment of chronic low back pain appears to be safe but only modestly effective in this patient group. These patients have only small functional improvements from the use of the medication, and are at risk for the adverse effects of opioid use including central nervous system depression, constipation, development of tolerance, and aberrant behavior. NSAIDs are perhaps the most commonly used single class of medications for back pain symptoms. NSAIDs are as effective as other medication classes but harbor the potential for gastrointestinal side effects. Their safety for long-term use in the setting of hypertension and/or cardiovascular disease has been questioned.

Adjunctive treatment options include physical therapy, a period of immobilization, and local treatment modalities that may include heat, ice, ultrasound, massage, and transcutaneous electrical nerve stimulation. Alternative treatment options may include spinal manipulation, acupuncture, yoga, and other exercise-based therapy programs.

These alternative therapies lack conclusive scientific evidence supporting their efficacy in the treatment of acute or chronic back pain. Despite this, there are patients who pursue these options, and many benefit to at least some extent. Physical therapy or exercise-based programs tend to focus on core muscle strengthening and aerobic conditioning. No differences have been found when comparing the effectiveness of supervised with home-based exercise programs.

Spinal injections have a limited role in the treatment of chronic, mechanical low back pain. There is some evidence that intralaminar epidural steroid injections may play a small role in the short-term treatment of this patient population. Some patients may also benefit from facet injections or facet blocks when other conservative treatment modalities have been exhausted.

For those unfortunate few who fail to improve and fall into the category of chronic back pain, modern medicine has failed to provide any effective treatments. Despite many advances in medicine, clinicians' ability to diagnose the exact source of a patient's axial back pain is extremely limited. Therefore, our ability to treat this clinical entity is poor. Many surgeons believe that there are some patients who suffer from chronic back pain who would improve with surgical treatment of their symptoms. The problem lies in our inability to determine which individual patient will benefit from surgery and which will be left with ongoing pain and disability. The goals of treatment for these patients should move away from a "cure" and focus on lessening symptoms and the effects they have on the patient, in addition to improving function.

SUMMARY

Back pain is an extremely common presenting complaint that occurs in upward of 80% of persons. The natural history of acute episodes of back pain is favorable in most patients. Numerous factors put patients at risk for the development of chronic back pain, including age, educational status, psychosocial factors, occupational factors, and obesity. Evaluation of these patients includes completing an appropriate history (including red-flag symptoms), performing a comprehensive physical examination, and, in some scenarios, obtaining imaging in the form of plain radiographs and MRI. Treatment of an acute episode of back pain includes relative rest, activity modification, NSAIDs, and physical therapy. Patient education is also imperative, as these patients are at risk for further episodes of back pain in the future. Chronic back pain (>6 months' duration) develops in a small percentage of patients. Clinicians' ability to diagnose the exact pathologic source of these symptoms is severely limited, making a cure unlikely. Treatment of these patients should be supportive, the goal being to improve pain and function rather than to "cure" the patient's condition.

REFERENCES

1. Hoy D, Brooks P, Blyth F, et al. The epidemiology of low back pain. Best Pract Res Clin Rheumatol 2010;24:769–81.
2. Chou R, Qaseem A, Snow V, et al, Clinical efficacy assessment Subcommittee of the American College of Physicians, American College of Physicians, American Pain Society Low Back Pain Guidelines Panel. Diagnosis and treatment of low back pain: a joint clinical practice guideline from the American College of Physicians and the American Pain Society. Ann Intern Med 2007;147(7):478–91.
3. Hart LG, Deyo RA, Cherkin DC. Physician office visits for low back pain. Frequency, clinical evaluation, and treatment patterns from a U.S. National Survey. Spine 1995;20:11–9.

4. Deyo RA, Mirza SK, Martin BI. Back pain prevalence and visit rates: estimates from U.S. national surveys, 2002. Spine 2006;31:2724–7.

5. Carey TS, Evans AT, Hadler NM, et al. Acute severe low back pain. A population-based study of prevalence and care-seeking. Spine 1996;21:339–44.

6. Lidgren L. The bone and joint decade 2000-2010. Bull World Health Organ 2003; 81(9):629.

7. Steenstra IA, Verbeek JH, Heymans MW, et al. Prognostic factors for duration of sick leave in patients sick listed with acute low back pain: a systematic review of the literature. Occup Environ Med 2005;62(12):851–60.

8. Kent PM, Keating JL. The epidemiology of low back pain in primary care. Chiropr Osteopat 2005;13:13.

9. Thelin A, Holmberg S, Thelin N. Functioning in neck and low back pain from a 12-year perspective: a prospective population-based study. J Rehabil Med 2008; 40(7):555–61.

10. Luo X, Pietrobon R, Sun SX, et al. Estimates and patterns of direct health care expenditures among individuals with back pain in the United States. Spine 2004;29: 79–86.

11. Andersson GB. Epidemiological features of chronic low-back pain. Lancet 1999; 354:581–5.

12. Dionne CE, Dunn KM, Croft PR. Does back pain prevalence really decrease with increasing age? A systematic review. Age Ageing 2006;35(3):229–34.

13. Jeffries LJ, Milanese SF, Grimmer-Somers KA. Epidemiology of adolescent spinal pain: a systematic overview of the research literature. Spine 2007;32(23): 2630–7.

14. Dionne CE, Von Korff M, Koepsell TD, et al. Formal education and back pain: a review. J Epidemiol Community Health 2001;55(7):455–68.

15. Linton SJ. A review of psychological risk factors in back and neck pain. Spine 2000;25(9):1148–56.

16. van Tulder M, Koes B, Bombardier C. Low back pain. Best practice & research. Clin Rheumatol 2002;16(5):761–75.

17. Matsui H, Maeda A, Tsuji H, et al. Risk indicators of low back pain among workers in Japan: association of familial and physical factors with low back pain. Spine 1997;22(11):1242–8.

18. Hoogendoorn WE, van Poppel MN, Bongers PM, et al. Systematic review of psychosocial factors at work and private life as risk factors for back pain. Spine 2000; 25(16):2114–25.

19. Webb R, Brammah T, Lunt M, et al. Prevalence and predictors of intense, chronic, and disabling neck and back pain in the UK general population. Spine 2003; 28(11):1195–202.

20. Pengel LH, Herbert RD, Maher CG, et al. Acute low back pain: systematic review of its prognosis. BMJ 2003;327:323.

21. Von Korff M, Saunders K. The course of back pain in primary care. Spine 1996; 21:2833–7 [discussion: 2838–9].

22. Deyo RA, Rainville J, Kent DL. What can the history and physical examination tell us about low back pain? JAMA 1992;268:760–5.

23. Bigos S, Bowyer O, Braen G, et al. Acute low back problems in adults. Clinical practice guideline No. 14. AHCPR Publication No. 95–0642. Rockville (MD): Agency for Health Care Policy and Research, Public Health Service, U.S. Department of Health and Human Services; 1994.

24. Devillé WL, van der Windt DA, Dzaferagić A, et al. The test of Lasègue: systematic review of the accuracy in diagnosing herniated discs. Spine 2000;25:1140–7.

25. Waddell G, McCullock JA, Kummel E, et al. Nonorganic physical signs in low-back pain. Spine 1980;5(2):117–25.
26. Hoppenfeld S. Physical examination of the spine and extremities. Norwalk (CT): Appleton-Century-Crofts; 1976. p. 164–229.
27. Malanga G, Wolff E. Evidence-informed management of chronic low back pain with nonsteroidal anti-inflammatory drugs, muscle relaxants, and simple analgesics. Spine J 2008;8(1):173–84.

Managing Chronic Pain in Special Populations with Emphasis on Pediatric, Geriatric, and Drug Abuser Populations

CrossMark

Kyle M. Baumbauer, PhD[a,b,c], Erin E. Young, PhD[a,c,d],
Angela R. Starkweather, PhD, ANCP-BC, CNRN, FAAN[a],
Jessica W. Guite, PhD[e,f,g,h], Beth S. Russell, PhD[i],
Renee C.B. Manworren, PhD, APRN, BC, PCNS-BC[a,e,h],*

KEYWORDS

- Chronic pain • Pain management • Multimodal treatment • Pediatric pain
- Geriatric pain

KEY POINTS

- The developmental status and genetic background of the patient should be considered during chronic pain treatment.
- Pediatric patients, geriatric patients, and patients who are drug abusers have unique demands for pain management.
- A multimodal treatment approach should be used for pain management.

INTRODUCTION

Pain serves as an evolutionarily adaptive tool to warn of tissue damage and allow for subsequent tissue repair. For unknown reasons, in some individuals the normally adaptive pain system is hijacked and chronic pain ensues. Numerous laboratories

[a] School of Nursing, The Center for Advancing Management of Pain, University of Connecticut, Storrs, CT 06269-4026, USA; [b] Department of Neuroscience, University of Connecticut Health Center, 263 Farmington Ave, Farmington, CT 06030, USA; [c] Institute for Systems Genomics, University of Connecticut Health Center, 400 Farmington Ave, CT 06030, USA; [d] Department of Genetics and Genome Sciences, University of Connecticut Health Center, 400 Farmington Ave, Farmington, CT 06030, USA; [e] Department of Pediatrics, University of Connecticut School of Medicine, 236 Farmington Ave, Farmington, CT 06030, USA; [f] Children's Center for Community Research (C3R), 12 Charter Oak Place, Hartford, CT 06106, USA; [g] Pediatric Psychology, Hartford Hospital/The Institute of Living, 100 Retreat, Suite 515, Hartford, CT 06106, USA; [h] Division of Pain and Palliative Medicine, Connecticut Children's Medical Center, 282 Washington St, Hartford, CT 06106, USA; [i] Human Development & Family Studies, University of Connecticut, 368 Mansfield Rd, Storrs, CT 06269-1058, USA
* Corresponding author. Division of Pain and Palliative Medicine, Department of Pediatrics, Connecticut Children's Medical Center, 282 Washington St, Hartford, CT 06106.
E-mail address: Rmanworren@connecticutchildrens.org

Med Clin N Am 100 (2016) 183–197
http://dx.doi.org/10.1016/j.mcna.2015.08.013
0025-7125/16/$ – see front matter © 2016 Elsevier Inc. All rights reserved.
medical.theclinics.com

are currently examining the neural and nonneural mechanisms that both initiate and support the persistence of pain in human and nonhuman models. Meanwhile, clinicians face the daunting task of treating patients with chronic pain based on incomplete information regarding the causative mechanisms and limiting options to facilitate resolution of pain. Multimodal treatment plans involve the use of analgesics that target the pharmacologic mechanisms underlying analgesia and nociception in conjunction with psychological and physical therapy. Although research indicates that these interventions reduce pain and improve function, a significant number of patients continue to have pain. Moreover, health care professionals face growing frustration in treating patients with chronic pain, largely because of the challenges involved in establishing personalized pain management strategies for those at greatest need. Identifying those individuals at the greatest risk for developing treatment-resistant chronic pain may lead to the development of novel strategies to mitigate suffering and disability.

The incidence of chronic pain is 20% to 25% worldwide and less than half of patients report experiencing adequate relief.[1] This prevalence can be substantially higher in the most vulnerable populations. For example, pediatric and geriatric patients are particularly susceptible to the development of chronic pain, as are individuals who are prone to substance abuse. This article highlights potential mechanisms of vulnerability for chronic pain during periods in which this risk may be most readily revealed: the extremes of age (ie, pediatrics and geriatrics). It proposes psychosocial, physiologic, and genetic mechanisms that may contribute to chronic pain susceptibility, and describes unique strategies for managing pain in geriatric and pediatric patients.

PEDIATRIC CHRONIC PAIN

Although chronic pain diagnoses are less frequent in pediatric compared with adult populations, their prevention and management may influence lifelong health outcomes. Chronic pediatric pain can have debilitating medical, emotional, social, functional, and economic consequences for youth and their families.[2–6] Up to 40% report significant effects on school attendance, social engagement, appetite, sleep, and health service use, which can continue into adulthood.[7–11] Moreover, periods of rapid development may represent times of enhanced vulnerability for chronic pain. Research from both human and animal models indicates that early life pain exposure may alter neurodevelopment and increase the likelihood of long-term, maladaptive changes on neurally mediated behaviors (eg, pain, cognition, social interactions, and emotional experiences).[12] Pediatric chronic pain prevalence estimates vary by pain location, with a high degree of variability in both location and prevalence of pain.[13] For example, headache is most prevalent and is reported in 8% to 83% of children, followed by abdominal pain (4%–53%), musculoskeletal pain (4%–40%), and back pain (14%–24%).

Children as young as 3 years of age may be able to provide a self-report of pain intensity with simple developmentally appropriate and validated tools.[14] When elicited, children and adolescents with chronic pain commonly report moderate to severe pain intensity, which often is much greater than expected. This discordance reflects the attenuation of overt behavioral signs of pain as pain becomes chronic. Social cues may trigger pediatric patients' behavioral expressions of pain, but there are no reliable or recommended observational measures of pediatric chronic pain.[14–17] By consensus, pediatric pain management experts recommend assessment of pain intensity, physical functioning, emotional functioning, role functioning, symptoms, and adverse events related to treatment and pain, global judgment of satisfaction with treatment, and sleep.[15] Obtaining self-report pain intensity ratings over time may be more valuable than single ratings and both paper and electronic pain diaries have been tested for developmental appropriateness and validity in children as young as 6 years.[15] At least 2 measures of physical functioning have been validated for children and adolescents with chronic pain: the Functional Disability Inventory[18,19] and the PedsQL.[20] The PedsQL is also a valid measure of emotional, social, and school functioning for children 2 to 18 years of age.[15] There are several other well-validated measures for emotional function, such as the Children's Depressive Inventory and the Revised Child Anxiety and Depression Scale. Role functioning can be assessed by school attendance and with the Pediatric Migraine Disability Assessment (PedMIDAS).[21] Additional measures, including measures of satisfaction with treatment and sleep, have emerging validity or are in development.[22] Assessment of pain quality, timing, location, aggravating factors, and alleviating factors may provide vital information for diagnosis and treatment. In addition, risk factors, such as pain catastrophizing and caregiver burden, may be valuable for developing a family centered multimodal pain management plan.

Despite recent approval by the US Food and Drug Administration (FDA) of OxyContin for children 11 to 16 years of age, opioids are rarely used in multimodal pediatric chronic pain management plans. Long-acting and extended release opioids are only indicated for daily around the clock treatment of severe pain for which alternative treatment options are inadequate. Alternative treatments commonly trialed in pediatric patients include traditional analgesics and other pharmacologic therapies that are not approved by the FDA for treatment of chronic pediatric pain; but are routinely used to treat chronic pain in adults.[23] A vital and uniquely pediatric component of the multimodal treatment plan for pediatric patients with chronic pain is pharmacologic strategies for managing acute procedurally based pain, such as topical dermal anesthetics before needle procedures. Optimal management for the discomfort and distress of even these short procedures should be coupled with coping strategies and biobehavioral therapies. These anxiety-provoking procedures are often necessary during a child's initial diagnostic work-up, but repeated and exhausted diagnostic testing is often not medically indicated and may be a barrier to pain treatment by delaying appropriate therapies and allowing catastrophizing to perseverate.

As pain in children and adolescents recurs, persists, and becomes chronic, resources for effective coping may be depleted. Therefore, the resulting disability associated with pediatric chronic pain (ie, pain-associated disability syndrome[2]) frequently becomes the primary focus of intervention. At the most basic level, the management of pain requires patients to contend with unpleasant physical and emotional experiences; those who manage these experiences adaptively use self-regulatory skills to modulate the intensity and duration of a given moment, often relying on psychological and behavioral coping skills to do so.[24,25] Coping is best described as the set of cognitive and behavioral efforts taken to manage distressing circumstances, which requires the perception of a situation as stressful and the effortful or planned steps to manage resulting emotions (emotion-focused coping) and/or the situation itself (problem-focused coping).[26] Hence coping with an uncomfortable sensation requires that the individual attends to the stimuli sufficiently to interpret the experience as unpleasant and to take steps to reduce the discomfort.

Although pediatric treatment plans are multimodal (eg, include medical, physical, psychological, and behavioral components), lack of engagement in treatment can result in school absenteeism, increased use of emergency departments, and hospital admissions. Increased parenting stress and interference in parent's regular roles/activities is a common challenge for families with a child with chronic pain. Hence, caregiver burden and parenting stress are markedly heightened in these families and subsequently pose risks to adaptive family functioning. Prior research has shown that threatening beliefs about pain such as pain catastrophizing influence the types of strategies used to cope with pain.[27–30] Parental catastrophizing about their child's pain further contributes to the child's disability as well as to parenting stress.[27,31,32] Our previous work documents significant agreement in adolescent-parent dyad reports of pain catastrophizing.[33] Moreover, we have found that parental protective responses to their child's pain are associated with disability indirectly through pain catastrophizing at an initial clinic visit and 2 months later.[34]

Social cognitive models of development[35,36] posit that a sense of competence in exerting control over circumstances results in patients' beliefs that they can take effective steps to mitigate their discomfort, stressing the importance of social reinforcement to develop a sense of personal efficacy in the presence of pain. Recent advancements in cognitive behavior therapies that target coping skills to improve distress tolerance have shown consistent benefit in pediatric patients with chronic pain.[37–40] Cognitive behavior mindfulness interventions are designed to bolster pediatric patients' abilities to self-monitor their physical and psychological states, maintain a nonjudgmental interpretive frame for their experiences, and to slow impulsive responses to discomfort.[41,42]

GERIATRIC CHRONIC PAIN

The risk for chronic pain conditions increases with age, making the geriatric population particularly vulnerable. National surveys of pain in older adults from North America, Europe, Asia, and Australia found that more than 50% of respondents reported bothersome pain in the last month.[43–46] The estimated incidence of chronic pain in adults is 4.69 per 100 person-years, and the prevalence of chronic pain in individuals more than 85 years old is as high as 79%.[47] Pain in older adults is a significant problem worldwide, and is associated with reduced activity, falls, mood disorders, sleep disturbances, isolation, and substantial disability; factors that compromise quality of life and well-being. Persistent pain may lead to frailty, compromising general health and functional status.[48,49] Although pain management can be successfully implemented for most older adults, pain remains undertreated in the oldest old, African Americans, and ethnic minorities, as well as in individuals with cognitive impairment.[50] Overall, older adults are less likely to receive analgesics compared with young adult patients despite the significant ramifications to general health and well-being.[51]

Neurophysiologic changes associated with aging seem to influence pain processing, with evidence to support a general increase in pain threshold and reduced pain tolerance from deterioration of the pathways involved in endogenous inhibition. An age-related increase in pain threshold to thermal stimuli may be related to loss in the structure and function of the peripheral (A delta fibers) and central nervous system (CNS) pathways implicated in the processing of noxious information.[52] Experimental pain studies provide some evidence of reduced sensitivity to mild pain with advancing age, particularly for thermal pain.[53] Other types of pain stimuli (ie, mechanical, electrical) are more equivocal, with reports of no change or decreased thresholds in older adults.[54] In contrast, results from 10 independent studies showed reduced pain tolerance as a function of age, irrespective of stimulus method.[53,54] In addition, temporal summation of noxious heat is enhanced in the CNS of older adults compared with younger individuals.[55] Age-related impairment in opioid and nonopioid mechanisms of the endogenous pain inhibitory systems have been described, showing less than a third of the strength of induced effects on sensitivity when compared with younger adults.[39,56] Collectively, these studies suggest that aging increases vulnerability to persistent severe pain owing to reduced pain tolerance and impaired endogenous pain-modulating capacities.

In concert with age-associated changes in somatosensory function, chronic comorbidities often contribute to pain, including musculoskeletal disorders, diabetes, and cancer, particularly with advanced stages of chronic disease. In addition, pain may result from treatments, such as surgery and chemotherapy.[57] In medically complex populations, such as older adults who are incarcerated, severe frequent pain is common and associated with difficulty in performing activities of daily living and limited independence.[58] Risk factors for chronic pain include advancing age, lower socioeconomic status, lower educational level, obesity, tobacco use, history of injury, strenuous job, childhood trauma, and psychological comorbidity, especially depression and anxiety.[57] The identification of risk factors that may influence long-term outcomes may be one avenue of informing the type and intensity of therapeutic modalities. For instance, at the initial presentation of musculoskeletal pain in older adults, 3 brief items have been shown to predict lack of patient improvement at 6 months: degree of interference from pain, pain in multiple body sites, and duration of pain.[59] An assessment of risk factors for persistent pain or poor clinical outcomes should be incorporated in the clinical examination and used to develop a multimodal treatment approach.

A comprehensive pain history and physical examination focused on cognitive, motor, and sensory assessments, as well as diagnostic tests when indicated, provides a foundation for the development of treatment approaches for older adults.[52] This foundation should include administering standardized pain assessment tools, identifying the impact of pain on mood and functioning, as well as identifying attitudes and beliefs about pain.[60] Input may be sought from family and/or caregivers when possible to assist in the sharing of information and implementation of the plan of care. In older adults with cognitive impairment or nonverbal individuals, pain assessment should include attempts at self-report, review of painful conditions, evaluation of pain behaviors, and family/caregiver interviews.[14] Well-established general principles for the management of pain have been published, including those of the American Geriatrics Society and American Pain Society.[61,62]

Specific physiologic changes in older adults need to be considered when selecting appropriate analgesic therapy.[52] Older adults have reduced intravascular volume and muscle mass, which may alter drug distribution resulting in increased plasma levels relative to younger individuals, and leading to increased volume of distribution of fat-soluble opioids (ie, fentanyl) because of greater fat/lean body mass ratio, whereas decreased total body water can result in increased plasma levels of hydrophilic opioids (ie, morphine). Renal clearance (glomerular filtration, tubular reabsorption, and secretion) decreases at a rate of 6% to 10% per decade beginning at age 30 years. Thus reduced renal function without underlying kidney disease is common in older adults. In addition, hepatic clearance is reduced because of decreased hepatic blood flow. Nonsteroidal antiinflammatory drugs are not recommended by the American Geriatrics Society, especially long-term use because of the high risk of adverse effects on the gastrointestinal, cardiovascular, and renal systems. Dosage reductions (25%–50%) of other medications used to treat pain in older adults are typically necessary, particularly at initiation of treatment.[63]

Although respiratory depression is rare in opioid-naive patients who are prescribed initial low-dose opioid therapy, the risk increases with older age, opioid dose, and underlying pulmonary conditions, particularly sleep apnea and chronic obstructive pulmonary disease. In addition the concomitant use of other CNS depressants, such as alcohol, benzodiazepines, or barbiturates, with opioids can significantly increase the risk of respiratory depression. Research on addiction and misuse in older adults is sparse; however, the prevalence is thought to be much lower than in younger populations. An approach of so-called universal precautions is recommended for any patient prescribed opioids, including the administration of opioid risk stratification tools and adherence monitoring.[64]

Multimodal approaches to pain management are encouraged, including cognitive behavior therapy, self-management programs, rehabilitation, and exercise programs. There are a growing number of well-designed geriatric chronic pain studies evaluating pharmacologic and nonpharmacologic therapies, although there are several factors that limit the ability to generalize these studies' findings. Longitudinal designs are needed to evaluate short-term and long-term outcomes with diverse study populations that include participants in the oldest-old category (>80 years). Data regarding treatment adherence including long-term safety and efficacy of different modalities, particularly multimodal approaches, are needed as well as identification of optimal strategies for the delivery of nonpharmacologic approaches. Understanding the neurophysiologic changes that influence pain in later life, including in patients with cognitive impairment, is important for ensuring adequate and ethical treatment at the end of life. Studies to test innovative treatment approaches will help to inform the delivery of multimodal treatment approaches that entail fewer adverse effects. Research on cost, quality, and safety outcomes of multidisciplinary approaches for the management of pain are also needed to inform policy decisions and standards of care.

SUBSTANCE ABUSERS: A SPECIAL POPULATION

Evidence suggests that approximately 10% of the population, 12 years of age and older, report recent substance use,[65] with an estimated 5.1 million of these individuals indicating misuse of prescription pain relievers. Prescription drug misuse is defined as use in a manner inconsistent with intended purpose or prescribed use; whereas prescription drug abuse or nonmedical use is defined as use for nontherapeutic or recreational purposes.[66] The estimated societal cost of drug misuse and/or diversion exceeds $500 billion annually.[67,68] Recent reviews of opioid abuse in the chronic pain population indicates that the potential risk factors for substance abuse in this population include genetic variation in opioid receptor and drug metabolism–associated genes, demographic factors (including age), pain severity, drug-related factors (eg, physician-reported aberrant use behavior), family history of substance use, and psychiatric comorbidity.[69] Other studies have consistently identified familial substance use and comorbid mental health diagnoses (eg, affective disorders including depression) as significant predictors of addiction in chronic pain samples and, further, that peer influence and substance use is of particular salience to models of use in younger samples.[70–73] Impulsivity and sensation-seeking personality traits have also been consistently identified as risk factors for substance abuse across the lifespan[74–77] and hold considerable value as intervention targets to stem the rates of substance abuse among patients with chronic pain.

The most prevalent motivation for medical misuse of opioids (84.2%) is to relieve pain.[78] Pain relievers are more commonly used for nonmedical reasons than any other class of prescription medications[79,80] and nonmedical use of prescription analgesics, specifically opioid analgesics like hydromorphone, has substantially increased in recent years.[65,68,81] Drug misuse is reported in approximately 40% of patients with pain with half (20%) of those identified as substance abusers and a much smaller proportion (2%–5%) identified as addicts.[82] However, health care professionals may overestimate the prevalence of those patients who seek prescription medication in response to addiction versus those who are seeking medication to relieve chronic pain.[83] Furthermore, health care professionals may perceive the development of an addiction as being a flip–of-the-switch phenomenon, but evidence suggests a slow developmental trajectory.[84,85] As a result of both societal and health care–specific beliefs about addiction, substance abusers/addicts may feel stigmatized and may be less likely to disclose their addictions.[86,87] However, the World Health Organization has identified pain relief as a fundamental human right. When diagnosed with a comorbid chronic pain condition, the medical management of these patients is particularly challenging given their prior history of substance abuse. The "American Society for Pain Management Nursing Position Statement on Pain Management in Patients with Substance Use Disorders" clearly supports maintenance of dignity, respect, and high-quality pain management in this population[88] despite their increased risk for subsequent misuse.

Beyond an understanding of the broad predictors of substance use and addiction in the chronic pain population, medical professionals are wise to consider the developmental and social context in which patients will use the recommended pain management plans. Compared with adult populations, choices about adolescent nonmedical drug use are especially informed by sociocultural contexts.[89,90] Currie and Wild[91] posit that adolescents may choose analgesics because they believe analgesics are safer given the pervasive marketing for pain medication in American culture. Consideration for the cognitive development of children and adolescents provides crucial elements to comprehensive models for substance use: beyond personality traits, including anxiety, impulsivity, and novelty-seeking tendencies, normative changes in future-oriented thinking, risk assessment, and perspective taking all contribute to adolescents' vulnerability to substance abuse; a vulnerability that is heightened during the normative neuroproliferation and subsequent synaptic pruning in the frontal lobes seen up to the early 20s.[92–94]

GENETICS AS A FUNDAMENTAL VULNERABILITY ACROSS THE LIFESPAN

Chronic pain can be described as a condition of complex etiology reflecting the interaction of environmental (eg, illness, injury) and genetic factors over the lifespan. With this in mind, genetic susceptibility to develop chronic pain is, arguably, one of the primary determinants of vulnerability across age, developmental status, and lifetime experience. Understanding the genetic underpinnings of chronic pain susceptibility may allow prevention and earlier diagnosis as well as the development of novel therapeutic interventions specifically targeting the fundamental mechanisms of vulnerability.

Twin studies and genetic association studies have both been used to shed light on the inherited nature of chronic pain risk. Twin studies provide evidence for heritability by determining how much of the variability in pain occurrence is caused by genetics and how much is caused by nongenetic factors, whereas genetic association studies are designed to identify and/or test the influence of individual genes on susceptibility to a given chronic pain condition. Twin studies offer the opportunity to evaluate polygenic inheritance without a priori hypotheses, which makes them a useful tool in the formation of subsequent specific empirical questions about mechanism. Data from twin studies estimate specific heritability for low back pain and neck pain to be ~60% and ~50% respectively.[95] Other chronic pain conditions, including migraine,[96] pelvic pain,[97] irritable bowel syndrome,[98,99] chronic widespread pain,[100] and osteoarthritis,[101,102] also show significant heritability, from 30% to 75%. Although these methods do not indicate a specific gene or set of genes that convey inherited risk for chronic pain, they do confirm that risk for these chronic conditions is heritable and encourage further investigation into the mechanisms by which risk is inherited.

Findings from candidate gene studies have shed light on the contribution of specific genetic variations to the risk of developing chronic pain. Reports from both animal models and clinical populations have identified genetic variations that convey chronic pain risk. Single nucleotide polymorphisms (SNPs) within several genes have been associated with risk or protection against the development of chronic pain, although some of the specific mechanisms remain to be fully elucidated. SNPs within the catechol O-methyltransferase (COMT) gene, known to play a role in inactivation of dopamine, norepinephrine, and epinephrine, have been linked with altered experimental pain sensitivity as well as susceptibility to chronic musculoskeletal and neuropathic pain.[103,104] Variation within ADRB2, encoding the beta2-adrenergic receptor, has been associated with variability in self-reports of the extent and duration of pain in patients with chronic widespread pain (CWP), in agreement with a previously reported association between ADRB2 haplotypes and an increased risk for Temporomandibular Disorder pain. Associations have also been revealed between polymorphisms within the serotonin transporter gene (SLC6A4), specifically the associated serotonin transporter linked promoter region (5-HTTLPR), and risk for developing fibromyalgia.[105] Along these same lines, a single SNP within HTR2A, the gene encoding the serotonin receptor 2A, has also been associated with an increased risk of chronic widespread pain diagnosis[106] and postsurgical pain burden.[107] Variations in signaling within both the serotonin and catecholamine systems have been linked with risk for depression, anxiety, and other psychological health issues, which may have implications for efficacy of treatment strategies targeting the negative cognitive and emotional aspects of chronic pain[108,109] and/or pain modulation.

Genetic polymorphisms unrelated to neurotransmission have also been associated with chronic pain susceptibility. Many of these genes are involved in ion channel function and directly affect the dynamics of the cellular response to noxious stimulation. SCN9A encodes the alpha subunit of the voltage-gated sodium channel NaV1.7 and evidence suggests a role for SCN9A in determining risk for chronic pain conditions, including sciatica, osteoarthritis, chronic pancreatitis, and phantom limb pain, as well as variation in pain responding within normal populations.[110] Rare gain-of-function mutations of this gene have been implicated in primary erythromelalgia and paroxysmal extreme pain disorder, whereas loss-of-function variants are shown to result in congenital insensitivity to pain (CIP, with or without anhidrosis).[110–112] These findings indicate a fundamental role for sodium channel function in the transmission of pain signals and confirm that this process must remain in delicate balance in order to prevent maladaptive changes conducive to chronic pain development. Other investigators have found that a single SNP within KCNS1, the gene encoding a voltage-gated potassium channel (subfamily S, member 1), increased risk for chronic pain in 5 separate clinical cohorts from patient populations with a high prevalence of pain reporting.[113] Variation within 2 genes related to calcium channel function, CACNA2D3 (encodes the alpha-2 delta-3 subunit of the voltage-dependent calcium channel) and CACNG2 (encodes the gamma-2 subunit of voltage-dependent calcium channel), have been shown to play a role in susceptibility to chronic back pain following lumbar discectomy and chronic postmastectomy pain, respectively.[114,115]

The responses to every injury, every surgery, and every illness are shaped by the context of people's genetic makeup. This framework shapes the physical and emotional response to a painful experience and creates the conditions for long-term changes that may be adaptive (recovery and return to normal function) or maladaptive (development of chronic pain and dysfunction). Taken together, these findings suggest that the future of personalized medicine may include genetic testing as part of the decision-making process between patient and healthcare provider. The ultimate goal is to develop a comprehensive list of chronic pain genes to be used for risk assessment in health care settings. This goal would be particularly important when the treatment plan includes procedures with high risk for developing chronic pain (eg, amputation, chemotherapy, surgical procedures). The frustration reported by medical professionals regarding the treatment of patients with chronic pain as well as the stigmatization of patients with chronic pain as being difficult could be decreased by further elucidation of the underlying mechanisms of chronic pain vulnerability.

SUMMARY

The geriatric, pediatric, and substance abuser populations represent groups with difficult-to-manage chronic pain. The therapeutic approach in each group should be multimodal, but include components that meet the unique needs of patients. Further research is required to fully understand how chronic pain develops and evolves in each of these patient groups. In particular, as understanding of the psychosocial, physiologic and genetic mechanisms underlying chronic pain in these understudied populations improves, advances in treatment options will also improve. Treatment will continue to use a multimodal approach and involve cooperative efforts between all health care professionals involved in the pain management team.

REFERENCES

1. Gold MS, Gebhart GF. Nociceptor sensitization in pain pathogenesis. Nat Med 2010;16(11):1248–57.
2. Bursch B, Walco GA, Zeltzer L. Clinical assessment and management of chronic pain and pain-associated disability syndrome. J Dev Behav Pediatr 1998;19(1): 45–53.
3. Kashikar-Zuck S, Goldschneider KR, Powers SW, et al. Depression and functional disability in chronic pediatric pain. Clin J Dev Behav Pediatr 2001;17: 341–9.
4. Palermo TM. Impact of recurrent and chronic pain on child and family daily functioning: a critical review of the literature. J Dev Behav Pediatr 2000;21(1):58–69.
5. Walker LS, Garber J, Greene JW. Psychosocial correlates of recurrent childhood pain: a comparison of pediatric patients with recurrent abdominal pain, organic illness, and psychiatric disorders. J Abnorm Psychol 1993;102(2):248–58.
6. Zernikow B, Wager J, Hechler T, et al. Characteristics of highly impaired children with severe chronic pain: a 5-year retrospective study on 2249 pediatric pain patients. BMC Pediatr 2012;12:54.
7. Fearon P, Hotopf M. Relation between headache in childhood and physical and psychiatric symptoms in adulthood: national birth cohort study. BMJ 2001; 322(7295):1145.
8. Hotopf M, Carr S, Mayou R, et al. Why do children have chronic abdominal pain, and what happens to them when they grow up? Population based cohort study. Br Med J 1998;316(7139):1196–200.
9. Hotopf M, Mayou R, Wadsworth M, et al. Childhood risk factors for adults with medically unexplained symptoms: results from a national birth cohort study. Am J Psychiatry 1999;156(11):1796–800.
10. Hotopf M, Wilson Jones C, Mayou R, et al. Childhood predictors of adult medically unexplained hospitalisations. Results from a national birth cohort study. Br J Psychiatry 2000;176:273–80.
11. Walker LS, Dengler-Crish CM, Rippel S, et al. Functional abdominal pain in childhood and adolescence increases risk for chronic pain in adulthood. Pain 2010;150(3):568–72.

12. Schneider M. Adolescence as a vulnerable period to alter rodent behavior. Cell Tissue Res 2013;354(1):99–106.

13. King S, Chambers CT, Huguet A, et al. The epidemiology of chronic pain in children and adolescents revisited: a systematic review. Pain 2011;152(12):2729–38.

14. Herr K, Coyne PJ, McCaffery M, et al. Pain assessment in the patient unable to self-report: position statement with clinical practice recommendations. Pain Manag Nurs 2011;12(4):230–50.

15. McGrath PJ, Walco GA, Turk DC, et al. Core outcome domains and measures for pediatric acute and chronic/recurrent pain clinical trials: PedIMMPACT recommendations. J Pain 2008;9(9):771–83.

16. Stinson JN, Kavanagh T, Yamada J, et al. Systematic review of the psychometric properties, interpretability and feasibility of self-report pain intensity measures for use in clinical trials in children and adolescents. Pain 2006; 125(1–2):143–57.

17. von Baeyer CL, Spagrud LJ. Systematic review of observational (behavioral) measures of pain for children and adolescents aged 3 to 18 years. Pain 2007; 127(1–2):140–50.

18. Walker LS, Greene JW. The Functional Disability Inventory: Measuring a neglected dimension of child health status. J Pediatr Psychol 1991;16(1):39–58.

19. Kashikar-Zuck S, Flowers SR, Claar RL, et al. Clinical utility and validity of the Functional Disability Inventory among a multicenter sample of youth with chronic pain. Pain 2011;152(7):1600–7.

20. Varni JW, Seid M, Rode CA. The PedsQL: measurement model for the pediatric quality of life inventory. Med Care 1999;37(2):126–39.

21. Hershey AD, Powers SW, Vockell ALB, et al. PedMIDAS: Development of a questionnaire to assess disability of migraines in children. Neurology 2001; 57(11):2034–9.

22. Zempsky WT, O'Hara EA, Santanelli JP, et al. Validation of the sickle cell disease pain burden interview-youth. J Pain 2013;14(9):975–82.

23. FDA. CDER Conversation: Pediatric pain management options. Available at: http://www.fda.gov/Drugs/NewsEvents/ucm456973.htm. Accessed August 14, 2015.

24. Gross JJ. The emerging field of emotion regulation: an integrative review. Rev Gen Psychol 1998;2(3):271–99.

25. Tennen H, Affleck G, Armeli S, et al. A daily process approach to coping: linking theory, research, and practice. Am Psychol 2000;55(6):626–36.

26. Lazarus RS, Folkman S. Stress, appraisal, and coping. New York: Springer; 1984.

27. Caes L, Vervoort T, Eccleston C, et al. Parental catastrophizing about child's pain and its relationship with activity restriction: the mediating role of parental distress. Pain 2011;152(1):212–22.

28. Guite JW. The relation of psychological and biomedical factors to children's experience of abdominal pain [doctoral dissertation]. Nashville (TN): Vanderbilt University; 2001.

29. Van Slyke DA. Parent influences on children's pain behavior [doctoral dissertation]. Nashville (TN): Vanderbilt University; 2001.

30. Walker LS, Smith CA, Garber J, et al. Testing a model of pain appraisal and coping in children with chronic abdominal pain. Health Psychol 2005;24(4):364–74.

31. Goubert L, Eccleston C, Vervoort T, et al. Parental catastrophizing about their child's pain. The parent version of the Pain Catastrophizing Scale (PCS-P): a preliminary validation. Pain 2006;123(3):254–63.

32. Vowles KE, Cohen LL, McCracken LM, et al. Disentangling the complex relations among caregiver and adolescent responses to adolescent chronic pain. Pain 2010;151(3):680–6.
33. Guite JW, Kim S, Chen CP, et al. Pain beliefs and readiness to change among adolescents with chronic musculoskeletal pain and their parents before an initial pain clinic evaluation. Clin J Pain 2014;30(1):27–35.
34. Welkom JS, Hwang WT, Guite JW. Adolescent pain catastrophizing mediates the relationship between protective parental responses to pain and disability over time. J Pediatr Psychol 2013;38(5):541–50.
35. Bandura A. Social cognitive theory of self-regulation. Organ Behav Hum Decis Process 1991;50(2):248–97.
36. Bandura A. Social cognitive theory; an agentic perspective. Annu Rev Psychol 2001;52:1–26.
37. Davis MC, Zautra AJ, Wolf LD, et al. Mindfulness and cognitive–behavioral interventions for chronic pain: differential effects on daily pain reactivity and stress reactivity. J Consult Clin Psychol 2015;83(1):24–35.
38. Lynch-Jordan AM, Sil S, Cunningham NR, et al. Measuring treatment response in an outpatient pediatric pain program. Clin Pract Pediatr Psychol 2015;3(1): 1–11.
39. Morley S, Eccleston C, Williams A. Systematic review and meta-analysis of randomized controlled trials of cognitive behaviour therapy and behaviour therapy for chronic pain in adults, excluding headache. Pain 1999;80(1–2): 1–13.
40. Reiner K, Tibi L, Lipsitz JD. Do mindfulness-based interventions reduce pain intensity? A critical review of the literature. Pain Med 2013;14(2):230–42.
41. Carlson M. CBT for chronic pain and psychological well-being: a skills training manual integrating DBT, ACT, behavioral activation and motivational interviewing. Hoboken (NJ): Wiley-Blackwell; 2014.
42. Day MA, Jensen MP, Ehde DM, et al. Toward a theoretical model for mindfulness-based pain management. J Pain 2014;15(7):691–703.
43. Henderson JV, Harrison CM, Britt HC, et al. Prevalence, causes, severity, impact, and management of chronic pain in Australian general practice patients. Pain Med 2013;14(9):1346–61.
44. Jackson T, Chen H, Iezzi T, et al. Prevalence and correlates of chronic pain in a random population study of adults in Chongqing, China. Clin J Pain 2014;30(4): 346–52.
45. Leadley RM, Armstrong N, Lee YC, et al. Chronic diseases in the European Union: the prevalence and health cost implications of chronic pain. J Pain Palliat Care Pharmacother 2012;26(4):310–25.
46. Patel KV, Guralnik JM, Dansie EJ, et al. Prevalence and impact of pain among older adults in the United States: findings from the 2011 National Health and Aging Trends Study. Pain 2013;154(12):2649–57.
47. Shi Y, Hooten WM, Roberts RO, et al. Modifiable risk factors for incidence of pain in older adults. Pain 2010;151(2):366–71.
48. Shega JW, Andrew M, Kotwal A, et al. Relationship between persistent pain and 5-year mortality: a population-based prospective cohort study. J Am Geriatr Soc 2013;61(12):2135–41.
49. Shega JW, Dale W, Andrew M, et al. Persistent pain and frailty: a case for homeostenosis. J Am Geriatr Soc 2012;60(1):113–7.
50. Malec M, Shega JW. Pain management in the elderly. Med Clin North Am 2015; 99(2):337–50.

51. Hwang U, Belland LK, Handel DA, et al. Is all pain is treated equally? A multicenter evaluation of acute pain care by age. Pain 2014;155(12):2568–74.

52. Hadjistavropoulos T, Herr K, Prkachin KM, et al. Pain assessment in elderly adults with dementia. Lancet Neurol 2014;13(12):1216–27.

53. Gibson SJ, Farrell M. A review of age differences in the neurophysiology of nociception and the perceptual experience of pain. Clin J Pain 2004;20(4): 227–39.

54. Lautenbacher S. Experimental approaches in the study of pain in the elderly. Pain Med 2012;2(13 Suppl):S44–50.

55. Edwards RR, Fillingim RB. Effects of age on temporal summation and habituation of thermal pain: clinical relevance in healthy older and younger adults. J Pain 2001;2(6):307–17.

56. Riley JL 3rd, King CD, Wong F, et al. Lack of endogenous modulation and reduced decay of prolonged heat pain in older adults. Pain 2010;150(1):153–60.

57. Reid MC, Eccleston C, Pillemer K. Management of chronic pain in older adults. BMJ 2015;350:h532.

58. Williams BA, Ahalt C, Stijacic-Cenzer I, et al. Pain behind bars: the epidemiology of pain in older jail inmates in a county jail. J Palliat Med 2014;17(12):1336–43.

59. Mallen CD, Thomas E, Belcher J, et al. Point-of-care prognosis for common musculoskeletal pain in older adults. JAMA Intern Med 2013;173(12):1119–25.

60. Makris UE, Abrams RC, Gurland B, et al. Management of persistent pain in the older patient: a clinical review. JAMA 2014;312(8):825–36.

61. American Geriatrics Society Panel on the Pharmacological Management of Persistent Pain in Older Persons. Pharmacological management of persistent pain on older persons. J Am Geriatr Soc 2009;57(8):1331–46.

62. American Pain Society. Principles of analgesic use in the treatment of acute and cancer pain. 6th edition. Glenview, IL: American Pain Society Panelists; 2009.

63. Gupta DK, Avram MJ. Rational opioid dosing in the elderly: dose and dosing interval when initiating opioid therapy. Clin Pharmacol Ther 2012;91(2):339–43.

64. Steinman MA, Komaiko KD, Fung KZ, et al. Use of opioids and other analgesics by older adults in the United States, 1999-2010. Pain Med 2015;16(2):319–27.

65. Substance Abuse and Mental Health Services Administration (SAMHSA). Drug abuse warning network, 2011: national stimats of drug-related emergency deparmtent visits. Rockville, MD; 2013. HHS Publication No (SMA) 13-4760, DAWN Series D-39. Available at: http://archive.samhsa.gov/data/2k13/DAWN2k11ED/DAWN2k11ED.htm.

66. Manworren RCB, Gilson AM. Nurses' role in preventing prescription opioid diversion. Am J Nurs 2015;115(8):34–40.

67. NCASA. 2011.

68. National Drug Intelligence Center. 2010.

69. Sehgal N, Manchikanti L, Smith HS. Prescription opioid abuse in chronic pain: a review of opioid abuse predictors and strategies to curb opioid abuse. Pain Physician 2012;15(3 Suppl):ES67–92.

70. Ewing BA, Osilla KC, Pedersen ER, et al. Longitudinal family effects on substance use among an at-risk adolescent sample. Addict Behav 2015;41:185–91.

71. Fergusson DM, Boden JM, Horwood LJ. The developmental antecedents of illicit drug use: evidence from a 25-year longitudinal study. Drug Alcohol Depend 2008;96(1–2):165–77.

72. Jamison RN, Ross EL, Michna E, et al. Substance misuse treatment for high-risk chronic pain patients on opioid therapy: a randomized trial. Pain 2010;150(3): 390–400.

73. Wasan AD, Butler SF, Budman SH, et al. Psychiatric history and psychologic adjustment as risk factors for aberrant drug-related behavior among patients with chronic pain. Clin J Pain 2007;23(4):307–15.
74. Acton GS. Measurement of impulsivity in a hierarchical model of personality traits: implications for substance use. Subst Use Misuse 2003;38(1):67–83.
75. McNamee RL, Dunfee KL, Luna B, et al. Brain activation, response inhibition, and increased risk for substance use disorder. Alcohol Clin Exp Res 2008; 32(3):405–13.
76. Staiger PK, Kambouropoulos N, Dawe S. Should personality traits be considered when refining substance misuse treatment programs? Drug Alcohol Rev 2007;26(1):17–23.
77. Young A, McCabe SE, Cranford JA, et al. Nonmedical use of prescription opioids among adolescents: subtypes based on motivation for use. J Addict Dis 2012;31(4):332–41.
78. McCabe SE, West BT, Boyd CJ. Motives for medical misuse of prescription opioids among adolescents. J Pain 2013;14(10):1208–16.
79. Viana AG, Trent L, Tull MT, et al. Non-medical use of prescription drugs among Mississippi youth: constitutional, psychological, and family factors. Addict Behav 2012;37(12):1382–8.
80. Young AM, Glover N, Havens JR. Nonmedical use of prescription medications among adolescents in the United States: a systematic review. J Adolesc Health 2012;51(1):6–17.
81. Miech R, Bohnert A, Heard K, et al. Increasing use of nonmedical analgesics among younger cohorts in the United States: a birth cohort effect. J Adolesc Health 2013;52(1):35–41.
82. Gourlay DL, Heit HA, Almahrezi A. Universal precautions in pain medicine: a rational approach to the treatment of chronic pain. Pain Med 2005;6(2): 107–12.
83. Baker K. Chronic pain syndromes in the emergency department: identifying guidelines for management. Emerg Med Australas 2005;17(1):57–64.
84. Ballantyne JC, LaForge KS. Opioid dependence and addiction during opioid treatment of chronic pain. Pain 2007;129(3):235–55.
85. Manworren RC. Pediatric nursing knowledge and attitude survey regarding pain. Pediatr Nurs 2014;40(1):50.
86. Arnstein P. Is my patient drug-seeking or in need of pain relief? Nursing 2010; 40(5):60–1.
87. McCaffery M. Stigma and misconceptions related to addictive disease. Am Nurse Today 2011;6(6). Available at: http://www.americannursetoday.com/stigma-and-misconceptions-related-to-addictive-disease/.
88. Oliver J, Coggins C, Compton P, et al. American Society for Pain Management nursing position statement: pain management in patients with substance use disorders. Pain Manag Nurs 2012;13(3):169–83.
89. Maccoun RJ. Competing accounts of the gateway effect: the field thins, but still no clear winner. Addiction 2006;101(4):473–4 [discussion: 474–6].
90. Olthuis JV, Darredeau C, Barrett SP. Substance use initiation: the role of simultaneous polysubstance use. Drug Alcohol Rev 2013;32(1):67–71.
91. Currie CL, Wild TC. Adolescent use of prescription drugs to get high in Canada. Can J Psychiatry 2012;57(12):745–51.
92. Schepis TS, Adinoff B, Rao U. Neurobiological processes in adolescent addictive disorders. Am J Addict 2008;17(1):6–23.

93. Stanger C, Budney AJ, Bickel WK. A developmental perspective on neuroeconomic mechanisms of contingency management. Psychol Addict Behav 2013; 27(2):403–15.

94. Stanger C, Elton A, Ryan SR, et al. Neuroeconomics and adolescent substance abuse: individual differences in neural networks and delay discounting. J Am Acad Child Adolesc Psychiatry 2013;52(7):747–55.e6.

95. MacGregor AJ, Andrew T, Sambrook PN, et al. Structural, psychological, and genetic influences on low back and neck pain: a study of adult female twins. Arthritis Rheum 2004;51(2):160–7.

96. Wessman M, Terwindt GM, Kaunisto MA, et al. Migraine: a complex genetic disorder. Lancet Neurol 2007;6(6):521–32.

97. Zondervan KT, Cardon LR, Kennedy SH, et al. Multivariate genetic analysis of chronic pelvic pain and associated phenotypes. Behav Genet 2005;35(2): 177–88.

98. Lembo A, Zaman M, Jones M, et al. Influence of genetics on irritable bowel syndrome, gastro-oesophageal reflux and dyspepsia: a twin study. Aliment Pharmacol Ther 2007;25(11):1343–50.

99. Levy RL, Jones KR, Whitehead WE, et al. Irritable bowel syndrome in twins: heredity and social learning both contribute to etiology. Gastroenterology 2001; 121(4):799–804.

100. Kato K, Sullivan PF, Evengard B, et al. Importance of genetic influences on chronic widespread pain. Arthritis Rheum 2006;54(5):1682–6.

101. Page WF, Hoaglund FT, Steinbach LS, et al. Primary osteoarthritis of the hip in monozygotic and dizygotic male twins. Twin Res 2003;6(2):147–51.

102. Spector TD, MacGregor AJ. Risk factors for osteoarthritis: genetics. Osteoarthritis Cartilage 2004;12(Suppl A):S39–44.

103. Belfer I, Segall S. COMT genetic variants and pain. Drugs Today 2011;47(6): 457–67.

104. Diatchenko L, Slade GD, Nackley AG, et al. Genetic basis for individual variations in pain perception and the development of a chronic pain condition. Hum Mol Genet 2005;14(1):135–43.

105. Buskila D, Neumann L. Genetics of fibromyalgia. Curr Pain Headache Rep 2005; 9(5):313–5.

106. Nicholl BI, Holliday KL, Macfarlane GJ, et al, European Male Ageing Study Group. Association of HTR2A polymorphisms with chronic widespread pain and the extent of musculoskeletal pain: results from two population-based cohorts. Arthritis Rheum 2011;63(3):810–8.

107. Aoki J, Ikeda K, Murayama O, et al. The association between personality, pain threshold and a single nucleotide polymorphism (rs3813034) in the 3'-untranslated region of the serotonin transporter gene (SLC6A4). J Clin Neurosci 2010;17(5):574–8.

108. Elder BL, Mosack V. Genetics of depression: an overview of the current science. Issues Ment Health Nurs 2011;32(4):192–202.

109. Helton SG, Lohoff FW. Serotonin pathway polymorphisms and the treatment of major depressive disorder and anxiety disorders. Pharmacogenomics 2015; 16(5):541–53.

110. Reimann F, Cox JJ, Belfer I, et al. Pain perception is altered by a nucleotide polymorphism in SCN9A. Proc Natl Acad Sci U S A 2010;107(11):5148–53.

111. Cox JJ, Sheynin J, Shorer Z, et al. Congenital insensitivity to pain: novel SCN9A missense and in-frame deletion mutations. Hum Mutat 2010;31(9):E1670–86.

112. Drenth JP, Waxman SG. Mutations in sodium-channel gene SCN9A cause a spectrum of human genetic pain disorders. J Clin Invest 2007;117(12):3603–9.
113. Costigan M, Belfer I, Griffin RS, et al. Multiple chronic pain states are associated with a common amino acid-changing allele in KCNS1. Brain 2010;133(9): 2519–27.
114. Neely GG, Hess A, Costigan M, et al. A genome-wide *Drosophila* screen for heat nociception identifies alpha2delta3 as an evolutionarily conserved pain gene. Cell 2010;143(4):628–38.
115. Nissenbaum J, Devor M, Seltzer Z, et al. Susceptibility to chronic pain following nerve injury is genetically affected by CACNG2. Genome Res 2010;20(9): 1180–90.

Emerging Treatment

Is Platelet-Rich Plasma a Future Therapy in Pain Management?

Nebojsa Nick Knezevic, MD, PhD[a,b], Kenneth D. Candido, MD[a,b], Ravi Desai, DO[a], Alan David Kaye, MD, PhD[c,d],*

KEYWORDS

- Platelet-rich plasma • Pain management • Future therapy • Chronic pain

KEY POINTS

- Platelet-rich plasma (PRP) has the potential to regenerate tissues through the effects of bioactive molecules and growth factors in the alpha granules of circulated platelets.
- Several PRP preparation systems exist on the market, but there is no universal protocol or standard dosing for PRP or its related growth factors.
- Although limited evidence in the form of prospective, randomized controlled trials exists, the popularity in PRP therapy has still increased in recent years.

INTRODUCTION

The practice of medicine relies on evidence-based clinical research, which prompts clinical researchers to search for alternative therapeutic modalities that are more efficacious and/or more tolerable than existing treatments. Platelet-rich plasma (PRP) has been around for decades, dating back to the 1950s through its use in dermatology and oral maxillofacial surgery, but interest in a role as an effective alternative treatment in many other clinical applications has increased greatly over the past several years.[1]

Platelets contain more than 1100 proteins, some of which include enzymes, enzyme inhibitors, growth factors, immune system messengers, and other bioactive compounds that play a role in tissue repair and wound healing.[2–5] These bioactive

Disclosure Statement: The authors have nothing to disclose.
[a] Department of Anesthesiology, Advocate Illinois Masonic Medical Center, 836 West Wellington Avenue, Suite 4815, Chicago, IL 60657, USA; [b] Department of Anesthesiology, University of Illinois, 1740 W. Taylor St, Chicago, IL 60612, USA; [c] Department of Anesthesiology, Louisiana State University School of Medicine, LSU Health Science Center, 1542 Tulane Avenue, Room 659, New Orleans, LA 70112, USA; [d] Department of Pharmacology, Louisiana State University School of Medicine, 1901 Perdido St, New Orleans, LA 70112, USA
* Corresponding author. Department of Anesthesiology, Louisiana State University School of Medicine, LSU Health Science Center, 1542 Tulane Avenue, Room 659, New Orleans, LA 70112.
E-mail address: alankaye44@hotmail.com

Med Clin N Am 100 (2016) 199–217
http://dx.doi.org/10.1016/j.mcna.2015.08.014   **medical.theclinics.com**

molecules and growth factors that stimulate the tissue healing process are actually found in the alpha granules of circulating platelets.[2-4] Basic science data suggest that platelet-related growth factors should have a beneficial role in enhancing connective tissue healing, but there have not been enough prospective, randomized, double-blinded, controlled studies documenting the positive effect of PRP growth factors on tissue healing.[6-8] Nonetheless, PRP has already been used extensively in various medical specialties, including dentistry, orthopedics, neurosurgery, ophthalmology, maxillofacial surgery, and cosmetic surgery for more than 3 decades.[5,9,10]

This review article clarifies what PRP consists of, how PRP is prepared, how the various PRP-related growth factors play a role in tissue healing and repair, and how the different PRP components affect wound healing. The use of PRP injections as an alternative treatment in pain management is highlighted through evidence-based research reporting the efficacy of PRP therapy in treating different pain conditions, including lateral epicondylitis, osteoarthritis, and surgical rotator cuff repair, as well as eliminating neuropathic pain and intervertebral disc degeneration (IDD).

WHAT IS PLATELET-RICH PLASMA AND HOW IS IT CREATED?

Classically, PRP is defined as a sample of plasma with a platelet concentration that is, 3 to 5 times greater than the physiologic platelet concentration found in healthy whole blood.[11] The normal range for platelet concentration in whole blood is between 150,000 and 450,000 platelets per microliter. However, owing to the large variety of PRP products that exist today, the term PRP has become more generic to account for these different end products. The typical process of obtaining PRP can take place in a clinic, or even an operating room, but it begins with collecting whole blood from a subject or patient through venipuncture.[11,12] There is usually a calcium-binding anticoagulant present when collecting the whole blood such that the conversion of prothrombin to thrombin is blocked, thereby inhibiting the initiation of the clotting cascade.[11] Although the use of an anticoagulant is not mandatory for obtaining PRP, the absence of a calcium-binding anticoagulant leads to rapid activation of the clotting cascade within 30 seconds to minutes.[13] Citrate dextrose-A and citrate phosphate dextrose are the only 2 anticoagulants that have been reported to safely separate platelets, while also supporting the metabolic needs of the platelets.[11]

Once whole blood is collected with or without the anticoagulant present, the most common technique to obtain PRP involves 1 or 2 rounds of centrifugation using a table-top centrifuge system.[5] Centrifugation is a process by which blood is separated into 3 layers (**Fig. 1**): with platelet-poor plasma as the top layer (specific gravity of 1.03), platelet concentrate with white blood cells (WBCs) as the middle layer (specific gravity of 1.06), and red blood cells as the bottom layer (specific gravity of 1.09).[14] The completion of the first centrifugation, often termed a "soft" spin (1200–1500 RPM with a low gravitational force), will result in separation of plasma and platelets from red blood cells and WBCs.[15] This plasma and platelet concentrate may still contain some WBCs that did not completely separate. A second centrifugation, often termed a "hard" spin (4000–7000 RPM), acts to further concentrate the platelets and plasma into PRP and platelet-poor plasma fractions.[14,15] The role of platelet-poor plasma in tissue healing is unclear currently.[15] Once PRP is collected via centrifugation, it is maintained in a sterile environment and used as needed for a particular procedure.[16] PRP remains stable in an anticoagulated state for 8 hours or longer, which is beneficial when performing lengthy procedures.[17]

The final concentration of platelets in the end PRP product is related directly to the amount of whole blood taken to create PRP, the volume of plasma that is used to suspend

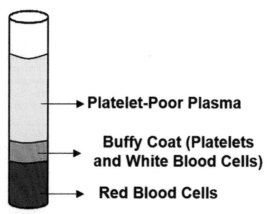

Fig. 1. Example of platelet-rich plasma (PRP) preparation. The buffy coat is the PRP, PRP-related growth factors.

these platelets, and the platelet recovery efficiency of the specific technique used to obtain PRP.[11] It is estimated that the final PRP volume is anywhere between approximately 10% and 16% the volume of whole blood originally obtained from a patient.[12,18]

As stated, the PRP growth factors (**Table 1**) that enhance wound healing are located in the alpha granules of circulating platelets. There have been multiple in vitro studies that have shown a dose–response relationship between the stimulation provided by PRP related growth factors and connective tissue cells.[4,11,19–21] However, most of these PRP growth factors do not have a linear dose–response relationship with connective tissue cells, and some can display an inhibitory effect on cellular function once a certain threshold concentration is reached.[19–21] The exact platelet concentration and the dose of associated growth factors required to optimize the numerous cell types involved in connective tissue healing in vivo remains unclear.[5] Moreover, through in vivo and in vitro research studies, it has been found that PRP actually induces the overexpression of endogenous growth factors in addition to the PRP-related growth factors found in the alpha granules of platelets.[22,23] It also remains unclear if the overexpression of endogenous growth factors offers an additional benefit in tissue healing.

Variety of Platelet-Rich Plasma End Products

Because there are numerous techniques available that create PRP, there is no universal PRP end product. The use of various existing techniques has resulted in a wide variety of PRP products. Currently, there are more than 40 commercial systems that create platelet-rich substance from autologous whole blood.[1] Individual patient factors such as age, circulation, and comorbidities can lead to a difference in PRP-related growth factors and overall content.[24] This PRP can vary in several ways, including the volume of whole blood that was harvested, the inclusion or exclusion of WBCs, the exogenous activation of platelets by thrombin, or the formation of a platelet-rich fibrin matrix.[14] Interestingly, even when specific PRP protocols are used implementing the same kits and centrifuges, the final platelet concentration can still vary greatly within a given technique.[24–27] There is no universal classification system for PRP, but there are 4 categories of PRP that are recognized including leukocyte poor or pure PRP, leukocyte PRP, pure platelet-rich fibrin clot, and leukocyte platelet-rich fibrin clot.[14]

Table 1
Growth factors identified within platelet-rich plasma and their biological functions

Name	Abbreviation	Function
Platelet-derived growth factor	PDGF	Stimulation of fibroblast production, chemotaxis, TGF-β1, collagen production; upregulation of proteoglycan synthesis of fibroblasts, smooth muscle cells, chondrocytes, osteoblasts and mesenchymal stem cells
Insulin-like growth factor-1	IGF-1	Promotion of cell growth, differentiation, recruitment in bone, blood vessel, skin, other tissues; upregulation of collagen synthesis with PDGF of fibroblasts
Transforming growth factor-beta 1	TGF-β1	Promotion of fibroblast proliferation, extracellular matrix formation, cell viability, production of collagen from fibroblasts; suppressed interleukin 1-mediated effects on proteoglycan synthesis in cartilage
Vascular endothelial growth factor	VEGF	Promotion of cell growth, migration, new blood vessel growth and antiapoptosis (anti-cell death) of blood vessel cells
Basic fibroblastic growth factor	bFGF	Stimulation of collagen production, angiogenesis and myoblast proliferation
Epidermal growth factor	EGF	Promotion of cell recruitment, proliferation, differentiation, angiogenesis, cytokine secretion by mesenchymal and epithelial cells
Connective tissue growth factor	CTGF	Promotion of angiogenesis, cartilage regeneration, fibrosis, platelet adhesion

From Wang SZ, Rui YF, Tan Q, et al. Enhancing intervertebral disc repair and regeneration through biology: platelet-rich plasma as an alternative strategy. Arthritis Res Ther 2013;15(5):220; with permission.

Platelet-Rich Plasma Containing White Blood Cells

Some of the techniques used to create PRP results in the inclusion of WBCs with the final PRP product. Currently, it remains unclear if PRP products containing WBCs are beneficial or harmful in tissue healing. PRP containing WBCs has been shown to not only increase healing in soft tissue injuries complicated by infection, but to also inhibit the growth of some bacteria causing infection.[12,28,29] Some studies have reported a positive correlation between increased WBC concentration in PRP and increased levels of the inflammatory cytokines interleukin-1β, tumor necrosis factor-α, interleukin-6, and interleukin-8, which leads to the current concept that WBCs in PRP could potentially inhibit healing in certain tissues or in certain phases of recovery.[2,30–37]

However, it can be stated that positive or negative effects cannot be generalized to all tissues or all clinical conditions and that PRP preparations with WBCs may be beneficial in some conditions.[27,30,31] Additionally, the presence of WBCs in PRP products could also be attributed to the fact that processing techniques are unable to separate these cells completely from the platelets and plasma concentrate.[5,14,26] Prospective clinical studies are therefore needed to prove whether PRP containing leukocytes is advantageous or deleterious.

Platelet-Rich Plasma Activated by Exogenous Thrombin

The half-life of circulating platelets is 7 days.[3] When these circulating platelets become activated by the forces of fluid flow, contact with fibrillar collagen, contact with thrombin, or contact with the basement membrane of cells, the cytokine contents and bioactive molecules present in the alpha granules of the platelets are released and subsequently secreted.[3,38] There are some PRP preparation techniques that implement exogenous bovine or autologous thrombin activation of platelets before injection of PRP because of the assumption that this makes the bioactive molecules in the alpha granules of platelets readily available to target cells.[38] However, it has yet to be proven clinically that the exogenous activation of platelets with thrombin improves connective tissue healing or that it is a recommended step in tissue repair. In fact, when PRP is injected into connective tissues, the platelets become activated by coming into contact with the collagen and tissue thromboplastin present in these tissues.[38] About 70% of the PRP growth factors are secreted within 10 minutes of platelet activation, and within 1 hour approximately 100% of the growth factors are secreted.[11] Thus, activating platelets with exogenous thrombin before injecting PRP leads to a rapid secretion of the platelet growth factors and therefore may shorten the time that target tissues are exposed to these growth factors.[11] Overall, the clinical impact of exogenous thrombin activation of platelets on tissue healing remains unclear because there is limited research at present.[39]

Platelet-Rich Fibrin Matrices

Fibrin serves a very important role in the initial stage of the healing process by acting as a scaffold to provide a surface for cell attachment, adhesion, and migration.[40] These fibrin scaffolds can be created via initiation of the clotting cascade during PRP preparations by adding calcium chloride and/or thrombin after the first centrifugation of whole blood.[24,41–43] The resultant platelet-rich fibrin matrices have the potential for acting as a conductive matrix for migration of cells involved in wound repair and as a reservoir for growth factors, thus serving to prolong growth factor activity, delivery, and availability.[44] Even though there has been a recent study demonstrating the ability of platelet-rich fibrin constructs to initiate healing in lower extremity ulcers, more prospective, randomized, blinded clinical trials are needed to study the role of such constructs in treating other tissues and areas.[45]

Current Clinical Applications of Platelet-Rich Plasma

There is not substantial scientific evidence available in the form of randomized, double-blind clinical studies that document the reliability and effectiveness of PRP therapy in various injuries, because PRP has become increasingly popular over time and its use has increased in similar degrees by orthopedists, primary care physicians, sports medicine physicians, dentists, and other medical specialists.[46,47] Some small, nonrandomized studies and anecdotal case reports have reported that PRP can reduce surgery-related swelling and pain, decrease wound infection rate, promote bone healing in a shorter period of time, increase bone strength, and decrease recovery time.[12,14] PRP has been documented to be used in heart bypass surgery, plastic surgery, maxillofacial surgery, dermatology, and orthopedic surgery.[16] Currently, PRP is used commonly to treat lateral epicondylitis, plantar fasciopathy, Achilles and patellar tendinopathies, acute muscle tears, medial collateral ligament tears, anterior cruciate ligament tears, and ankle sprains.[16]

Platelet-Rich Plasma Injection in Lateral Epicondylitis (Tennis Elbow)

PRP use in tennis elbow has been rather extensively studied. In fact, a recent large double-blinded randomized controlled trial (n = 100)[48] that compared PRP injections with corticosteroid injections concluded that there was a statistically and clinically significant difference in tennis elbow–specific quality of life in pain scores favoring the PRP group.[48] Criteria to participate in the study included having lateral epicondylitis for longer than 6 months with a pain score of at least 50 on a visual analog score (0–100), and excluded patients age younger than 18 years and a history of cervical radiculopathy or carpal tunnel syndrome.[48] As part of the double-blind approach, 27 mL of whole blood was collected from both the PRP group and the corticosteroid (control) group into a 30-mL syringe containing 3 mL sodium citrate.[48] After 3 mL of PRP was obtained from this blood, all the tubes were masked with opaque tape, then 3 mL of PRP was injected in each patient in the PRP group and 3 mL of corticosteroid was injected in each patient in the control group.[48] The study suggested that progressive healing could be playing a significant role in the clinical improvement of the PRP group based on the finding that the PRP group progressively improved at the 1- and 2-year follow-up visits in comparison with the corticosteroid group, which only showed short-term clinical improvement followed by a decline.[48,49] Mishra and Pavelko[50] did a controlled trial with 20 patients comparing PRP injections containing WBCs with bupivacaine local injections for treating chronic elbow epicondylar tendinosis. They found that the PRP group had a 93% reduction in pain at an average follow-up of 25.6 months ($P<.0001$). Additionally, after 8 weeks of treatment with PRP, there was a significant clinical improvement in the visual analog scale and Mayo elbow scores ($P = .001$ and $P = .008$, respectively). Based on the results of these studies, it is suggested that PRP injections provide better clinical outcomes than local anesthetic and corticosteroid injections in treating pain related to tennis elbow.

Osteoarthritis and Articular Cartilage Healing

Overall, through the results of several studies, it seems that PRP may offer therapeutic benefits for repairing cartilage in patients with joint disease secondary to arthritic changes. A particular prospective, double-blind, randomized trial that randomized 78 patients with bilateral knee osteoarthritis to receive either a single saline injection, a single WBC-filtered PRP injection, or 2 PRP injections 3 weeks apart, concluded that both of the PRP groups had significantly better clinical outcomes than the control group 6 months status post treatment.[51] Cerza and colleagues[52] performed a prospective, double-blind, randomized controlled trial that showed better outcomes 24 weeks after treatment in a group receiving a single PRP injection when compared with a group receiving a single injection of hyaluronic acid ($P<.001$). In another prospective, double-blind, randomized controlled trial that involved 109 patients, Filardo and colleagues[53] reported that the group receiving intraarticular PRP injections had significant clinical improvement 1 year after treatment, but their improvement was not better than the group receiving a single hyaluronic acid injection. Although the benefits of PRP injections in treating osteoarthritis is highlighted by these 3 studies, a group of authors of a Clinical Practice Guideline sponsored by the American Academy of Orthopedic Surgeons were "unable to recommend for or against growth factor injections and/or PRP for patients with symptomatic osteoarthritis of the knee."[54]

Mei-Dan and colleagues[55] performed a prospective, nonrandomized controlled trial comparing the effects of PRP and hyaluronic intraarticular injections in 32 patients with symptomatic osteochondral lesions of the talus. The results of the study at 28 week follow-up showed that the PRP group had significantly greater clinical improvements in pain, stiffness, and function scores when compared with the hyaluronic acid group ($P<.0001$). Overall, 87% of the patients in the PRP group obtained good results. These findings led the authors of the study to state that PRP should be a first-line treatment for symptomatic osteochondral lesions of the talus.[55]

Even though these studies reveal that PRP offers clinical benefits in the treatment of osteoarthritis, further research still needs to be done to determine just how effective PRP is in treating damaged articular cartilage related to arthritic changes.

Platelet-Rich Plasma as an Adjunct Therapy to Surgical Rotator Cuff Repair

Based on the results of 5 level I and II controlled studies, there seems to be some potential benefit of using PRP therapy as an adjunct to the surgical repair of rotator cuffs; however, further evidence is still needed before PRP therapy can actually be recommended as a routine treatment with rotator cuff repairs.

Three of these studies did not show a significant benefit from using PRP therapy. Castricini and colleagues[56] reported that PRP does not have a significant benefit for small to medium sized rotator cuff tears. Likewise, in a different study consisting of 79 patients, Rodeo and colleagues[57] found that the group with platelet-rich fibrin matrix sutured in the tendon–bone interface did not show any difference in clinical scores at a 1-year follow-up when compared with the control group.[57] Furthermore, there was also a prospective cohort study with 42 patients done by Jo and colleagues[58] that studied the effects of PRP gel applied to arthroscopic rotator cuff repairs. The authors of this study concluded that the PRP group did not have accelerated recovery with respect to pain, motion, strength, or overall patient satisfaction at any time point beginning with 16 months status post surgery.

On the other hand, the remaining 2 clinical trials did document a potential benefit of using PRP in rotator cuff repair surgeries. The first of these studies, done by Randelli and colleagues,[59] consisted of a double-blind randomized controlled trial of 53 patients in which the experimental group had PRP with autologous thrombin applied during arthroscopic rotator cuff repair. The findings of this study demonstrated that using PRP in grade 1 and 2 rotator cuff tears led to significantly higher strength in external rotation scores at 3, 6, 12, and 24 months postoperatively ($P<.05$) and a lower rate of rerupture ($P = .08$). Randelli and colleagues[59] used a different commercial preparation of PRP than Castricini and colleagues[56] and Rodeo and colleagues[57] Moreover, another randomized trial consisting of 40 patients with subacromial decompression also concluded that the PRP group had significantly decreased pain scores and improved shoulder range of motion after surgery when compared with the control group ($P<.001$).[11]

HOW PLATELET-RICH PLASMA CAN HELP TO RELIEVE NEUROPATHIC PAIN

PRP was found to promote axon regeneration in studies involving animal models.[60–65] In this regard, Cho and colleagues[64] conducted a prospective, controlled study investigating the effects of PRP and neural-induced human mesenchymal stem cells (MSC) on axonal regeneration from a facial nerve axotomy injury in 24 albino guinea pigs. The guinea pigs were anesthetized with pentobarbital sodium by intraperitoneal injection and surgery was performed under an operating microscope.[64] The guinea pigs were randomly divided into 4 groups: group I received microsuture only, group II received microsuture with 5 μL PRP, group III received microsuture with 1×10^5 cells in 5 μL of neural-induced human MSCs, and group IV received microsuture with 5 μL PRP and 1×10^5 cells in 5 μL of neural-induced human MSCs.[64] This 6-week study concluded that the combined use of PRP and neural-induced MSCs promoted facial nerve regeneration and was of greater benefit for facial nerve regeneration than using either treatment alone.[64]

Studying tissue cultures, PRP was also seen to promote axon growth by spinal cord tissue and PRP related factors insulin-like growth factor (IGF)-1 and vascular endothelial growth factor.[60,66] Although, there exists 1 study that did not find axonal regeneration in the presence of PRP, this result may have been attributed to the methods in which PRP was prepared.[67] A specific component in PRP that might play a pivotal role in axonal regeneration is multipotent MSCs.[68–70] Axonal regeneration occurred in 1 series of experiments after MSCs were applied to the end of transected peripheral nerves.[71] The means by which this axonal regeneration occurs in the presence of MSCs may be related to the promotion of angiogenesis and secretion of nerve growth factor and brain-derived neurotrophic factor by MSCs.[72–76] The importance of MSCs remains unclear, because in another study involving a series of experiments, axonal regeneration was not enhanced in the presence of MSCs.[64] However, in this same study, axonal regeneration increased when MSCs were combined with PRP compared with the impact of PRP alone on axonal regeneration.[64]

Clinical Evidence That Platelet-Rich Plasma Has the Potential for Relieving Neuropathic Pain

A recent small clinical study was performed by Kuffler[77] using PRP therapy in patients suffering from mild to severe neuropathic pain secondary to a damaged nonregenerated nerve. The purpose of this study was to determine whether the neuropathic pain in these patients would decrease or resolve as a result of PRP's promotion of axonal regeneration and target reinnervation. The surgical procedure used in this study involved refreshing the central and distal nerve stumps of damaged nerves, followed by inserting these stumps into a collagen tube, and then filling each tube with autologous PRP. The results of this procedure actually caused resected axons to regenerate across long gaps, up to 16 cm in length. Further, neuropathic pain in 94% of the patients, including 1 patient with severe neuropathic pain, was eliminated. Additionally, the neuropathic pain of another patient who had severe pain decreased to a tolerable level. The neuropathic pain of the patients in this study remained eliminated or reduced for a minimum of 6 years after the operative procedure. In fact, every single patient noticed their pain start to decrease within 3 weeks of the surgery, which was weeks before target reinnervation could even begin. Owing to this fact, a correlation cannot be made between the number of axons that reinnervated their targets and the extent to which neuropathic pain decreased. The data from this study suggest that a single PRP injection can lead to a long-term decrease in or elimination of neuropathic pain. It remains unclear whether the actual application of autologous PRP, the reestablishment of axon contact with Schwann cells, or the reinnervation of target tissues was the key factor leading to the reduction of neuropathic pain.[77]

More prospective clinical studies are warranted to confirm the results of this study, determine its reliability, and determine the various nerve conditions under which it is effective. If future clinical studies can demonstrate that autologous PRP therapy is in fact effective at decreasing or eliminating neuropathic pain, then this could pave the way for PRP therapy as a superior treatment approach for neuropathic pain when compared with other treatments and drugs currently available.

INTERVERTEBRAL DISC DEGENERATION AND THE ROLE OF PLATELET-RICH PLASMA AS A THERAPEUTIC OPTION

IDD is a leading cause of lower back pain. This degeneration may be owing to aging, biomechanical loading, genetics, or an individual's daily activity and overall condition. PRP therapy has the potential for reversing IDD and relieving the lower back pain attributed to IDD. PRP may slow or reverse IDD by upregulating the synthesis of aggrecan and collagen and by directly stimulating MSC to differentiate into mature intervertebral disc cells.[78] In an in vitro study, it was proven that PRP increased human

MSC proliferation and MSC chondrogenic differentiation.[79] Aggrecan and collagen are 2 main components of the extracellular matrix of intervertebral discs so an increase in their production through the synergistic effects of PRP growth factors may help to maintain the function of these discs.[78] Aggrecan, as the major proteoglycan, leads to an increase in water absorption and hydration of the disc.[80–82] Collagen anchors tissue to bone and acts to provide tensile strength.[80] The various growth factors secreted by activated platelets all play significant roles in the proliferation of tissues. These growth factors include platelet-derived growth factor, IGF-1, transforming growth factor (TGF)-β, vascular endothelial growth factor, basic fibroblastic growth factor, epidermal growth factor, and connective tissue growth factor.[83,84] Platelets may also be able to absorb, store, and transfer molecules that regulate tissue regeneration.[4] In comparison with other bioactive peptides and growth factors involved in tissue healing, autologous PRP seems to be a superior choice. Because autologous PRP is obtained via centrifugation of an individual's own whole blood, disease transmission and immunologic reactions are avoided.[85] However, because of the nature in which PRP is obtained, it is only suitable for patients without hematologic diseases.

In general, PRP injection into intervertebral discs is less invasive than other therapeutic procedures, such as surgery. However, caution is still required when using PRP injection. It is most beneficial to use smaller needles and fewer injections because needle puncture into the intervertebral disc could induce cell death and disc degeneration.[86–88] A few studies using animal models have actually shown that a single PRP injection into the degenerated intervertebral disc has been effective in healing the disc via regeneration. For example, Obata and colleagues[87,88] used a rabbit IDD model to conclude that a single intradiscal injection of PRP had the ability to restore disc height and lead to cell proliferation. Gullung and colleagues[86] concluded that 1 PRP injection in the intervertebral discs of Sprague-Dawley rats was enough to maintain fluid content on MRI. The evidence of the benefits of single PRP injections with small needles in these animal studies may be enough to pave way for clinical application of autologous PRP injections in humans with low back pain attributed to IDD.

The Efficacy of Platelet-Rich Plasma Therapy in Intervertebral Disc Degeneration Seen Through In Vivo and In Vitro Studies

There have been several in vivo and in vitro studies demonstrating the efficacy of PRP therapy in treating IDD. Through culturing intervertebral disc cells, specifically human nucleus pulposus cells isolated from volunteers of different ages, with TGF-β1 in PRP for 6 weeks, Chen and colleagues[89] concluded that PRP significantly increased disc height index, increased levels of messenger RNAs involved in matrix accumulation and chondrogenesis, and promoted nucleus pulposus regeneration. They determined that the most effective dose for human nucleus pulposus proliferation was 1 ng/mL of TGF-β1 in PRP.[89] A study from Akeda and colleagues[90] concluded that locally administering PRP mildly stimulates intervertebral disc repair by increasing the accumulation of glycosaminoglycan, type II collagen, and aggrecan. Interestingly enough, Akeda and colleagues suggested that directly injecting the intervertebral disc could lead to uncontrolled release of growth factors at variable rates. Nagae and colleagues[91] focused on this unstable release of growth factors and slowed down the release of growth factors through a study using a rabbit IDD model that implemented PRP implanted within gelatin hydrogel microspheres. They concluded that this combination therapy led to a sustained release of the PRP growth factors, resulting in a significant suppression of the degeneration of intervertebral discs over an 8-week period. Furthermore, Sawamura and colleagues[92] strengthened the effectiveness of the same combination therapy through noting results of increased messenger RNA expression of proteoglycan and type II collagen and maintenance of disc height and signal intensity on MRI.

A study from Gullung and colleagues[86] used PRP injection on Sprague-Dawley rats to compare early intervention and late intervention in IDD. They found that while injecting PRP early in disease and late in disease both resulted in greater intervertebral disc fluid content on MRI, there was a superior effect in the early PRP injection group. Similarly, in a degenerative murine caudal disc compression model, Walsh and colleagues[93] concluded that early intervention during disc degeneration could potentially slow down degeneration. This early intervention makes sense because many viable cells remain and few phenotypic changes are seen during the early stages of disc degeneration.

There have been several studies demonstrating the positive effects of PRP growth factors on intervertebral discs (**Table 2**). The cytokines and growth factors of PRP help

Table 2
The effects of platelet-rich plasma growth factors on intervertebral discs

Author(s), Year	Growth Factor	Cell Type	Results
Liu et al,[117] 2010	CTGF	Rhesus monkey lumbar intervertebral disc nucleus pulposus cells	Enhanced synthesis of proteoglycan and collagen II
Thompson et al,[118] 1991	EGF	Mature canine intervertebral disc cells	Enhanced proliferation
Thompson et al,[118] 1991	bFGF	Mature canine intervertebral disc cells	Increased matrix synthesis and cell proliferation
Pratsinis & Kletsas,[119] 2007	bFGF	Bovine coccygeal nucleus pulposus and annulus fibrosus cells	Enhanced proliferation
Fujita et al,[120] 2008	VEGF	Mouse nucleus pulposus cells	Promotion of nucleus pulposus survival
Walsh et al,[93] 2004	IGF-1	Mouse caudal disc compression model	Upward trend of cell density, but not statistically significant (single injection); trend of increased disc height, but not statistically significant (multiple injections)
Walsh et al,[93] 2004	TGF-β1	Mouse caudal disc compression model	Greater percentage of proliferating cells, but not statistically significant (single injection); increased population of annular fibrochondrocytes (multiple injections)

Abbreviations: bFGF, basic fibroblastic growth factor; CTGF, connective tissue growth factor; EGF, epidermal growth factor; TGF, transforming growth factor; VEGF, vascular endothelial growth factor.

From Wang SZ, Rui YF, Tan Q, et al. Enhancing intervertebral disc repair and regeneration through biology: platelet-rich plasma as an alternative strategy. Arthritis Res Ther 2013;15(5):220; with permission.

to maintain intervertebral disc homeostasis through shifting from catabolism to anabolism.[94] TGF-β1, IGF-1, and platelet-derived growth factor are 3 important growth factors that have been reported to play a role in this shift to anabolism. For example, Gruber and colleagues[95] reported that TGF-β1 stimulates the proliferation of human annulus fibrosus cells after 4 days of exposure. Lee and colleagues[96] also saw the proliferative effect of TGF-β1 on annulus fibrosus cells through culturing rabbit annulus fibrosus cells with TGF-β1. Additionally, Hayes and Ralphs[97] concluded that TGF-β1 and IGF-1 in combination or alone stimulate annulus cells to synthesize type I collagen, type II collagen, and sulfated glycosaminoglycan. IGF-1 and platelet-derived growth factor have been shown to actually reduce the percentage of apoptotic annulus fibrosus cells.[98] These studies all suggest that the PRP growth factors contribute greatly to the regeneration of intervertebral discs.

INFORMATION FOR PHYSICIANS USING PLATELET-RICH PLASMA THERAPY

It is suggested that sterile technique should be used when administering PRP injections.[16] Currently, it remains unclear as to what effect, if any at all, local anesthetic has on PRP.[16] Therefore, the use of local anesthetic in the region of PRP injection is typically avoided.[16] The method by which PRP is commonly injected consists of using either a 20-G or 22-G needle under ultrasound guidance.[16] Imaging such as ultrasonography or fluoroscopy can be useful to not only guide PRP injections to the proper location of target tissues, but to also observe tissue healing over time.[16] Additionally, diagnostic imaging before applying PRP injections may be valuable in establishing a diagnosis and a baseline clinical condition. Having a baseline clinical condition of target tissues helps to evaluate tissue healing after PRP injection.

Patient Disclosure, Potential Side Effects, and Costs of Treatment

Just like any other procedure, an informed consent is required of any patient receiving PRP injections. The informed consent includes the risks related to PRP injections, which are infection, bleeding, and soft tissue injury.[16] Because PRP causes local inflammation, it is normal for there to be pain at the injection site for 24 to 48 hours after the procedure. However, nonsteroidal anti-inflammatory drugs should be avoided 2 weeks before and at least 2 weeks after the procedure so that they do not inhibit the healing process or the PRP growth factors that play a role in the tissue healing.[16] Currently, no postprocedure guidelines exist that may lead to optimization of PRP therapy.[16]

Because PRP treatment is still considered experimental, it is not usually covered by insurance companies. It is important to disclose this information to patients and make them aware that they will most likely be paying the costs of treatment out of pocket. This information should also be discussed in the informed consent process before administering PRP injections.[16] A physician is restricted from billing for imaging guidance, harvesting, and preparation of PRP separately, because these 3 are grouped under the 0232T billing code, which is a category III temporary code for emerging technologies, services, and procedures.[99] Even though the market for PRP is expected to grow to $126 million by 2016, there is not enough clinical evidence to do a cost–benefit analysis for the use of PRP in orthopedic conditions.[100] However, if PRP therapy eventually leads to a decreased need for further intervention with regard to pain control or has a greater patient satisfaction during follow-up visits in comparison with other treatment modalities used to achieve pain relief, such as corticosteroid injections, it will likely lead to lower total costs for the patients seeking treatment.

Gosens and colleagues[49] actually suggested that in the long run PRP therapy may be less expensive than corticosteroid therapy based on a double-blind randomized controlled trial comparing the positive effects of PRP injection with corticosteroid injection in lateral epicondylitis with 2-year follow-up visits. The recurrence rate of pain from lateral epicondylitis and the need for repeated injection was greater in the corticosteroid group than in the PRP group.[49] On a short-term basis, PRP is not cost effective compared with corticosteroid injections, but if the costs of patients failing on corticosteroid therapy who proceed to surgery are taken into account, the differences in cost effectiveness may level out.[49]

FUTURE CONSIDERATION/SUMMARY

PRP, through the action of its related growth factors, has the potential to stimulate tissue healing and repair.[39] However, no standard procedure for PRP production exists, which leads to varying concentration of platelets produced, varying number of growth factors within the PRP, and thus varying clinical results from PRP therapy.[78] It remains unclear whether PRP containing WBCs or the activation of PRP by exogenous thrombin has a beneficial effect on tissue healing.[39] Platelet-rich fibrin matrices have the ability to increase the migration of cells involved in tissue repair and can lead to the prolongation of PRP growth factor activity, availability, and delivery by serving as a reservoir for these growth factors.[44]

Regardless of the limited clinical-based evidence that currently exists, PRP injections have already been applied clinically to initiate healing and decrease pain associated with lateral epicondylitis, osteoarthritis, rotator cuff tears, and ligament and tendon injuries.[55,101–111] Based on the most recent randomized controlled clinical trial data, PRP therapy seems to be beneficial for treating chronic tendinopathy.[48,50,112]

It is also determined that PRP leads directly to the elimination of neuropathic pain through a full cascade of wound healing, beginning with the induction of enhanced inflammation and its complete resolution, followed by tissue remodeling and wound repair, and concluding with axon regeneration and target tissue reinnervation.[77] This complex cascade of events allows axons to take up target-released factors that will eliminate nociceptive neuron hyperexcitability.[77]

Furthermore, PRP shows promise for reversing disc degeneration via its promotion of wound healing and tissue repair.[113–115] Moreover, steroid injections continue to be a common clinical therapy for pain relief from back pain and other injuries, but studies have demonstrated that the pain relief from these steroids is only temporary and that there is no impact on the actual underlying pathophysiology causing the pain.[116] Corticosteroid therapy tends to have side effects, especially with repeat injections. Based on current research studies, there have been no reported complications associated with PRP injections.[12,48,112]

PRP likely will not be a primary or mainstream therapy until further prospective, randomized controlled clinical trials in human patients are completed documenting its benefits and positive influence on tissue healing. Further research and clinical trials are also needed to study the undesirable effects induced by PRP, to determine optimal dosing of growth factors in PRP for tissue healing, and to determine possible interactions between these growth factors.[78] According to evidence-based literature, the success of PRP therapy will depend on the method of preparation and composition of PRP, the patient's medical condition, anatomic location of the injection, and the type of tissue that is injected.

REFERENCES

1. Hsu WK, Mishra A, Rodeo SR, et al. Platelet-rich plasma in orthopaedic applications: evidence-based recommendations for treatment. J Am Acad Orthop Surg 2013;21:739–48.

2. Toumi H, Best TM. The inflammatory response: friend or enemy for muscle injury? Br J Sports Med 2003;37:284–6.
3. Blair P, Flaumenhaft R. Platelet α-granules: basic biology and clinical correlates. Blood Rev 2009;23:177–89.
4. Leslie M. Beyond clotting: the power of platelets. Science 2010;328:562–4.
5. Arnoczky SP, Delos D, Rodeo SA. What is platelet-rich plasma? Oper Tech Sports Med 2011;19:142–8.
6. Gullota LV, Rodeo SA. Growth factors for rotator cuff repair. Clin Sports Med 2009;28:13–23.
7. Vavaken P, Saad FA, Murray MM. Age dependence of expression of growth factor receptors in porcine ACL fibroblasts. J Orthop Res 2010;28:1107–12.
8. Sprugel KH, McPherson JM, Clowes AW, et al. Effects of growth factors in vivo. Am J Pathol 1987;129:601–13.
9. Kingsley CS. Blood coagulation: evidence of an antagonist to factor VI in platelet-rich human plasma. Nature 1954;173:723–4.
10. Sampson S, Gerhardt M, Mandelbaum B. Platelet-rich plasma injection grafts for musculoskeletal injuries: a review. Curr Rev Musculoskelet Med 2008;1:165–74.
11. Marx RE. Platelet-rich Plasma (PRP). What is PRP and what is not PRP? Implant Dent 2001;10:225–8.
12. Alsousou J, Thompson M, Hulley P, et al. The biology of platelet-rich plasma and its application in trauma and orthopaedic surgery: a review of the literature. J Bone Joint Surg Br 2009;91:987–96.
13. Steine-Martin EA, Lotspeich-Steininger CA, Koepke JA. Clinical hematology: principles, procedures, correlations. 2nd edition. Philadelphia: Lippincott Williams & Wilkins; 1998.
14. Dohan Ehrenfest DM, Rasmusson L, Albrektsson T. Classification of platelet concentrates: from pure platelet-rich plasma (P-PRP) to leukocyte- and platelet-rich fibrin (L-PRF). Trends Biotechnol 2009;27:158–67.
15. Mazzocca AD, McCarthy MB, Chowaniec DM, et al. Platelet-rich plasma differs according to preparation method and human variability. J Bone Joint Surg Am 2012;94:308–16.
16. Lee KS. Platelet-rich plasma injection. Semin Musculoskelet Radiol 2013;17:91–8.
17. Marx RE, Carlson ER, Eichstaedt RM, et al. Platelet rich plasma: growth factor enhancement for bone grafts. Oral Surg Oral Med Oral Pathol Oral Radiol Endod 1998;85:638–46.
18. Kuffler DP, Reyes O, Sosa IJ, et al. Neurological recovery across a 12-cm-long ulnar nerve gap repaired 3.25 years post trauma: case report. Neurosurgery 2011;69:E1321–6.
19. Mooren R, Hendriks EJ, van der Beuken J, et al. The effect of platelet-rich plasma in vitro on primary cells: rat osteoblast-like cells and human endothelial cells. Tissue Eng Part A 2010;16:3159–72.
20. Alberts B, Bray D, Lewis J, et al. Molecular biology of the cell. 3rd edition. New York: Garland Publishing Inc; 1994.
21. Ranly DM, McMillan J, Keller T, et al. Platelet-derived growth factor inhibits demineralized bone matrix-induced intramuscular cartilage and bone formation. A study of immune-compromised mice. J Bone Joint Surg Am 2005;87:2052–64.
22. de Mos M, van der Windt AE, Jahr H, et al. Can platelet-rich plasma enhance tendon repair? A cell culture study. Am J Sports Med 2008;36:1171–8.
23. Lyras DN, Kazakos K, Agrogiannis G, et al. Experimental study of tendon healing early phase: is IGF-1 expression influenced by platelet rich plasma gel? Orthop Traumatol Surg Res 2010;96:381–7.

24. Mazzucco L, Balbo V, Cattana E, et al. Not every PRP-gel is born equal: evaluation of growth factor availability for tissues through four PRP-gel preparations: Fibrinet®, RegenPRP-Kit®, Plateltex®, and one Manual Procedure. Vox Sang 2009;97:110–8.

25. Weibrich G, Hansen T, Kleis W, et al. Effect of platelet concentration in platelet-rich plasma on peri-implant bone regeneration. Bone 2004;34:665–71.

26. Mei-Dan O, Mann G, Maffulli N. Platelet-rich plasma: any substance to it? Br J Sports Med 2010;44:618–9.

27. Leitner GC, Gruber R, Neumuller J, et al. Platelet content and growth factor release in platelet-rich plasma: a comparison of four different systems. Vox Sang 2006;91:135–9.

28. Bielecki TM, Gazdzik TS, Arendt J, et al. Antibacterial effect of autologous platelet gel enriched with growth factors and other active substances: an in vitro study. J Bone Joint Surg Br 2007;89:417–20.

29. Cieslik-Bielecka A, Bielecki T, Gazdzik TS, et al. Autologous platelets and leukocytes can improve healing of infected high energy soft tissue injury. Transfus Apher Sci 2009;41:9–12.

30. McCarrel TM, Minas T, Fortier LA. Optimization of leukocyte concentration in platelet-rich plasma for the treatment of tendinopathy. J Bone Joint Surg Am 2012;94:1–8.

31. Dragoo JL, Braun HJ, Durham JL, et al. Comparison of the acute inflammatory response of two commercial platelet-rich plasma systems in healthy rabbit tendons. Am J Sports Med 2012;40:1274–81.

32. Muylle L, Joos M, Wouters E, et al. Increased tumor necrosis factor alpha (TNF alpha), interleukin 1, and interleukin 6 (IL-6) levels in the plasma of stored platelet concentrates: relationship between TNF alpha and IL-6 levels and febrile transfusion reactions. Transfusion 1993;33:195–9.

33. Stack G, Snyder EL. Cytokine generation in stored platelet concentrates. Transfusion 1994;34:20–5.

34. Aye MT, Palmer DS, Giulivi A, et al. Effect of filtration of platelet concentrates on the accumulation of cytokines and platelet release factors during storage. Transfusion 1995;35:117–24.

35. Palmer DS, Aye MT, Dumont L, et al. Prevention of cytokine accumulation in platelets obtained with the COBE spectra apheresis system. Vox Sang 1998; 75:115–23.

36. Martin P, Leibovich SJ. Inflammatory cells during wound healing: the good, the bad, and the ugly. Trends Cell Biol 2005;15:599–607.

37. Schneider BS, Tiidus P. Neutrophil infiltration in exercise-injured muscle: how do we solve the controversy? Sports Med 2007;37:837–56.

38. Mann KG. Biochemistry and physiology of blood coagulation. Thromb Haemost 1999;82:165–74.

39. Arnoczky SP, Shebani-Rad S. The basic science of platelet-rich plasma (PRP): what clinicians need to know. Sports Med Arthrosc Rev 2013;21:180–5.

40. Ahmed TA, Dare EV, Hincke M. Fibrin: a versatile scaffold for tissue engineering applications. Tissue Eng Part B Rev 2008;14:199–215.

41. Visser LC, Arnoczky SP, Caballero O, et al. Platelet-rich fibrin constructs elute higher concentrations of TGF-β1 and increase tendon cell proliferation over time when compared to blood clots: a comparative in vitro analysis. Vet Surg 2010;39:811–7.

42. Lucarelli E, Beretta R, Dozza B, et al. A recently developed bifacial platelet-rich fibrin matrix. Eur Cell Mater 2010;20:13–23.

43. Anitua E, Sanchez M, Nurden AT, et al. New insights into and novel applications for platelet-rich fibrin therapies. Trends Biotechnol 2006;24:227–34.
44. Macri L, Silverstein D, Clark RA. Growth factor binding to the pericellular matrix and its importance in tissue engineering. Adv Drug Deliv Rev 2007;59:1366–81.
45. O'Connor SM, Impeduglia T, Hessler K, et al. Autologous platelet-rich fibrin matrix as cell therapy in the healing of chronic lower-extremity ulcers. Wound Repair Regen 2008;16:749–56.
46. Foster TE, Puskas BL, Mandelbaum BR, et al. Platelet-rich plasma: from basic science to clinical applications. Am J Sports Med 2009;37:2259–72.
47. Jeong GK, Sandhu HS, Farmer J. Bone morphogenic proteins: applications in spinal surgery. HSS J 2005;1:110–7.
48. Peerbooms JC, Sluimer J, Bruijn DJ, et al. Positive effect of an autologous platelet concentrate in lateral epicondylitis in a double-blind randomized controlled trial: platelet-rich plasma versus corticosteroid injection with a 1-year follow-up. Am J Sports Med 2010;38:255–62.
49. Gosens T, Peerbooms JC, van Laar W, et al. Ongoing positive effect of platelet-rich plasma versus corticosteroid injection in lateral epicondylitis: a double-blind randomized controlled trial with 2-year follow-up. Am J Sports Med 2011;39:1200–8.
50. Mishra A, Pavelko T. Treatment of chronic elbow tendinosis with buffered platelet-rich plasma. Am J Sports Med 2006;34:1774–8.
51. Patel S, Dhillon MS, Aggarwal S, et al. Treatment with platelet-rich plasma is more effective than placebo for knee osteoarthritis: a prospective, double-blind, randomized trial. Am J Sports Med 2013;41:356–64.
52. Cerza F, Carni S, Carcangiu A, et al. Comparison between hyaluronic acid and platelet-rich plasma, intra-articular infiltration in the treatment of gonarthrosis. Am J Sports Med 2012;40:2822–7.
53. Filardo G, Kon E, Di Martino A, et al. Platelet-rich plasma vs hyaluronic acid to treat knee degenerative pathology: study design and preliminary results of a randomized controlled trial. BMC Musculoskelet Disord 2012;13:229.
54. American Academy of Orthopaedic Surgeons. Treatment of osteoarthritis of the knee: evidence-based guideline. 2nd edition. Available at: http://www.aaos.org/research/guidelines/TreatmentofOsteoarthritisoftheKneeGuideline.pdf. Accessed October 3, 2013.
55. Mei-Dan O, Carmont MR, Laver L, et al. Platelet-rich plasma or hyaluronate in the management of osteochondral lesions of the talus. Am J Sports Med 2012;40:534–41.
56. Castricini R, Longo UG, De Benedetto M, et al. Platelet-rich plasma augmentation for arthroscopic rotator cuff repair: a randomized controlled trial. Am J Sports Med 2011;39:258–65.
57. Rodeo SA, Delos D, Williams RJ, et al. The effect of platelet-rich fibrin matrix on rotator cuff tendon healing: a prospective, randomized clinical study. Am J Sports Med 2012;40:1234–41.
58. Jo CH, Kim JE, Yoon KS, et al. Does platelet-rich plasma accelerate recovery after rotator cuff repair? A prospective cohort study. Am J Sports Med 2011;39:2082–90.
59. Randelli P, Arrigoni P, Ragone V, et al. Platelet rich plasma in arthroscopic rotator cuff repair: a prospective RCT study, 2-year follow-up. J Shoulder Elbow Surg 2011;20:518–28.
60. Emel E, Ergun SS, Kotan D, et al. Effects of insulin-like growth factor-I and platelet-rich plasma on sciatic nerve crush injury in a rat model. J Neurosurg 2011;114:522–8.

61. Elgazzar RF, Mutabagani MA, Abdelaal SE, et al. Platelet-rich plasma may enhance peripheral nerve regeneration after cyanoacrylate reanastomosis: a controlled blind study on rats. Int J Oral Maxillofac Surg 2008; 37:748–55.

62. Yu W, Wang J, Yin J. Platelet-rich plasma: a promising product for treatment of peripheral nerve regeneration after nerve Injury. Int J Neurosci 2011;121: 176–80.

63. Wu CC, Wu YN, Ho HO, et al. The neuroprotective effect of platelet-rich plasma on erectile function in bilateral cavernous nerve injury rat model. J Sex Med 2012;9:2838.

64. Cho HH, Jang S, Lee SC, et al. Effect of neural-induced mesenchymal stem cells and platelet-rich plasma on facial nerve regeneration in an acute nerve injury model. Laryngoscope 2010;120:907–13.

65. Farrag TY, Lehar M, Verhaegen P, et al. Effect of platelet-rich plasma and fibrin sealant on facial nerve regeneration in a rat model. Laryngoscope 2007;117: 157–65.

66. Takeuchi M, Kamei N, Shinomiya R, et al. Human platelet-rich plasma promotes axon growth in brain-spinal cord coculture. Neuroreport 2012;23:712–6.

67. Piskin A, Kaplan S, Aktas A, et al. Platelet gel does not improve peripheral nerve regeneration: an electrophysiological, stereological, and electron microscopic study. Microsurgery 2009;29:144–53.

68. Duan J, Kuang W, Tan J, et al. Differential effects of platelet rich plasma and washed platelets on the proliferation of mouse MSC cells. Mol Biol Rep 2011; 38:2485–90.

69. Pak J. Autologous adipose tissue-derived stem cells induce persistent bone-like tissue in osteonecrotic femoral heads. Pain Physician 2012;68:22–4.

70. Tischler M. Platelet rich plasma. The use of autologous growth factors to enhance bone and soft tissue grafts. N Y State Dent J 2002;68:22–4.

71. Goel RK, Suri V, Suri A, et al. Effect of bone marrow-derived mononuclear cells on nerve regeneration in the transection model of the rat sciatic nerve. J Clin Neurosci 2009;16:1211–7.

72. Wang Y, Jia H, Li WY, et al. Synergistic effects of bone mesenchymal stem cells and chondroitinase abc on nerve regeneration after acellular nerve allograft in rats. Cell Mol Neurobiol 2012;32:361–71.

73. Wang X, Luo E, Li Y, et al. Schwann-like mesenchymal stem cells within vein graft facilitate facial nerve regeneration and remyelination. Brain Res 2011; 1383:71–80.

74. Singh K, Masuda K, An HS. Animal models for human disc degeneration. Spine J 2005;5:267S–79S.

75. Adams MA, Roughley PJ. What is intervertebral disc degeneration, and what causes it? Spine 2006;31:2151–61.

76. Freemont AJ. The cellular pathobiology of the degenerate intervertebral disc and discogenic back pain. Rheumatology 2009;48:5–10.

77. Kuffler DP. Platelet-rich plasma and the elimination of neuropathic pain. Mol Neurobiol 2013;48:315–32.

78. Wang SZ, Rui YF, Tan Q, et al. Enhancing intervertebral disc repair and regeneration through biology: platelet-rich plasma as an alternative strategy. Arthritis Res Ther 2013;15:220.

79. Mishra A, Tummala P, King A, et al. Buffered platelet-rich plasma enhances mesenchymal stem cell proliferation and chondrogenic differentiation. Tissue Eng 2009;15:431–5.

80. Urban JP, Roberts S. Degeneration of the intervertebral disc. Arthritis Res Ther 2003;5:120–30.
81. Johnstone B, Bayliss MT. The large proteoglycans of the human intervertebral disc. Changes in their biosynthesis and structure with age, topography, and pathology. Spine 1995;20:674–84.
82. Urban JP, Maroudas A, Bayliss MT, et al. Swelling pressures of proteoglycans at the concentrations found in cartilaginous tissues. Biorheology 1979;16:447–64.
83. Brass L. Understanding and evaluating platelet function. Hematology Am Soc Hematol Educ Program 2010;2010:387–96.
84. Knighton DR, Hunt TK, Thakral KK, et al. Role of platelets and fibrin in the healing sequence: an in vivo study of angiogenesis and collagen synthesis. Ann Surg 1982;196:379–88.
85. Marx RE. Platelet-rich plasma: evidence to support its use. J Oral Maxillofac Surg 2004;62:489–96.
86. Gullung GB, Woodall JW, Tucci MA, et al. Platelet-rich plasma effects on degenerative disc disease: analysis of histology and imaging in an animal model. Evid Based Spine Care J 2011;2:13–8.
87. Obata S, Akeda K, Morimoto R, et al. Intradiscal injection of autologous platelet-rich plasma-serum induces the restoration of disc height in the rabbit annular needle puncture model: 12 [abstract]. Spine Aff Soc Meet Abstr 2010;15.
88. Obata S, Akeda K, Imanishi T, et al. Effect of autologous platelet-rich plasma-releasate on intervertebral disc degeneration in the rabbit annular puncture model: a preclinical study. Arthritis Res Ther 2012;14:R241.
89. Chen WH, Lo WC, Lee JJ, et al. Tissue-engineered intervertebral disc and chondrogenesis using human nucleus pulposus regulated through TGF-beta1 in platelet-rich plasma. J Cell Physiol 2006;209:744–54.
90. Akeda K, An HS, Pichika R, et al. Platelet-rich plasma (PRP) stimulates the extracellular matrix metabolism of porcine nucleus pulposus and annulus fibrosus cells cultured in alginate beads. Spine 2006;31:959–66.
91. Nagae M, Ikeda T, Mikami Y, et al. Intervertebral disc regeneration using platelet-rich plasma and biodegradable gelatin hydrogel microspheres. Tissue Eng 2007;13:147–58.
92. Sawamura K, Ikeda T, Nagae M, et al. Characterization of in vivo effects of platelet-rich plasma and biodegradable gelatin hydrogel microspheres on degenerated intervertebral discs. Tissue Eng 2009;15:3719–27.
93. Walsh AJ, Bradford DS, Lotz JC. In vivo growth factor treatment of degenerated intervertebral discs. Spine 2004;29:156–63.
94. Masuda K, Oegema TR Jr, An HS. Growth factors and treatment of intervertebral disc degeneration. Spine 2004;29:2757–69.
95. Gruber HE, Fischer EC Jr, Desai B, et al. Human intervertebral disc cells from the annulus: three-dimensional culture in agarose or alginate and responsiveness to TGF-Beta 1. Exp Cell Res 1997;235:13–21.
96. Lee KI, Moon SH, Kim H, et al. Tissue engineering of the intervertebral disc with cultured nucleus pulposus cells using atellocollagen scaffold and growth factors. Spine 2012;37:452–8.
97. Hayes AJ, Ralphs JR. The response of foetal annulus fibrosus cells to growth factors: modulation of matrix synthesis by TGF-β1 and IGF-1. Histochem Cell Biol 2011;136:163–75.
98. Gruber HE, Norton HJ, Hanley EN Jr. Anti-apoptotic effects of IGF-1 and PDGF on human intervertebral disc cells in vitro. Spine 2000;25:2153–7.

99. CPT Category III Codes. American Medical Association Web site. Available at: http://www.ama-assn.org/resources/doc/cpt/x-pub/cpt3codes.pdf. Accessed March 10, 2015.

100. Hibner M, Castellanos ME, Drachman D, et al. Repeat operation for treatment of persistent pudendal nerve entrapment after pudendal neurolysis. J Minim Invasive Gynecol 2012;19:325–30.

101. Thanasas C, Papadimitriou G, Charalambidis C, et al. Platelet-rich plasma versus autologous whole blood for the treatment of chronic lateral elbow epicondylitis: a randomized controlled clinical trial. Am J Sports Med 2011;39: 2130–4.

102. Kanno T, Takahashi T, Tsujisawa T, et al. Platelet-rich plasma enhances human osteoblast-like cell proliferation and differentiation. J Oral Maxillofac Surg 2005;63:362–9.

103. Sanchez M, Gaudilla J, Fiz N, et al. Ultrasound-guided platelet-rich plasma injections for the treatment of osteoarthritis of the hip. Rheumatology 2012;51: 144–50.

104. Hechtman KS, Uribe JW, Botto-vanDemden A, et al. Platelet-rich plasma injection reduces pain in patients with recalcitrant epicondylitis. Orthopedics 2011; 34:92.

105. Scudeller L, Del Fante C, Perotti C, et al. N of 1, Two contemporary arm, randomized controlled clinical trial for bilateral epicondylitis: a new study design. BMJ 2011;343:d7653.

106. Li M, Zhang C, Ai Z, et al. Therapeutic effectiveness of intra-knee-articular injection of platelet-rich plasma on knee articular cartilage degeneration. Zhongguo Xiu Fu Chong Jian Wai Ke Za Zhi 2011;25:1192–6.

107. Kon E, Mandelbaum B, Buda R, et al. Platelet-rich plasma intra-articular injection versus hyaluronic acid viscosupplementation as treatments for cartilage pathology: from early degeneration to osteoarthritis. Arthroscopy 2011;27: 1490–501.

108. Andia I, Sanchez M, Maffuli N. Platelet rich plasma therapies for sports muscle injuries: any evidence behind clinical practice? Expert Opin Biol Ther 2011;11: 509–18.

109. Andia I, Sanchez M, Maffuli N. Joint pathology and platelet-rich plasma therapies. Expert Opin Biol Ther 2012;12:7–22.

110. Bava ED, Barber FA. Platelet-rich plasma products in sports medicine. Physician Sports Med 2011;39:94–9.

111. Araki J, Jona M, Eto H, et al. Optimized preparation method of platelet-concentrated plasma and noncoagulating platelet-derived factor concentrates: maximization of platelet concentration and removal of fibrinogen. Tissue Eng Part C Methods 2012;18:176–85.

112. De Vos RJ, Weir A, van Schie HT, et al. Platelet-rich plasma injection for chronic Achilles tendinopathy: a randomized controlled trial. JAMA 2010;303:144–9.

113. Lemont H, Ammirati KM, Usen N. Plantar fasciitis: a degenerative process (fasciosis) without inflammation. J Am Podiatr Med Assoc 2003;93:234–7.

114. Kalaci A, Cakici H, Hapa O, et al. Treatment of plantar fasciitis using four different local injection modalities: a randomized prospective clinical trial. J Am Podiatr Med Assoc 2009;99:108–13.

115. Alfredson H, Lorentzon R. Chronic Achilles tendinosis: recommendations for treatment and prevention. Sports Med 2000;29:135–46.

116. Gottlieb NL, Riskin WG. Complications of local corticosteroid injections. JAMA 1980;243:1547–8.

117. Liu Y, Kong J, Chen BH, et al. Combined expression of CTGF and tissue inhibitor of metalloprotease-1 promotes synthesis of proteoglycan and collagen type II in Rhesus monkey lumbar intervertebral disc cells in vitro. Chin Med J (Engl) 2010; 123:2082–7.
118. Thompson JP, Oegema TR Jr, Bradford DS. Stimulation of mature canine intervertebral disc by growth factors. Spine 1991;16:253–60.
119. Pratsinis H, Kletsas D. PDGF, bFGF and IGF-1 stimulate the proliferation of intervertebral disc cells in vitro via the activation of the ERK and Akt signaling pathways. Eur Spine J 2007;16:1858–66.
120. Fujita N, Imai J, Suzuki T, et al. Vascular endothelial growth factor-A is a survival factor for nucleus pulposus cells in the intervertebral disc. Biochem Biophys Res Commun 2008;372:367–72.

Index

Note: Page numbers of article titles are in **boldface** type.

Med Clin N Am 100 (2016) 219–235
http://dx.doi.org/10.1016/S0025-7125(15)00219-9
0025-7125/16/$ – see front matter © 2016 Elsevier Inc. All rights reserved.

Printed and bound by CPI Group (UK) Ltd, Croydon, CR0 4YY

07/10/2024

01040498-0009